Toohey's
Medicine for Nurses

Toohey's
Medicine for Nurses

BY
Arnold Bloom M.D., F.R.C.P.
Physician, Whittington Hospital, London

THIRTEENTH EDITION

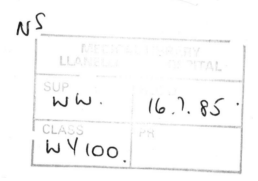

CHURCHILL LIVINGSTONE
EDINBURGH LONDON MELBOURNE AND NEW YORK 1981

CHURCHILL LIVINGSTONE
Medical Division of Longman Group Limited

Distributed in the United States of America by
Churchill Livingstone Inc., 1560 Broadway, New York,
N.Y. 10036 and by associated companies, branches
and representatives throughout the world.

First edition 1953
Second edition 1955
Third edition 1957
Fourth edition 1959
Fifth edition 1960
Sixth edition 1963
Seventh edition 1965
Eighth edition 1967
Ninth edition 1969
Tenth edition 1971
Eleventh edition 1975
Twelfth edition 1978
Thirteenth edition 1981
   Reprinted 1982
   Reprinted 1983

ISBN 0 443 02201 1

British Library Cataloguing In Publication Data
Toohey, M
   Toohey's medicine for nurses.—13th ed.
   1. Pathology
   I. Bloom, Arnold   II. Medicine for nurses
   616'.002'4613   RT65   80-41159

Printed in Singapore by Huntsmen Offset Printing Pte Ltd.

Preface to the Thirteenth Edition

The appearance of the thirteenth edition of this textbook emphasises its continuing value to the modern nurse. The book is designed to help the nurse to enjoy her profession and to look after her patients with a better understanding of the nature of their illnesses and the aims of treatment. It contains the information necessary for her training and her examinations, and it should serve as a reference book later in her career.

Opportunity has been taken in this edition to incorporate new treatments, new methods of diagnosis and new attitudes that have arisen since the previous edition. It is good to be able to record that smallpox has been eradicated and is now mentioned only for its historical interest.

It is a pleasure to express my appreciation to the publishers for their valued advice in preparing this edition, to Mrs Joyce Toohey for her continuing interest and to those authors and publishers whose material has been used again.

1981   Arnold Bloom

Preface to the First Edition

In writing this textbook of medicine for nurses I have tried to make it as comprehensive as possible so that it may not only help the nurse during her training but also serve as a reference book afterwards.

The basic physiological and pathological facts which are needed for the understanding of the various diseases and their treatment have accordingly been dealt with in some detail.

Perhaps a special word about the illustrations may be useful. Apart from the photographs, there are many original diagrams intended to emphasise in a simple and effective fashion the salient facts relating to the most important diseases.

1953   M. Toohey

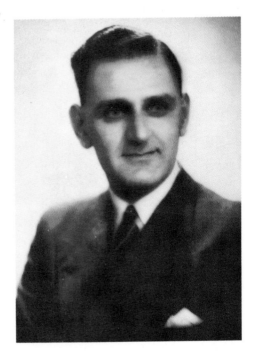

Extract from the Preface to the Sixth Edition

It is a melancholy duty to record that Dr Toohey died shortly before the appearance of the fifth edition of this textbook, which now becomes a memorial to him. He set out to provide a book which would help the nurse to understand the nature of the various diseases encountered in her profession. How well he succeeded can be seen by the fact that this now celebrated textbook has achieved six editions since it first appeared less than ten years ago. Dr Toohey was a physician wholeheartedly devoted to his profession. He was an acknowledged authority on anticoagulants, and had made many important and original contributions in this field. In every way a fine man, his untimely death was a great loss and a sad blow to all who knew him.

It is my aim to sustain the high standard set by him in creating a textbook that provides rational explanation of diseases and their management. No nurse today should be expected to perform her duties without the opportunity to understand their purpose.

1963   Arnold Bloom

Contents

1 Introduction. Clinical Observations

The nurse will make her first real contact with her patients in the ward of a hospital and will soon realize that the nurse is part of a team, a team organised with one objective, the welfare of the patient. Many hospitals are large and forbidding, many old and gloomy, some new and impersonal, but all of them depend on the people who work in them. The porters and the clerical staff, the gardeners, the laundry workers, the telephonists, the electricians and plumbers, the administrative staff, the cooks and the kitchen staff: they all play an important part in the efficient running of a modern hospital and in creating an atmosphere that is friendly and encouraging. Medicine today has become so complex that the physician alone could not diagnose or treat without the help of his colleagues and the paramedical services. He needs the radiologist and the pathologist to reach his diagnosis, and they in turn must have radiographers and technicians to help them provide the answers the physician requests. In treatment, the physician will need to call on the physiotherapist, the chaplain, the occupational therapist, speech therapist, chiropodist, dietitian, the pharmacist and the social worker. But above all, the physician depends on the co-operation of the nurse: for it is the nurse, male or female, who can play the greatest part in providing physical and emotional comfort to the patient in the hour of his need and in supervising that the treatment prescribed is properly administered.

Faced with a ward of patients lying in their beds, it is easy to forget that each is an individual with his family and his friends, with anxieties relating to his illness, his children, his job and his future. The nurse will observe the patient's attitude and response to his illness and his surroundings so that she can help the patient and communicate her observations to the doctors.

NURSE–PATIENT RELATIONSHIP

Our patients come from all walks of life and with widely differing backgrounds. To a few, the hospital represents a standard of luxury not previously experienced; to some it involves a terrifying loss of personal privacy and an affront to a fastidious nature. Some are frightened by the atmosphere and size of the hospital and by the significance of their illness; others have been in hospital often before and feel a sense of comfort in escaping from the struggle and discomfort of their existence outside. Of course, all patients cannot be treated the same; but in different ways we want to do the best we can to help them all, and this entails an understanding and a perception of the needs of others.

It is easy to be kind and helpful to patients who are pleasant and appreciate our efforts. It is much less easy with patients who are grumpy, aggressive and ungrateful. We have to seek an understanding of these attitudes so that we can help more efficiently and give comfort where it is needed. Sometimes aggression in a patient is a manifestation of fear and anxiety, and sometimes these emotions can be found in the context of his family background, in his uncertainty about the nature of the illness, or about his future. Often a quiet talk, with questions directed to the patient's background and his health, will reveal the reason for his attitude and enable help to be offered to restore his self-esteem. Few patients remain hostile when it is made clear that the nurse is genuinely anxious to be helpful.

Explanation and reassurance of the patient as to the nature of his illness is essentially the responsibility of the doctor, and the nurse has to be most circumspect in offering medical advice or explanation that might be counter to the doctor's intentions. Certainly the nurse can do much to calm the fears of a patient due for a barium meal or a liver biopsy, for example. She can explain what these routine examinations entail in a reassuring way and so remove the fear of the unknown and the unexpected. The arrival of the porters and the wheelchair to take a patient to X-ray, so commonplace and so routine to those who work in hospital, may be a source of fear and stress to the uninitiated patient.

Diet

In most hospitals today food is prepared in central kitchens and brought to the wards in trollies. In some modern hospitals, the patient states his requirements on a menu card supplied the day before and each individual meal is sent up from the central kitchens in a heated trolley with a compartment for every patient's tray. Very little is now available on the ward itself. The disadvantage of this system is that it lacks flexibility. If a patient unexpectedly falls ill, the food ordered the day before may be totally inappropriate in the changed situation and facilities are not always available to prepare a light meal on the ward.

It is important to the patient that meals should be served in as attractive a manner as possible, and that the food should not be lukewarm or served on cold plates. The nurse must observe and record the patient's appetite and particularly whether all the food is eaten or whether most of it is left on the plate. Of course, it is fundamental to assist those whose incapacities make it difficult for them to eat or drink on their own.

Hospital catering today has reached a good standard and the nurse can often pass on to the catering staff patients' comments, be they laudatory or critical.

Special diets are usually provided under supervision of a dietitian. The nurse will be aware of which patients require a special diet and will keep an eye open for would-be helpful friends and relatives who bring in extras. The diabetic patient should not be offered the temptation of chocolates, for example.

Smoking

Cigarette smoking is a harmful habit which seriously diminishes the expectation of health and life. Patients on the ward should be discouraged from smoking, particularly when this is to the discomfort of non-smokers, and if possible, areas of the ward should be set aside where smoking is absolutely forbidden. Similarly, visitors should not be allowed to smoke. Having said this, it may be regarded as unreasonable to deny ill patients the demands of a lifelong addiction at a time when their courage and resistance are at a low ebb.

Elderly patients

Partly thanks to better nutrition and better social conditions, and partly thanks to improved medical treatment, the population contains an ever-increasing proportion of elderly people. The large majority lead independent existences, either in their own homes or with their families, but this is the section of the community most likely to need hospital care when ill-health supervenes. Geriatrics is the term used for the special medical and nursing care of old people and many hospitals today have separate geriatric departments. But in practice these facilities are inadequate to the needs and most elderly people who require hospital treatment are admitted to an acute medical or surgical ward. Indeed, a high proportion of patients in any general medical ward today are over the age of 65.

Many special nursing and medical problems apply to the care of the elderly apart from those associated with the treatment of the particular disorder which occasioned admission to hospital. The prime aim of management must be to mobilise and rehabilitate the elderly patient as soon as possible. Lying in bed is potentially dangerous to the old and frail. It promotes the development of incontinence of bladder and bowel, it disposes to pressure sores and it leads to apathy.

The admission to hospital of an elderly patient should be regarded as the first step towards returning him back into the community. A proposed date for discharge should be decided as soon as possible after admission so that relatives and friends can plan accordingly. The help of the ancillary services should be sought. The dietitian can advise as to suitable food for a patient who may be without teeth, for example. The physiotherapist may be enlisted to help with mobilisation and exercises. The occupational therapist will assess the ability of patients to perform the daily tasks necessary for an independent existence and, if need be, to retrain patients who have been incapacitated by illnesses such as a stroke. The social workers will have the opportunity to prepare a social report, describing the home background and the facilities available when the patient is ready to leave hospital. In doubtful cases, the patient may be allowed home for a day or a weekend to see how well he can manage, and whether there are unexpected difficulties to be overcome before he is able finally to be discharged from hospital.

Many services are available to help the elderly in their homes, and indeed a team is available, the Primary Care Team, built round the family doctor in this respect. The district nurse (home nurse) can provide a nursing service such as dressings and injections; she can supervise progress and inform the family doctor of any problems; and she can organise the supply of special aids such as walking frames or commodes. The health visitor has specialised knowledge of community facilities available to the elderly and may visit the patient in his home to see if help is needed. The home help, provided by the local authority, is available for the housework and shopping, and may provide company and friendship as well. The Meals-on-Wheels service ensures that elderly people can get a regular hot meal at low cost and helps to keep the elderly in touch with the community.

Social workers may visit the elderly in their homes and advise them on such matters as pensions, laundry services, libraries, telephone, old peoples' clubs and holidays.

CLINICAL OBSERVATIONS

The nurse is responsible for various clinical observations and much depends on the conscientious recording of the findings.

Temperature

The temperature chart is of prime importance to the physician. In infections, a decline in fever suggests that the treatment is proving effective and the infection is being overcome. A rise of temperature alerts the physician to the possibility of an unexpected bacterial infection.

The thermometer is placed under the tongue with the lips closed, and allowed to remain for at least two minutes. The normal reading is about 36·9°C (98·4°F). A falsely elevated temperature will be obtained if the patient has just taken a hot drink. The temperature is usually slightly higher in the evening than in the morning. In women the temperature is elevated after ovulation in the latter part of the menstrual cycle and indeed this fact is used as a test of ovulation in cases of amenorrhoea. With a comatose or unco-operative patient the temperature can be taken by placing the thermometer in the axilla and holding the patient's arm to his side: the normal temperature taken in this way is less than the mouth temperature, usually 36·7°C (98°F) after two minutes. When a very low temperature is suspected (hypothermia) especially in elderly patients found in unheated rooms in the winter, the thermometer should be inserted in the rectum and allowed to remain for at least two minutes.

A temperature raised above normal is referred to as a *pyrexia* and with some exceptions is associated with a quickened pulse rate (*tachycardia*). Pyrexia without tachycardia suggests the likelihood of a false reading. Neurotic patients sometimes like to draw attention to themselves by surreptitiously warming the thermometer in a cup of tea or a hot pipe near the bed, or by other ways, and so falsely appear to have a high temperature.

A sudden rise of temperature may be due to a bacterial invasion into the blood stream and is associated with *rigors*. The patient in a rigor feels intensely cold and shivers violently, often shaking the bed. As the temperature rises, the rigor eases off, the patient sweats profusely and wants to throw off the bedclothes. Rigors are a characteristic feature of septicaemia and in malaria.

The pulse

The heart is a powerful pump and each time it contracts it sends a surge of blood through all the arteries. The pressure in the arteries increases with each beat of the heart and falls again when the heart relaxes between contractions. The pulse is the wave of distension in the artery after each heart beat, and it can be felt by the nurse in any large artery that is easily accessible.

The radial artery is the pulse most frequently palpated. It is easily felt at the wrist and is convenient both for the nurse and the patient.

The brachial artery can be felt at the bend of the elbow and should be identified when taking the blood pressure to see where to place the stethoscope.

The carotid pulses can be felt on either side of the neck and may be helpful when the patient is so collapsed that the radial pulse is difficult to find.

The temporal arteries, just in front of the ear, are often used by the anaesthetist during an operation when other pulses are not accessible.

The femoral arteries can be felt in the groins, about midway across, and are of great importance when the circulation to the legs is impaired or obstructed: when the femoral artery is partially ob-structed, listening over it with a stethoscope may reveal a loud murmur caused by the blood passing through the narrowed lumen.

Two pulses can normally be palpated in the feet. The dorsalis artery is found on the front of the foot and the posterior tibial pulse behind the medial malleolus.

Taking the pulse is an important observation because it reveals so much about the action of the heart. The rate, the rhythm and volume should all be noted and the rate should be recorded as a routine.

RATE

A rapid heart rate is called *tachycardia* while a slow heart rate is called *bradycardia*. In most healthy people the heart rate at rest is between 70 and 80 to the minute, but some have a heart rate of only 50 while others have a heart rate of 90. The heart is under the control of the nervous system and responds to the needs of the body, quickening when there is a need for greater effort and slowing at rest. Thus after exercise or an emotional disturbance the heart rate quickens, while during sleep the heart rate slows.

They are many causes of tachycardia and bradycardia (see p. 99).

RHYTHM

The pulse is normally as regular as a clock but in children and young adults the heart rate often quickens with inspiration (breathing in) and slows with expiration (breathing out). Particularly in older people, extra beats of the heart are not uncommon but the basic rhythm is regular. However, in the condition known as atrial fibrillation (see p. 97), the pulse rate is totally irregular and, indeed, often the heart beat is so rapid that not all contractions are transmitted to the pulse. Listening with a stethoscope to the heart itself is the only way to determine the heart rate in such cases; the difference between the heart rate and the pulse rate is known as the *pulse deficit*.

VOLUME

This describes the strength and character of the pulse, whether it is full and bounding or weak and thready. It gives an indication of the state of the circulation. Thus after a severe haemorrhage or a serious myocardial infarction the pulse volume may be so low that the radial pulse is scarcely palpable.

Respiration

An adult at rest has a respiration rate of about 16 to 20 a minute, and this rate of breathing can be observed and recorded while the temperature is being taken.

The term *dyspnoea* means difficult or painful breathing, such as is seen in pleurisy where every deep breath or cough causes pain; but often the word dyspnoeic is merely used to mean rapid breathing or breathlessness (see p. 155).

Orthopnoea occurs particularly in heart failure and signifies that the patient can only breathe with any comfort when propped up: orthopnoeic patients usually feel easier when sitting up in a high armchair than in bed.

Breathing may be quiet or noisy. In asthma, expiration is wheezy; after a stroke, the breathing may be sterterous with a snore-like quality; and where there is obstruction to the upper airway tract, stridor may be heard, a coarse crowing sound on inspiration.

Blood pressure

The blood pressure is a most important observation and may be difficult to determine, especially in a collapsed patient. Every nurse must practise taking the blood pressure until complete competence is attained.

The blood pressure is measured by an instrument known as the sphygmomanometer. This consists of: (i) an inflatable cuff to be wrapped around the upper arm; (ii) a mercury manometer, attached by a tube to the cuff, which measures the pressure in the cuff.

The arm should be bared to the shoulder so that when the cuff is applied to the upper arm sufficient room is left for the stethoscope to be placed over the brachial pulse.

When the cuff has been securely wrapped round and attached to the manometer, the brachial pulse must be identified, conveniently by the thumb of the right hand. The stethoscope head is now applied over the brachial pulse below the cuff and the cuff is pumped up sufficiently to obliterate the artery pulsation. The pressure in the cuff is now slowly released by turning the screw. When the thumping of the artery can be heard through the stethoscope, the pressure is read on the manometer. This is the *systolic pressure*. The pressure in the cuff is now further reduced until the thumping over the pulse dies away. The reading on the manometer now records the *diastolic pressure*.

The systolic pressure represents the maximum pressure of blood in the artery as the ventricle contracts. The diastolic pressure is the lower pressure when the ventricle relaxes between beats.

The normal systolic blood pressure in adults at rest is about 110 to 140 mm of mercury (mmHg) on the manometer. The diastolic pressure varies from about 60 to 80 mmHg. Thus a healthy young adult might have a systolic pressure of 120 mmHg and a diastolic pressure of 70. This would be recorded as 'BP 120/70'. The blood pressure tends to be higher as we get older and the arteries harden. A man of 70 in good health might have a blood pressure of 170/90.

Normally the blood pressure in an individual is lowest when warm and comfortable in mind and body and in the recumbent position. It rises somewhat on sitting up or standing. However, in many patients receiving drugs for the treatment of high blood pressure the blood pressure falls when the patient stands up and rises when he lies down. Hence it is advisable to record the position in which the blood pressure is taken, lying down, sitting or standing.

Particularly in patients receiving intravenous fluids, it is important to the physician not only to know the blood pressure in the arteries but in the veins as well. The pressure in the veins can be estimated by observation of the jugular veins in the neck. When the patient is lying in the semirecumbent position, with the head and shoulders about 30 degrees above the horizontal, the pulsation of the jugular vein can be seen just above the clavicle. But in congestive heart failure, when the heart is unable completely to sustain the circulation, the right atrium is not emptied at each beat and the pressure in the veins rises accordingly. The veins in the neck are distended and the venous pulsation may be seen well above the clavicle. Precise measurement of venous pressure may be needed in patients when they are receiving fluid intravenously since, if the heart is weak, the circulation may become overloaded. A catheter is introduced into the internal jugular vein and attached to a water manometer reading up to 10 cm of water. The reading on the manometer is called the central venous pressure and will help determine the rate and volume of administered fluid that the heart can tolerate.

Cough and sputum

A cough is a reflex mechanism to expel irritants, foreign material and secretion from the respiratory tract. It is a protective mechanism. Elderly or debilitated patients with bronchopneumonia may be too feeble to cough adequately and the smaller bronchioles become clogged with thick secretions which they are unable to expel; physiotherapy and suction by a pump may be required to clear the airway. On the other hand, a cough may be due to irritation of the mucous membrane lining the upper respiratory tract and serves no useful purpose since there is nothing to cough up. A dry cough of this sort may keep the patient awake and cause needless distress; a cough suppressant medicine may be prescribed in such cases.

A productive cough is one in which sputum is brought up and waxed cartons with screw tops are provided for the collection of sputum by the bedside. These cartons, which are easily destroyed by burning, allow inspection of the sputum and this provides valuable information as to the nature of the respiratory illness. The nature and the amount of sputum coughed up should be noted. When infection is minimal, the sputum is usually mucoid: it is clear, viscid and not profuse. When infection is present, the sputum becomes purulent: it may be very profuse and foetid (foul smelling), as occurs in bronchiectasis or lung abscess: or it may form round blobs, the so-called nummular sputum of pulmonary tuberculosis. The extent to which the sputum is profuse and purulent offers the physician a guide to progress and treatment.

Coughing up blood is called haemoptysis and is seen particularly in pulmonary tuberculosis and in bronchial carcinoma, due to the rupture of small vessels in the affected area. More common than pure blood is sputum with streaks of blood in it due to inflammation of the bronchial wall and sometimes to the strain of coughing (see p. 154).

Sputum may be sent to the laboratory for two important investigations. (1) It will be examined and cultured for bacteria so that the nature of the infection can be determined and, if need be, appropriate antibiotic prescribed. (2) It can be examined microscopically to see if malignant cells are present as a test for bronchial carcinoma.

Urine

Examination of the urine is a most important routine which is always undertaken for each new patient. It is easy to do and may give valuable information.

VOLUME

The amount of urine passed is modified by the amount of fluid drunk and the amount lost in perspiration, in the breath and from the bowel. An average daily output of urine for a normal adult is about 1200 ml but it can vary from as little as 400 ml to as much as 3000 ml according to circumstances. A significantly increased output of urine is described as *polyuria*, a diminished output as *oliguria* and a complete absence of urine as *anuria*.

Especially in severely ill patients or in those receiving intravenous fluids, an intake and output chart must be kept. This records all the fluid taken by mouth or drip over 24 hours and all the fluid lost by urine, vomit or bowel over the same time. Normally fluid intake will exceed output by about 500 ml because no record can be kept of fluid lost in the breath or in perspiration.

REACTION

The urine is normally slightly acid and turns blue litmus paper red. If excess alkalis have been taken or if the urine is infected or has been allowed to stand, the reaction becomes alkaline and red litmus paper turns blue.

SPECIFIC GRAVITY

The specific gravity of urine depends on the weight of substances dissolved in it compared with water. The specific gravity of water is 1000 and that of urine usually 1012 to 1024 as measured by a hydrometer: this partially floats in urine and the depth to which it sinks is calibrated to give the reading. After a large intake of fluid, the urine is dilute with a low specific gravity. When fluid intake is restricted, the urine should be concentrated with a high specific gravity if the kidneys are healthy. In diabetes, although a lot of urine is passed, the presence of sugar in the urine leads to a high specific gravity.

NORMAL DEPOSITS

Healthy urine may often show a deposit on standing. This may be due to mucous secretion or to urates or phosphates from certain foods; it disappears on adding acid.

Protein (albumin). Occasionally protein (albumin) appears in the urine in healthy young adults after exercise or prolonged standing and this is known as *orthostatic proteinuria*. However, usually the glomerular filter (see p. 364) is too fine to allow molecules of protein to pass through into the urine and the presence of albumin in the urine suggests kidney disease. Since the urine test may provide the first indication of a renal disorder, the test is of great importance.

Albustix test. This is a simple, rapid and reliable test for protein in the urine. The test end of the strip is dipped in the urine, and the colour compared with the colour strip provided. The greater the amount of protein, the deeper green on the strip.

Salicylsulphonic acid test. Eight drops of salicylsulphonic acid are added to approximately 5 ml of urine in a test-tube. If protein is present, a white cloud forms.

Boiling test. Urine is boiled in a test-tube. If albumin is present, a turbidity appears which does not clear when dilute acetic acid is added. If the turbidity clears after acidification, it is not due to albumin but to phosphates.

Sugar (glucose). The presence of any appreciable amount of sugar (glucose) in the urine suggests that diabetes may be present. In many cases of diabetes developing in older people, there may be no symptoms of the disorder and the diagnosis is only suspected on routine testing of the urine.

Clinistix test. This is a specific test for glucose. The pink end of the strip is dipped in the urine and if sugar is present, the moistened end turns mauve in 10 seconds. If the strip remains pink, sugar is absent. The test is valuable for demonstrating the presence or absence of glucose but not reliable as a quantitive guide as to how much sugar is present.

Clinitest tablets. In this test five drops of urine from a standard dropper are placed in a clean test-tube and ten drops of water are then added. A Clinitest tablet is dropped into the test-tube whereupon a boiling reaction takes place. Fifteen seconds after the boiling has ceased, the tube is shaken. If sugar is present the fluid changes colour, turning green, yellow or deep orange, according to the amount of sugar present. If there is no sugar, the fluid remains blue. A deep orange colour represents more than 2 per cent sugar to be present and as a refinement the test can be repeated but using only two drops of urine. If the test again shows orange, this means that 5 per cent sugar is present. Hence this test offers a guide not only to whether sugar is present in the urine but to what degree. It is most useful for diabetics needing insulin as a guide to control (see p. 424).

The Clinitest tablets readily absorb moisture, which turns them blue, so that care must be taken to keep them dry by screwing the bottle top firmly after use. The tablets should be mainly white with speckled blue and should be discarded if they become mostly blue. As they contain caustic soda, they must be handled with care.

Benedict's test is an older, but less expensive test. Five millilitres of clear-blue Benedict's reagent are placed in a test-tube and eight drops of urine are added. The mixture is boiled for 2 minutes. If sugar is present, a green, yellow or brick-red precipitate forms according to the amount of sugar present.

Ketone bodies (acetone). Acetone is derived from the abnormal or rapid burning up of fat and it appears in the urine when it is produced in excess. This happens after starvation (perhaps to reduce weight) or after persistent vomiting. It also occurs in diabetics when the diabetes is poorly controlled (see p. 426).

Ketostix. The test end of the strip is dipped in the urine and read after 15 seconds. A lavender colour develops when ketones are present, the depth of the colour depending on the degree of ketosis.

Other tests

Tests are also available for blood, bile and pus and these are dealt with in the appropriate chapters.

It should be added that compound strips are available which combine more than one test in the same strip. For example, Labstix is a clear plastic strip with five test areas which tests the reaction of the urine as well as detecting protein, glucose, ketones and blood.

Faeces

Inspection of the stools may provide valuable information as to the condition of the bowel.

In severe constipation the bowel may only be evacuated after a suppository or an enema and the stool may consist of small hard balls of faeces known as *scybalae*. Sometimes impaction of scybalae in the rectum occurs in elderly dehydrated patients and only manual evacuation by doctor or nurse can relieve the patient of his misery.

Diarrhoea means frequent loose stools. When this is due to an intestinal infection, the stools are watery. In the malabsorption syndrome (see p. 234), the motions are large, bulky and pale. In thyrotoxicosis (see p. 438) although the motions are very frequent, they are usually small but normally formed.

Melaena is the term applied to blood in the motions. When the bleeding occurs in the stomach or duodenum, the blood is altered in its passage through the bowel and the motions are black and sticky, the so-called tarry stool: there may be a characteristic smell of blood. It should not be forgotten that iron preparations taken for anaemia colour the stools black and this can be confused for melaena. When bleeding occurs in the lower bowel, perhaps from a carcinoma in the rectum or from haemorrhoids, the blood is bright red and often appears as streaks of blood in the faeces.

In ulcerative colitis, diarrhoea may be very severe, the motions may be loose or watery and may contain blood and mucus.

The normal brown colour of the motion is due to the presence of stercobilin, a derivative of bile. Hence in conditions in which the flow of bile into the intestine is obstructed, as occurs in gallstones or severe hepatitis, the stools may be pale or clay-coloured.

The stools should also be inspected for the presence of worms. Threadworms, roundworms or tapeworms may be seen (see p. 238).

2 Causes of Disease

Medicine is the study and treatment of disease and we usually classify ailments according to the part of the body that is mainly affected. Thus there are disorders which affect the heart, while others involve the blood or the nervous system. But before looking at the various disorders of the different parts of the body, we should first consider the factors in general which can lead to ill-health and how the body reacts to protect itself.

GENERAL CAUSES OF DISEASE

The cause of a disease is referred to as its *aetiology*. Sometimes the aetiology of a disorder is environmental and induced by factors outside the body. For example, infected food can cause enteritis or intense cold can lead to frostbite. In other cases, however, the disease is due to the inheritance of a genetic disorder, sometimes manifesting itself in childhood, sometimes not until later in life. Some ailments are partly environmental and partly inherited. Thus, although a tendency to diabetes may be inherited, in many cases the ailment will only become manifest after prolonged overeating. Indeed, there is nearly always an interplay between the environment and the bodily constitution. An elderly man in a state of poor nutrition is more prone to bacterial infection than someone young and healthy. Furthermore, the body is endowed with a complex system to rebuff and repel noxious agents which invade and threaten it. This is called the *immunity system*. Disease can occur when the immunity system functions improperly. So although a classification of causes of disease now follows, it should be regarded as a simplification which ignores the interaction of environment and constitution, the seed and the soil.
1. Hereditary disorders.
2. Physical and chemical agents:
    (a) Drugs, including cigarettes and alcohol
    (b) Excess of heat or cold
    (c) Electricity and radioactive substances
    (d) Injury (trauma).

3. Unknown causes leading to cancer.
4. Living organisms (microbes):
    (a) Bacteria
    (b) Viruses
    (c) Fungi
    (d) Parasites (protozoa and helminths). } Chapter 3
5. Disorders of the immunity system.
6. Deficiency diseases:
    (a) Malnutrition and vitamins (Chapter 12)
    (b) Hormonal.

HEREDITY

Parents transmit certain characteristics to their children, so that a child inherits qualities from each parent. A boy may be tall and dark like his father but he may inherit his mother's ability to play tennis well. These characteristics are transmitted by the germ cells at the moment of union of the male sperm and female ovum. Each sperm and each ovum contains 23 chromosomes.

CHROMOSOMES AND GENES

Chromosomes lie within the nucleus of every human cell. They are threads of basic material known as DNA (deoxyribonucleic acid). Sited along the length of each chromosome are a series of genes, and it is these genes which are responsible for reproducing all the different characteristics of the child-to-be. If a gene is faulty, the result is termed a *genetic disorder*.

The fertilised ovum contains 46 chromosomes, i.e. two sets of 23 chromosomes, one set from the sperm and one set already in the ovum. This fertilised ovum, containing chromosomes and genes from both parents, is the blueprint from which all cells in the growing fetus will be patterned.

Of the 23 chromosomes, the ovum has one special sex chromosome designated X. The sperm also has a sex chromosome which may either be X, as in the ovum, or a smaller chromosome designated Y. The sex of the offspring will depend on whether the union yields XX or XY.

Sperm X + ovum X yields female XX
Sperm Y + ovum X yields male XY

Occasionally abnormalities of the sex chromosomes may occur. Thus the ovum may contain an extra sex chromosome XX. If junction occurs with a sperm having a sex chromosome Y, this now yields XXY. Males born with this abnormality of their sex chromosomes do not develop properly. They are sterile with small genitalia and may be mentally retarded.

Chromosomes other than sex chromosomes are known as *autosomes* and these have been identified and enumerated by special radioactive staining techniques. It is now known that certain diseases in man are associated with abnormalities of the autosomes. Thus Down's syndrome (mongolism) (see p. 321) is due to an extra autosome. At the time of conception the ovum has 47 chromosomes instead of 46. As a result, every cell produced in the growing fetus carries this abnormality and a mentally subnormal child is born with characteristic physical defects.

Many different types of metabolic and blood disorders are due to abnormalities of various genes. Genes control the way in which proteins are formed from basic amino acids. As an example, normal blood clotting requires the presence of a particular protein known as antihaemophiliac globulin. In haemophilia, this globulin is not formed because of an inherited genetic defect. Consequently, in this disorder (see p. 355) bleeding from a minor injury can lead to death unless the missing globulin is administered.

There are many other genetic disorders, some common, some rare, all of them inherited to a lesser or greater degree. An abnormal gene may be passed on from a parent or parents. This defect may continue to be transmitted from generation to generation. These hereditary defects are more likely to be seen when there is any inbreeding in families, as when near cousins marry. The reason for this is that many of the defects passed on to the future generation are *recessive* (quiescent or dormant). Such a gene may only cause disease if it links up with a similar recessive gene. The mating of two recessive defects is much more likely to occur in marriage between people in the same family. Other hereditary genes are known as *dominant* because they give rise to disease in future generations without having to link up with other similar genes.

Some common diseases appear to have a genetic factor as part of the aetiology. These ailments are very much more prone to be present in some families than in others. Diabetes mellitus, hypertension and peptic ulcer are examples of ailments in which heredity plays a part in the aetiology. When both parents have diabetes, for example, their children are much more likely to develop diabetes than the children of parents without diabetes. But even when both parents have diabetes, only about a quarter of their children in fact develop the disease, so other factors play an important role.

PHYSICAL AND CHEMICAL AGENTS
Drugs

Drugs are prescribed:
1. For the treatment or prevention of illnesses and infections.
2. For the alleviation of pain and discomfort.
3. For the relief of anxiety, depression and sleeplessness.

Other preparations sometimes included under the heading of drugs really replace substances normally present in food, such as vitamins, or are normally produced within the body, such as hormones.

Although vitamins and hormones may be prescribed as replacement treatment where these are deficient, they may also be used in the treatment of other unrelated disorders.

Drugs are prescribed very widely and indeed many people have such faith in drugs that they would feel cheated if they were not given tablets after a visit to the doctor. If no drug is indicated, the doctor may respond by prescribing a *placebo*. A placebo is a preparation without any pharmacological effect, designed to give the patient confidence and help him by suggestion.

Properly prescribed and properly taken, drugs play an important role in the treatment of ill-health and the alleviation of suffering. But it must be realised that different people react differently to the same drug and that drugs exert effects on the body other than those for which they have been prescribed. Furthermore, since drugs of all sorts are readily available, deliberate or accidental overdosage is becoming a common cause of admission to hospital. Consequently, although drug treatment can be a powerful aid to better health, drugs can also be a frequent cause of illness.

Before any new drug is released for general prescription it has to undergo stringent trials, at first on animals. When no untoward effects are found, clinical trials are then undertaken with volunteers, usually patients suffering from the disorder which the drug is designed to cure. Finally, if these trials show the drug to be safe and effective, it has to be approved by the Committee on Safety of Drugs before it can be released for general use.

Drug-induced illness is sometimes described as *iatrogenic* and may be due to different causes.

DRUG SENSITIVITY

Not all patients react the same way to the same drug. Most people tolerate penicillin without trouble but some develop troublesome skin rashes, for example. This sort of sensitivity is common and liable to be more serious if it occurs a second time. Hence, if a patient has had a reaction to a particular drug, he should be warned to avoid this preparation in future and the fact should be recorded, preferably on the front of the case paper in a hospital patient.

Perhaps the most dangerous type of drug sensitivity is that which affects the blood. Many drugs are liable to depress the action of the bone marrow in producing blood cells. *Aplastic anaemia* means complete suppression of blood cell production and becomes fatal unless the bone marrow recovers. *Agranulocytosis* means suppression of the white cells and this disposes to infection. Many drugs in current use are liable to cause these blood disorders. The justification for prescribing them is that they are effective in treating the ailment for which they are used and the incidence of sensitivity reaction is excessively rare. The onus is on the physician to weigh up the advantage of using the drug as against the remote danger of a reaction. Having prescribed the drug, he will be on the lookout for trouble. As an example, myocrisin is a gold preparation used in the treatment of rheumatoid arthritis. It occasionally leads to kidney damage. Hence the urine must be tested for protein before each administration of myocrisin: if protein is seen, no further gold treatment can be administered.

SIDE-EFFECTS

No drug has a single pharmacological action. It may be prescribed effectively for one purpose but it may have other undesirable effects as well. Aspirin may be effective in relieving pain but it causes unwanted constipation. Some diuretics successfully relieve oedema but also deplete the system of potassium. Cortisone relieves inflammation but leads to obesity. Consequently, in prescribing any drugs for one purpose, the physician has to consider the possible side-effects in other directions and how to minimise them.

DRUG OVERDOSE

Accidental. Very few households today do not have drugs available, sometimes carefully kept in a closed cupboard for emergencies, more often lying around in bottles, half-full and forgotten. These tablets are an attraction and a deadly danger to small children. Every day some child is admitted to hospital having taken a dangerous dose of his mother's tablets, and nurse has a duty to remind parents of their responsibility in this respect. Bottles containing drugs should be firmly closed and kept out of the reach of small children.

Apart from mistakes in prescribing the wrong strength or dose of tablets, another potent cause of overdosage occurs in elderly people who are becoming forgetful. Having taken a sleeping tablet and pottered about, they may well forget and take another one. If an elderly person is on regular tablets, it is best to leave out the day's ration each morning.

Deliberate overdosage (acute poisoning) with dangerous drugs is becoming more and more common. Hypnotics and tranquillisers are freely prescribed for those who are anxious, harassed or depressed and this is the sort of person most likely to attempt suicide. Not all cases of deliberate drug overdosage really mean to commit suicide. More often the taking of the tablets is a gesture to demonstrate to others the depth of misery or despair that is being experienced. The tablets most commonly taken are aspirins, barbiturates and various tranquillisers, all easily available on prescription or in the case of aspirin, at any chemist's shop. However, almost any drug for whatever prescribed may be taken in large quantities with the intention of self-destruction. Indeed, any substance thought to be harmful may be taken by the desperate or the deluded, including paraffin, bleach, cosmetic preparations or weedkiller. Combinations of drugs are often taken if they are available and often alcohol as well.

Carbon monoxide poisoning. Coal gas contains carbon monoxide and was a common cause of poisoning, either accidental or deliberate, when coal gas was used for heating and cooking. Since coal gas has been replaced for domestic purposes by natural gas, the risks in this respect have been greatly reduced. It still can be a danger in badly ventilated garages since the exhausts of motor cars contain carbon monoxide. Carbon monoxide combines with haemoglobin to form carboxyhaemoglobin and prevents the proper uptake of oxygen.

General management of acute poisoning and drug overdosage
1. Urgent information must be sought from relatives or friends as to the nature of the drugs that have been taken. Often the ambulancemen will bring in any empty bottles lying by the bedside, although the labels on the bottles may be misleading.
2. The airway must be kept clear. Dentures are removed and the mouth cleared of phlegm or vomit. If the complexion is not cyanosed and the breathing is unimpaired, the patient can be kept in the left lateral position with the foot of the bed elevated to avoid the risk of inhaling mucus or vomit. If the breathing sounds obstructed or if the patient is too unconscious to clear the chest by coughing, it will be necessary to insert an endotracheal tube into the trachea. Oxygen can be administered through this tube or suction can be applied to clear it of secretions.
3. Gastric lavage. The stomach should be emptied as soon as possible to prevent further absorption of ingested tablets or other poisonous material.

In conscious patients vomiting can be induced by encouraging the patient to drink about 500 ml of warm water and then stimulating the back of the throat with a spatula or with the fingers. This is then followed by gastric lavage. A Jacques tube (30 English gauge) is lubricated with liquid paraffin and passed gently but firmly into the stomach, in an adult a distance of about 50 cm.

Five hundred ml of warm water is introduced into the stomach via the tube and then immediately siphoned out by inverting and lowering the funnel attached to the end of the tube. The first washout is likely to contain the maximum amount of drug or poison and should be set aside and kept separate from all subsequent washings. The washout is then continued using 300 ml water at a time, until 2 or 3 litres have been used.

All stomach washings, with the first washing kept separately, must be labelled with the name of the patient, date and time and sent to the laboratory for analysis.
4. Forced diuresis. Especially in barbiturate and salicylate poisoning, acceleration of renal excretion of the drug from the blood stream can be achieved by forced diuresis. Alkaline fluids are given intravenously with a diuretic: this leads to a large output of urine from the kidneys. The rate of the infusion can be controlled by watching

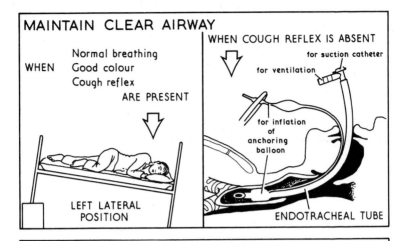

MAINTAIN CLEAR AIRWAY

WHEN
Normal breathing
Good colour
Cough reflex
ARE PRESENT

LEFT LATERAL POSITION

WHEN COUGH REFLEX IS ABSENT

for suction catheter
for ventilation
for inflation of anchoring balloon

ENDOTRACHEAL TUBE

SEEK INFORMATION TO IDENTIFY DRUG

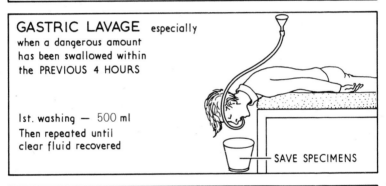

GASTRIC LAVAGE especially
when a dangerous amount has been swallowed within the PREVIOUS 4 HOURS

1st. washing — 500 ml
Then repeated until clear fluid recovered

SAVE SPECIMENS

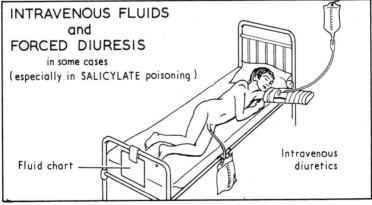

INTRAVENOUS FLUIDS and
FORCED DIURESIS
in some cases
(especially in SALICYLATE poisoning)

Fluid chart

Intravenous diuretics

FIG. 2.1 The treatment of drug overdosage.

the central venous pressure (if it rises too high the rate must be reduced) and by the urinary volume.

SOME DRUGS COMMONLY TAKEN IN OVERDOSE CASES

1. Salicylates (aspirin). Main features are nausea, vomiting, tinnitus, overbreathing and sweating. Blood should be taken for salicylate levels.
2. Paracetamol. Particularly dangerous since it can cause irreversible liver damage.
3. Carbon monoxide. Patient often pale and cyanosed with respiratory depression. Examination of the blood will reveal the presence of carboxyhaemoglobin.
4. Barbiturates. Mental confusion followed by deep sleep and coma.
5. Morphine. Pinpoint pupils, slow pulse, shallow breathing, cyanosis and hypotension.

Cigarette smoking

This is a harmful habit which reduces the expectation of good health and shortens life. Cigarette smokers absorb into the lungs:
1. Nicotine. This is a habit-forming drug with a mild stimulatory effect. It causes constriction of small blood vessels and a rise in blood pressure.
2. Carcinogenic tars. These tars isolated from cigarette smoke have been shown to cause cancer in experimental animals.
3. Carbon monoxide. Cigarette smokers have raised blood levels of carboxyhaemoglobin. If the mother smokes during pregnancy, carboxyhaemoglobin passes through into the fetal circulation.

The following ailments are prone to occur in cigarette smokers:

Cancer of the lung. Heavy cigarette smokers are 30 times as liable to develop cancer of the lung as non-smokers. There is overwhelming evidence that lung cancer is caused by cigarette smoking.

Bronchitis and emphysema. Prolonged cigarette smoking commonly leads to progressive cough and breathlessness, ultimately leading to respiratory incapacity.

Coronary thrombosis and intermittent claudication (see p. 144) are more prone to occur in those who smoke cigarettes.

Gastric and duodenal ulcers take longer to heal in cigarette smokers.

Pregnant women who smoke cigarettes have smaller babies than non-smokers, with a higher incidence of fetal abnormalities.

Alcohol

Alcohol is the basis of wine, beer and spirits. Taken in moderation, with a meal, or in the company of friends, it can be regarded as one of the pleasures of life. But as with any drug, there are dangers as well as advantages associated with alcohol.

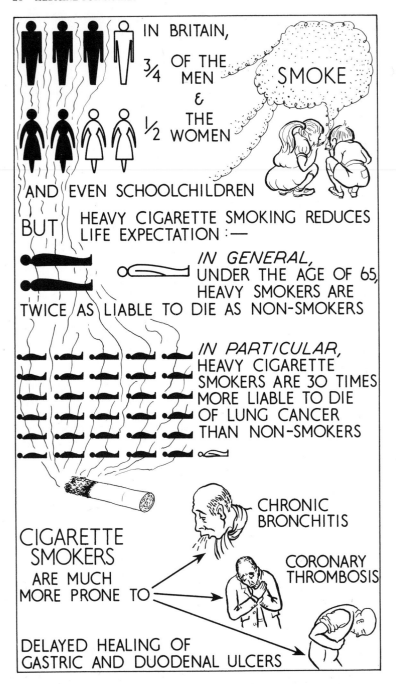

FIG. 2.2   Dangers of smoking.

Alcohol is rapidly absorbed from the stomach and intestine and soon appears in the blood. As the blood circulates through the lungs, alcohol diffuses into the air in the alveoli. The higher the concentration of alcohol in the blood, the higher the concentration in the breath. This is the basis of the breathalyser test used by the police in motorists suspected of driving while under the influence of drink. Alcohol can also be measured in the blood. It is metabolised (broken down) by the liver so that after 6 to 8 hours none can be detected in the blood or breath.

Apart from the pleasures to the palate, the main social reason for drinking is that it removes inhibitions of shyness and restraint, so enabling conversation to flow more easily. But judgement and prudence are also diminished as are technical skills demanding accuracy and co-ordination. This is particularly dangerous when driving a car, and it has been abundantly demonstrated that even a moderate intake of alcohol can diminish critically the driver's ability to deal with the unexpected.

Many men and women are ill-equipped to cope with the stringencies of life. Alcohol offers a temporary escape and an easement of depression and stress. But unfortunately alcohol is an addictive drug and more and more has to be taken to achieve the same effect. The term *alcoholic* is used to describe a person who has become dependent on alcohol. Alcoholism has become a serious health problem. Its onset is gradual and leads to a disintegration of the personality and of the physical health.

Delirium tremens in the alcoholic can be induced by a sustained high intake of spirits or by sudden deprivation of alcohol. It is characterised by a delusional state, often of a terrifying nature, by restlessness and by tremor: the behaviour may become aggressive and violent.

In the long term alcoholism can lead to:

1. Korsakoff's psychosis. This develops gradually with disordered behaviour, confabulation (telling plausible accounts of imaginary events), disorientation (not sure of place or time), hallucinations and emotional disturbances.
2. Polyneuritis (see p. 289).
3. Cirrhosis of the liver (see p. 256).

The treatment of alcoholism is difficult and demands the willingness of the patient to co-operate. Hospital treatment is often necessary during the period of alcohol withdrawal since tranquillising drugs are necessary to suppress intolerable symptoms. Supportive treatment by a psychiatrist or trained social worker is necessary on leaving hospital, and the organisation 'Alcoholics Anonymous' can play an important role in restoring confidence and self-esteem.

Drug addiction

Many commonly prescribed drugs if taken regularly and for long periods may lead to drug-dependence or addiction. The list will include sedatives, tranquillisers, weight reducers, stimulants, pain relievers and hypnotics, so that great care must be taken when prescribing such helpful medicaments that the patient is not allowed to take them indefinitely unless under medical supervision and for good purpose. When a patient becomes addicted to a drug he feels an overwhelming need to continue to take the drug and will make any excuse to get further supplies. He becomes physically and psychologically dependent on it, so that if the drug is not available he will suffer symptoms of withdrawal. Often the dose of the drug has steadily to be increased to make life bearable, and this leads to changes detrimental to physical and mental health. Doctors, dentists and nurses are liable to become addicted when they take drugs because such drugs are easily accessible to them, but the risk is only serious where the personality is unstable or neurotic.

Unfortunately, the problem of addiction has increased alarmingly in recent years, not as a result of medical treatment but as a result of obtaining drugs from illicit sources for self-indulgent purposes. Alcohol and tobacco are two habit-forming drugs widely used and socially acceptable, though carrying serious hazards to health. Many other drugs are being taken illegally, often by young people and with tragic results. These include:

1. Morphine, heroin and cocaine. These are known as narcotics or 'hard drugs' and form the core of the addiction problem. Opium is a mixture of compounds obtained from poppy seeds, and morphine is obtained from it. Heroin, or diamorphine, is itself a derivative of morphine. Used medically as a powerful pain reliever, it induces a drowsy sensation which may be pleasurable to some people, though not all. Dependence on the drug soon follows regular administration. Intolerable symptoms occur when the drug is withdrawn including shivering, watering of the eyes and nose, stomach contractions, violent vomiting, diarrhoea, twitching and complete physical and mental collapse. Prolonged usage leads to organic brain damage and disintegration of personality, so that the addict becomes untrustworthy and obsessed with the need to obtain the next dose. Hard-drug addicts usually die young. Cocaine is derived from the leaves of the coca plant and is a stimulant. It is usually injected by addicts together with heroin, at first subcutaneously and later intravenously. Since no precautions are taken to ensure sterility, infection is liable to follow.

2. Cannabis indica, also known as hashish, is obtained from the flowering top of the Indian hemp plant which grows wild in many countries. It is usually smoked in cigarette form, the so-called 'reefers', and its sale is illegal. It induces a sense of excitement and unreality. It is less likely to lead to addiction than the hard drugs and is much less harmful to health. The danger lies in the fact that since it can only be obtained from

illegal sources, access is made available to more vicious narcotics. Many heroin addicts have started with cannabis.

3. Amphetamine groups, including 'purple hearts', are taken because they lead to an elevation of the mood with a sense of being able to think and act more quickly, though in reality this does not occur. When under the influence of amphetamines, behaviour becomes erratic and irresponsible. Emotional dependence on the drug develops after a time, and bigger doses may be needed to achieve the desired effect.

4. Lysergic acid, or LSD, produces hallucinogenic effects so that those under its effect develop a heightened and distorted sense of their surroundings, which seem to attain unusual significance. The experience, which is not uniform in its effect, may last several hours and may lead to self-inflicted harm.

Treatment

Many or most drug addicts have unstable personalities and take to drugs because they are unable to resolve or accept the problems and difficulties of modern city life. Often they are unwilling to be treated, requesting only a regular supply of drugs. If these drugs are not supplied through legal channels, illicit sale of narcotics is encouraged by a network of unscrupulous 'pushers' who sell drugs for profit. Consequently, hospital centres are available for the treatment and supervision of drug addicts, who must be registered in order to obtain treatment of drugs. In this way, some control over the situation is maintained.

Treatment is in two directions. Firstly, the drug of addiction is slowly withdrawn, often by weaning the addict on to an alternative drug such as the synthetic narcotic methadone which is an easier drug to control. Secondly, an attempt must be made at mental rehabilitation, perhaps by group psychotherapy, and at social rehabilitation, to fit the addict for a place in society. Unfortunately, the success rate of methods currently employed is not high and there is urgent need for more knowledge and research before the problem can be tackled more successfully.

EFFECTS OF HEAT OR COLD

Extremes of heat or cold, if prolonged, can lead to serious metabolic and electrolytes disturbances.

Heat stroke

This is most likely to occur in individuals subjected to high temperatures to which they are unacclimatised. It may be provoked by prolonged exercise or by heavy clothing which prevents evaporation of sweat.

The patient may become restless and confused- and sometimes convulsions occur. The skin is hot and dry. The oral temperature exceeds 41°C (106°F) and the pulse is rapid with a poor volume.

Effective cooling is essential, usually by spraying the exposed body with cold water and by using fans to promote active air movement. Intravenous saline fluids may be given to replace salt loss from perspiration.

Hypothermia

Serious lowering of the body temperature is now recognised as a common cause of stupor or coma, particularly in elderly patients during the winter months. The ordinary clinical thermometer does not record temperatures below 35°C (95°F), and every ward should now possess a special low-reading thermometer for recording the rectal temperature in suspected cases. In elderly people, particularly those living on their own, various circumstances dispose to hypo-thermia—

1. Inadequate room heating, a meagre food intake, unsuitable clothing, and cold weather.
2. Immobilisation, due to a fracture or a stroke, for example, which prevents the summoning of help.
3. Overdosage with drugs or alcohol and falling asleep in an unheated room without adequate covering; the unconscious patient loses heat very quickly.
4. Myxoedema (see p. 444).

In the early stages of exposure to cold, the skin goes white, the extremities are cold and shivering occurs. This is followed by stiffness of the muscles, the shivering ceases and a stuperose state supervenes. The breathing becomes slow and shallow and the blood pressure falls. At this stage the rectal temperature may be less than 30°C (86°F). With further lowering of the temperature, the patient loses consciousness and coma ensues.

Prevention

Poverty, poor housing and insufficient heating are not easily eradicated but awareness by local authorities and social workers of this problem may do much to help. Regular visiting, meals-on-wheels and advice as to forms of heating may all be necessary.

Treatment

No attempt should be made to heat the patient rapidly, since this causes the skin vessels to dilate. Fluid is then lost from the general circulation. It is best to wrap the patient in a warm blanket in a warm room or hospital ward and ensure that the rectal temperature is recorded regularly. Since dehydration is often present, a slow drip of warmed 5 per cent dextrose may be given intravenously.

Electricity

Most cases of electric shock occur in the home or at work due to faulty electrical apparatus, inadequately earthed. The passage of electricity through the body causes burning of the skin and if the current is large enough it may lead to cardiac arrest (see p. 117).

Radiation

Natural radiation exists in small amounts in the atmosphere, some in the form of cosmic rays from the sun and the stars, some from radioactive materials in the earth. Manmade radiation comes from the products of nuclear energy, from the use of X-rays and in radiotherapy.

Excess radiation can do irreparable damage to various tissues of the body, particularly the skin, hair, blood and reproductive organs and can give rise to cancer. Hence those working in X-ray departments must be protected by stringent safety regulations to avoid any possible long-term dangers. Techniques are adopted to minimise the patients' exposure to radiation, particularly as some investigations, such as a barium meal, involve more lengthy exposure and may have to be repeated on several occasions. The adoption of safety standards is routine in all X-ray departments.

Radiotherapy can be used to control the spread of certain malignant growths. The cells of the growing tumour are particularly vulnerable to the burning effect of deep X-rays directed on them, while the healthy surrounding tissues are largely unaffected. Superficial X-ray therapy can be used for malignant skin disorders.

Radioactive forms of normal elements are also used in the treatment of various disorders. Radioactive iodine, for example, when given by mouth is taken up by the thyroid gland. It suppresses the metabolism of overactive thyroid cells and so can be used in the treatment of disorders of the thyroid (see p. 437).

TUMOUR FORMATION

The various organs and tissues of the body grow and are maintained in an orderly and disciplined manner. A tumour is an abnormal growth of tissue which has no useful function.

Some tumours are called benign because their growth is restricted and local: they may compress surrounding structures, but they do not invade them. Examples of benign tumours are lipomas under the skin, papillomata in the nose or bowel and fibroids in the uterus.

Malignant tumours grow in size and invade and destroy neighbouring tissues: cells from this growth enter the lymphatics and the blood vessels and so are carried to the lymph nodes and to other organs. These cells which spread to other organs form similar malignant growths and are called *secondary deposits* or *metastases*.

Malignant tumours are known as cancer. A malignant tumour of epithelial cells is called a *carcinoma* and a malignant tumour of connective tissue, such as bone or muscle, is called *sarcoma*. Thus we talk of a carcinoma of the bronchus or a sarcoma of the femur. The malignant process is referred to as *neoplasia* and, especially in front of patients, a cancer is often referred to as a *neoplasm* (which means new growth).

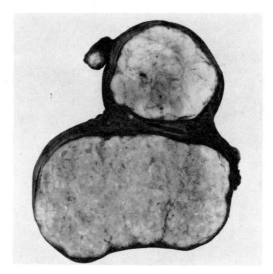

FIG. 2.3   Benign tumour (fibroid) of the uterus.

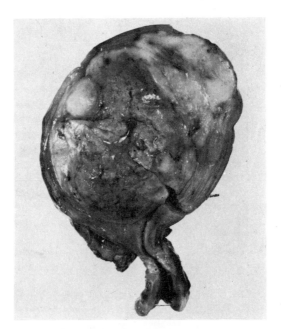

FIG. 2.4   Malignant tumour (carcinoma) of the uterus. It can be seen that, in contrast with Fig. 2.3, there is marked invasion and destruction of the walls of the uterus and gross ulceration. Severe haemorrhage from the uterus occurred.

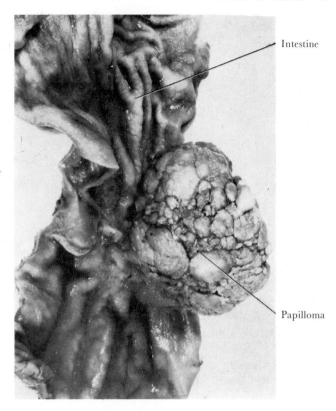

Intestine

Papilloma

FIG. 2.5 Benign tumour (papilloma) growing from the intestinal mucous membrane.

The study and management of malignant growth is known as *oncology* and the physician who specialises in this subject is an *oncologist*.

The cause of neoplasia is unknown in many cases. However some forms of cancer can be brought about by—

Radiation (see above).

Various industrial chemicals and tars, including cigarettes.

Certain viruses can probably cause cancer in animals and possibly in man.

Malignant growths cause harm in different ways—

1. They invade and destroy neighbouring tissues, including blood vessels.

2. They spread to more remote organs and tissues. Malignant cells enter the blood vessels and lymphatics and settle in other areas. These secondary deposits (metastases) themselves begin to grow and invade local structures. Thus a carcinoma of the bronchus can cause metastases in the liver and brain.

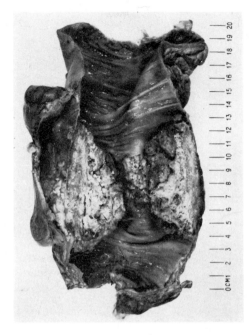

FIG. 2.6 Malignant tumour (carcinoma) of the rectum. When compared with Fig. 2.5 it can be seen that there is invasion of the intestinal wall with ulceration of the tissues. In addition it can be seen how the growing tumour is causing obstruction of the intestinal canal.

3. They produce toxic substances which can damage the function of the nervous system, including the brain and the peripheral nerves.
4. They can produce hormones such as ACTH (see p. 457) which lead to symptoms due to excess hormonal effect.
5. They lead to metabolic disorders and a general malaise, wasting and exhaustion known as *cachexia*.

Management of malignancy

The successful treatment of most cases of carcinoma and sarcoma depends on early diagnosis and surgical treatment, either by operative removal or by radiotherapy. However, particularly when surgical treatment has failed to prevent the spread of carcinoma, administration of drugs (chemotherapy) may be considered. Drugs used for this purpose are called *cytotoxic* drugs: malignant cells are sensitive to their destructive action and healthy tissues are not seriously affected. Some forms of neoplasm often respond very well to chemotherapy, particularly Hodgkin's disease, carcinoma of the prostate, and acute leukaemia in children.

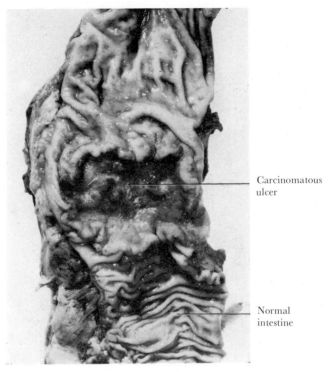

Carcinomatous
ulcer

Normal
intestine

FIG. 2.7 Another example of a carcinoma of the intestine showing the marked ulceration of the tissues. Intestinal haemorrhage was a feature of this case.

Cytotoxic drugs act by interfering with the growth processes of the malignant cells. Since they may also exert harmful effects on healthy tissue, particularly the bone marrow, they have to be administered with great care. Usually combinations of different types of cytotoxic drugs are administered, sometimes intravenously and in intermittent courses. Close supervision is obligatory where this form of treatment is used. Particularly in the treatment of leukaemia, steroids (see p. 357) may be given in addition to the cytotoxic drugs to help reduce complications of the treatment on healthy blood cells. In carcinoma of the prostate, and in some forms of breast cancer, the malignant cells seem to be influenced by hormones, and oestrogens in the form of stilboesterol can be effective in suppressing the growth and spread of the cancer.

3 Infection, Immunity and Chemotherapy

INFECTION

Many types of living organisms can invade and damage the human body:

1. Bacteria. These are single-celled forms of life, visible under the microscope They exist all around us, in the air, in the earth, in our food. They are present on our skin, in the mouth and in the bowel. They are not all harmful or disease-producing (*pathogenic*). Most are *non-pathogenic* and indeed may be beneficial. Bacteria normally present in the bowel may prevent the growth of pathogenic organisms and they help to produce vitamins.

2. Viruses. Viruses are too small to be seen under the microscope. They can only survive inside living cells since they depend on the nutriment of the cell for their growth and replication. Viruses are resistant to the action of antibiotics.

3. Fungi (mycoses). Numerous fungi or moulds exist in the soil, in decaying vegetation and in the excreta of birds. Fungi can be regarded as a form of vegetation and sometimes are antagonistic to the growth of bacteria—penicillin is derived from one such mould. Other fungi, known as mycoses, can infect the skin (see p. 483), the mouth (commonly known as thrush), and the lungs.

4. Protozoa. These are single-celled parasites, bigger than bacteria and changing form during their life cycle. Malaria and amoebic dysentery are two widespread tropical diseases caused by protozoa.

5. Metazoa. These are many-celled organisms, the majority visible to the naked eye. They include such parasites as lice, scabies (see p. 481) and intestinal worms (see p. 237).

BACTERIA

There are a large number of different types of bacteria, some of more importance than others in both the seriousness and the frequency with which they cause disease. Only the most common and important bacteria will be discussed here.

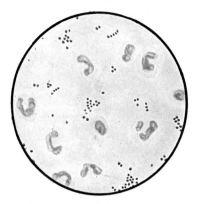

FIG. 3.1   Staphylococci after staining appear under the microscope in clusters.

Bacteria are usually divided up into different groups known as cocci, bacilli and spirochaetes.

Cocci

These are rounded organisms and, according to the manner in which they grow, they are divided up into different groups. When they grow in bunches or clusters they are spoken of as *staphylococci*. If they form chains as they grow they are called *streptococci*, and if they grow in pairs they are called *diplococci*.

These main groups are further divided into classes according to various factors. For example, certain important streptococci, when they grow in a special medium containing blood, cause the red cells to be destroyed, or, as it is said, the blood is haemolysed. For this reason these are called *haemolytic* streptococci, to distinguish them from other forms of streptococci which do not cause haemolysis when they grow on blood.

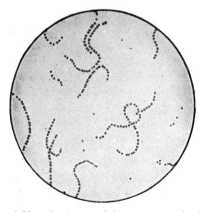

FIG. 3.2   Streptococci. Note the characteristic arrangement in chains.

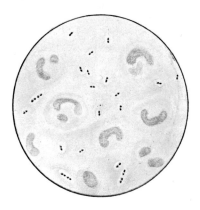

FIG. 3.3 Pneumococci are in pairs.

TABLE I The cocci

Name	Pathological effects	Diseases
Staphylococci	Acute inflammation with pus formation. Lesions tend to remain localised with the development of abscesses	Skin conditions; boils, carbuncles, impetigo Bone lesions: osteo-myelitis Otitis media, meningitis, pneumonia, acute bacterial endocarditis, septicaemia
Streptococci. (a) Haemolytic	Acute inflammation with pus. Lesions usually spread	Skin conditions: cellulitis, erysipelas and impetigo. Acute tonsillitis, scarlet fever, otitis media, meningitis, pneumonia, acute bacterial endocarditis, septicaemia
(b) Non-haemolytic	Subacute inflammation	Subacute bacterial endo-carditis
Pneumococci	Acute inflammation with pus	Pneumonia of both lobar and broncho types. Otitis media, meningitis, peritonitis
Meningococci	Acute inflammation with pus	Meningitis (cerebro-spinal fever)
Gonococci	Acute and chronic inflammation with pus	Gonorrhoea, causing acute urethritis, epididymo-orchitis and prostatitis in the male; acute eurethritis, vaginitis and salpingitis in the female. Ophthalmia in the newborn. Arthritis

Again, some cocci are called by the name of the disease they set up in the body. The common disease of the lungs known as pneumonia is usually due to a certain group of cocci which are given the name of *pneumococci*. Some cocci and bacilli in causing disease usually set up an inflammation with pus formation, and for this reason they are often

TABLE II The bacilli

Name	Pathological effects	Diseases
Tubercle bacilli	Specific type of subacute and chronic inflammation. Tubercles form which often break down to a cheesy material (caseation). Ulceration with cavity formation is also a feature. Healing by fibrosis	Tuberculosis, which affects many organs and tissues. Especially important are: pulmonary tuberculosis, tuberculous meningitis, glandular tuberculosis, tuberculosis of the bones (N.B. spine), joints, kidneys and skin
Coliform bacilli	Acute and chronic inflammation with pus.	Pyelitis, cystitis, peritonitis, cholecystitis, meningitis, puerperal sepsis
Pertussis bacilli	Specific acute infectious fever mainly involving the lungs	Whooping-cough
Diphtheria bacilli	Specific localised lesion, the diphtheritic membrane, and a powerful toxin with widespread effects	Diphtheria, with the membrane in the throat, nose, or larynx. Toxin causes albuminuria, acute myocarditis and neuritis
Typhoid and paratyphoid bacilli	Specific infectious fevers with acute inflammation and ulceration. General invasion of the body including the blood stream, but marked local changes in the small intestine	Typhoid and paratyphoid fever (enteric fever)
Dysentery bacilli	Specific acute inflammation with ulceration of the intestinal tract. Toxin also produced	Acute bacillary dysentery
Salmonella bacilli	Acute inflammation of the intestinal tract. Toxin	Food poisoning
Influenza bacilli	Acute inflammation with pus	Influenzal meningitis
Abortus and melitensis bacilli	Specific inflammation of a subacute type mainly involving the joints, glands and spleen	Undulant fever (brucellosis)
Tetanus bacilli	Powerful toxin produced which has a selective effect on the nerve cells	Tetanus

classed together as *pyogenic organisms*. These include, especially, staphylococci, streptococci, pneumococii, meningococci and the coliform bacilli.

Table I gives the names, main types of lesion or pathological change, and finally the most common diseases caused by the more important cocci.

Bacilli

Bacilli instead of being rounded bodies are rod-shaped and are mainly classified according to the type of disease which they cause.

Table II gives the commonest bacilli and the diseases caused by them.

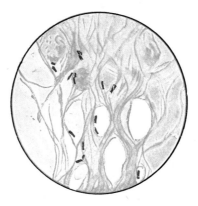

FIG. 3.4   Tubercle bacillus is slender, straight or curved with rounded ends.

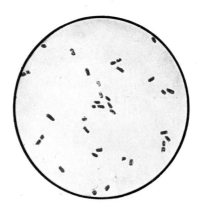

FIG. 3.5   *Bacillus coli.*

Spirochaetes

The last important group of bacteria is the spirochaetal group. These organisms are larger than either cocci or bacilli and their bodies have several curves. Fewer diseases are caused by spirochaetes than by the two preceding groups. The most important disease in man due to a spirochaete is syphilis.

Table III lists the few well-known diseases caused by the spirochaetes.

TABLE III   The spirochaetes

Name	Pathological effects	Diseases
Treponema pallidum	Chronic inflammation with fibrosis and ulceration. Widespread lesions, with the heart, arteries and nervous system particularly affected	Syphilis
Leptospira icterohaemorrhagiae	Toxin which particularly affects the liver to cause a hepatitis and jaundice	Weil's disease (spirochaetal jaundice)
Borrelia vincentii	Acute inflammation and ulceration of the throat and gums	Vincent's angina

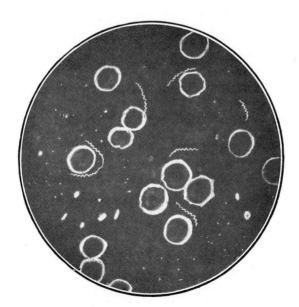

FIG. 3.6   The spirochaete of syphilis.

VIRUSES

Viruses are responsible for such widespread ailments as influenza and the common cold. Many acute infectious fevers, which include measles, rubella, mumps, and chickenpox, are due to viruses. More serious viral infections include poliomyelitis, encephalitis and viral pneumonia.

Unlike infections due to bacteria, viral infections do not respond to antibiotics or sulphonamides so there is no effective treatment to overcome these ailments. Happily in most viral infections the body's immunity system overcomes the virus. However, occasionally very severe strains of viruses become rampant, as occurred in the influenzal epidemic in 1918, when thousands of deaths occurred.

The diagnosis of most viral illnesses is evident from the typical signs and symptoms. In bacterial infections, the white cells in the blood are greatly increased (leucocytosis), but this does not occur with most infections due to a virus. Confirmation of the diagnosis of a virus infection is much more difficult and takes much longer than with bacterial infections.

Special techniques are required to culture viruses present in infected material. Viral antibodies can be demonstrated in the blood but usually this investigation takes several weeks.

SPECIMENS FOR BACTERIOLOGICAL EXAMINATION

The primary object of practical bacteriological methods is to find out what part a particular organism plays in causing a particular disease. Of course to do this it is essential to obtain the particular organism: therefore if a disease is suspected of being caused by bacteria, certain methods are adopted to try to obtain the organism. From experience it is known that in certain diseases the responsible organism can be found in specific excretions or tissues; these are accordingly examined for presence of the organism.

In general the common specimens or material examined for the presence of bacteria are as follows:

Throat swabs

A swab is a piece of sterile cotton-wool wrapped round the end of a stick. The sterile wool is rubbed over the surface or area from which the specimen is to be taken. Swabs are often taken from the throat, as in many diseases the causative organism is to be found in the throat. Fresh swabs should be delivered to the laboratory as soon as possible after taking

Diseases in which throat swabs are normally taken are:

(a) Acute tonsillitis or any 'sore throat'
(b) Diphtheria
(c) Scarlet fever
(d) Rheumatic fever.

Nasal swabs

These are less important than throat swabs but are taken in suspected nasal diphtheria.

Sputum

In most diseases in which sputum is being coughed up it is sent for bacteriological examination, but this is of special importance in the following:

(a) Pulmonary tuberculosis
(b) Pneumonia.

Sputum examination for the presence of *tubercle bacilli*, the bacteria causing pulmonary tuberculosis, is of great importance. Firstly, it establishes the diagnosis of the case as one of active pulmonary tuberculosis; and secondly, it denotes that the case is infectious and should be treated with full isolation procedure. In pneumonia, examination of the sputum for bacteria is often carried out to determine what is the causative organism.

Faeces

Many bacteria cause lesions in the intestinal tract and the organisms in these cases can often be found in the faeces. Diseases in which this examination of faeces for organisms is most commonly performed are:

(a) All cases of acute diarrhoea
(b) Dysentery
(c) Food poisoning
(d) Typhoid and paratyphoid fevers
(e) Tuberculosis of the intestinal tract.

Urine

The urine is frequently examined for the presence of bacteria and, if sent for this examination, it must be obtained with aseptic precautions. A specimen is obtained after washing the genitalia with soap and water and discarding the first urine passed (*midstream specimen*). Urine examination for bacteria is of importance in the following diseases:

(a) Acute pyelitis and cystitis
(b) Acute urethritis
(c) Tuberculosis of the renal tract.

Blood

In cases where it is suspected that the bacteria may be actually growing in the blood stream (that is, in septicaemia) a small quantity of blood, usually 2 to 3 ml, is put into a special bottle known as a *blood culture* bottle. This bottle contains a special medium, usually glucose broth or cooked meat, which helps the organisms to grow. It is of the utmost importance that the blood should be collected under strict aseptic technique, as otherwise contaminating organisms will get into the blood culture bottle and confuse the result of the test.

A properly sterilised syringe must be used.

Blood cultures are usually taken in the following diseases:

(a) All cases of suspected septicaemia
(b) Bacterial endocarditis
(c) Typhoid and paratyphoid fevers
(d) All cases of prolonged undiagnosed fever.

Pleural and cerebrospinal fluid

When fluid is present in the chest a sample is frequently aspirated in order to isolate any organism that may be present. Such organisms include pneumococci, streptococci, staphylococci and tubercle bacilli. All these organisms commonly cause disease of the lungs and pleura with resulting fluid in the pleural cavity.

Cerebrospinal fluid is withdrawn by doing a lumbar puncture. It is examined for bacteria in all cases of meningitis (inflammatory disease of the meninges). The bacteria often found include, in particular, meningococci, pneumococci, and tubercle bacilli.

Any discharge of pus from any abscess, sore, or other lesion
Swabs from the genital regions

In all cases of a discharge from the vagina or urethra a swab is taken and an examination for the presence of organisms, particularly the gonococcus, made.

If there is a sore on the genital organs, a scraping from the sore is taken for examination for the presence of the spirochaete of syphilis.

Eye swabs

In many cases of inflammation of the eyes, and also before any operation on the eyes, swabs are taken. Before eye operations are performed it is essential that no organisms should be present in the conjunctiva.

METHODS OF IDENTIFICATION OF ORGANISMS

The usual way in which material is obtained for bacteriological examination has just been described. The material so obtained is treated in the laboratory by many different methods so that the organism may be identified.

Staining of smears

In some cases the material obtained is smeared on to a slide and various stains or dyes are applied to colour and show up the organisms. By means of these stains we can differentiate between certain organisms, as some turn one colour while others turn another. For example, one important and commonly used stain is known as

Gram's stain. By means of this most of the common organisms can be divided into two groups:
1. Gram-positive organisms, which turn blue on application of the stain.
2. Gram-negative organisms, which turn red.

The cocci (except for the meningococci and gonococci) are usually Gram-positive, whilst many of the more important bacilli (but not the tubercle bacilli or *Bacillus diphtheriae*) are Gram-negative.

Again, by washing out the stain with acid most organisms are distinguished from the tubercle bacillus which resists the action of acid and is thus called an *acid-fast bacillus*.

Cultures

Most specimens taken are put on a special plate containing suitable material, such as blood, which will enable the organism to grow to the best advantage and, as far as possible, in a pure state. The plate is placed in a special box, known as an *incubator*, which is kept at a temperature of 37°C (body temperature); most organisms grow best at body temperature. After 24 to 48 hours the plate is examined for growth of the organism. This method of examination is spoken of as a culture. Smears or films are then taken from the culture plate and stained for examination under the microscope as outlined above. The culture plate yields very useful information on the identity of the organisms, as in their growth certain characteristics are shown. For instance, the haemolytic streptococcus, an important organism causing several diseases, can be distinguished from the non-haemolytic streptococcus. As the names imply, the latter does not cause haemolysis on a blood culture plate while the haemolytic streptococcus does.

Agglutination reactions

To explain what is meant by an agglutination reaction it is best to take a particular example, e.g. the *Widal reaction,* a typical agglutination reaction, which is used in the diagnosis of typhoid fever. If a patient is suffering from typhoid fever, antibodies are developed in the body against the typhoid bacilli as part of the body's protective mechanism to fight the disease. If serum from the patient is mixed with known typhoid bacilli in a test-tube the bacilli become clumped or agglutinated owing to the action of the antibodies on the bacilli. No agglutination would occur if serum and organisms other than typhoid bacilli were mixed together. In this way the agglutination reaction can be used for diagnosis in certain infections. This test is of value where it is difficult to isolate the actual organisms and is mostly used in cases of the enteric fevers. Agglutination reactions only become positive after the illness has lasted approximately a week, as it takes this time for the antibodies to form in the body.

HOW BACTERIA ENTER THE BODY

Organisms must enter the body if they are to set up a disease. The ways in which the organisms can do so are often referred to as the modes of spread.

Droplet infection. If organisms are present in the upper air passages they are expelled into the air on speaking and especially on sneezing and coughing, and they can then be readily inhaled by others. Infection can thus easily spread through close proximity to the infected person; direct contact is not necessary. In some cases the infected droplets can contaminate dust, and inhalation of the dust can cause infection. Fortunately most organisms soon die outside the body, but an important exception is the tubercle bacillus which can remain alive in dust for many months. The majority of the acute infectious diseases, such as measles, whooping-cough, diphtheria, etc., are contracted in this way through the respiratory tract.

Infection may spread through *handling articles* which have become infected with the organism, e.g. clothes, bedlinen, toys, pencils, etc. Neglect in washing the hands thoroughly is very likely to spread infection from patient to patient.

The infecting organism may be present in the *faeces* and *urine* and, if the hands are not washed properly after visits to the toilet, food can become contaminated and the infection may thus spread to others. Contamination of water supplies from leaking drains was also formerly a common cause of large epidemics. *Flies* which feed on excreta are another common means by which food can become contaminated.

The diseases which are spread through contamination of food, milk or water are the intestinal infections such as food poisoning, dysentery and typhoid fever.

Certain organisms, especially gonococci and the syphilitic spiro-chaete, require actual *direct contact* between the infected person and the one to be infected.

Infecting organisms may be conveyed by means of a *blood-sucking insect*, e.g. by mosquitoes carrying the malarial parasites and lice carrying the typhus organisms.

Finally, infection may spread to man from contact with *animals*, e.g. rabies from dogs and anthrax from sheep.

HOW BACTERIA CAUSE DISEASE

We have now seen how bacteria can enter the body. Before going further it must be realised that bacteria exist all around us but they do not necessarily cause disease. Why is this? It is because to cause disease, even after entry of the organism into the body, certain conditions must prevail:

1. The bacteria must be present in *sufficient* numbers.

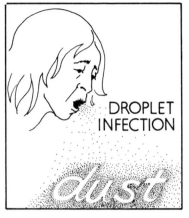
DROPLET INFECTION

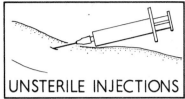
UNSTERILE INJECTIONS

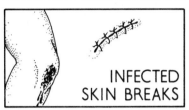
INFECTED SKIN BREAKS

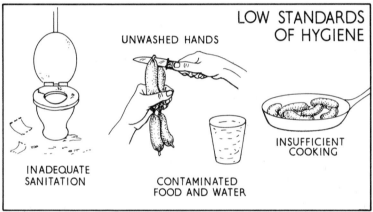
LOW STANDARDS OF HYGIENE

UNWASHED HANDS

INADEQUATE SANITATION

CONTAMINATED FOOD AND WATER

INSUFFICIENT COOKING

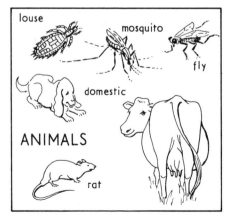
louse

mosquito

fly

domestic

ANIMALS

rat

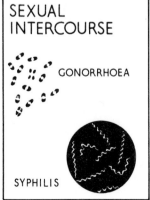
SEXUAL INTERCOURSE

GONORRHOEA

SYPHILIS

Fig. 3.7 Some common modes of infection.

2. The bacteria must be *virulent*, that is, of a sufficient degree of activity.
3. The organisms must have entered the body by the *proper pathway*, e.g. gonococci if swallowed are destroyed and do not cause disease, while dysentery organisms cause disease only if swallowed.
4. The person infected must be *susceptible* to the organism, that is, must not be resistant (immune). This subject is discussed further under Immunity.

Given the above suitable conditions, the organisms entering the body will multiply and produce toxins, which are poisonous substances that react on tissues and cells. The nature of these reactions varies with different bacteria, some toxins causing inflammation, either acute or chronic, whilst others cause degeneration of cells. Many toxins tend to have specific selective action on particular tissues or cells, e.g. diphtheria toxin on the nerves and heart. These specific actions will be described more fully under the individual diseases.

HOW THE BODY RESISTS AND OVERCOMES INFECTION (IMMUNITY)

So far in our discussion we have considered:
1. The identification of bacteria causing disease.
2. How these bacteria get into the body.
3. The conditions necessary before these bacteria, having entered the body, can give rise to disease.
4. How these bacteria set up their toxic effects to cause disease.

In discussing the conditions necessary before bacteria can cause disease we saw that the person infected must be sensitive or susceptible to the organisms. In many cases the infected person is not susceptible and does not suffer from the disease even though he or she is harbouring the organism in the body. In these circumstances the person is said to be immune to the disease.

Immunity to a particular disease may be acquired naturally, or it may be acquired deliberately by artificial immunisation.

THE DEFENCE AGAINST INFECTION

The body defends itself against infection by bacteria and viruses both locally and constitutionally. The local response to an infection is by the process of *inflammation* and the constitutional reaction by the *immunity system.*

INFLAMMATION

This is the reaction of local tissues in response to an infection or traumatic agent.

(*a*) **Acute**

Acute inflammation is characterised by redness, swelling and heat of the area involved. There is often considerable pain and impairment or loss of function. These features are caused by dilatation of the small blood vessels which then exude fluid.

(*b*) **Chronic**

The white cells now appear on the scene. Polymorphonuclear leuco-cytes (polymorphs) engulf foreign material or bacteria; there may be so many polymorphs present that an abscess is formed. Lymphocytes produce antibodies which neutralise any toxins present and prevent the bacteria from spreading. Fibrous tissue cells form strands of dense tough tissue which wall off the infected area and lead to scar formation. If this is extensive, distortion and deformity of the area occur.

The nature and degree of the inflammation depend mainly on the type of agent or bacteria responsible. Some diseases, such as tuberculosis, cause gradual and chronic inflammation. Others, such as staphylococcal infections, can cause acute and severe inflammation. Sometimes an inflamed area can give rise to a discharge or exudate. This may be:

(i) SEROUS. Often when the pleura or peritoneum is inflamed, there is an effusion of clear yellow fluid.

(ii) PURULENT. Here the exudate is purulent since it contains infective organisms, masses of polymorphs and debris of dead tissue cells.

(iii) HAEMORRHAGIC. A bloodstained exudate occurs sometimes with bacterial infections, but it is particularly common with malignant growths (carcinoma).

(*c*) **Repair**

If the inflammation is mild, then the protective forces of the body can overcome the disease and healing can occur with very little per-manent change in the affected area. If it is more severe, permanent changes, principally fibrosis or scarring, may occur. It can be seen that if this scarring is extensive, owing to severe inflammation, then it can interfere with the proper function of the part. This may be a serious disability, perhaps with fatal results, if the part affected is a vital organ. For example, disease causing a chronic inflammation of the valves of the heart can give rise to scarring and deformity, with the result that the heart cannot function properly, so that after a period it fails and death occurs.

IMMUNITY

Most organisms, though not all, on getting into the body stimulate the lymphocytes to produce substances which react with these toxic invading organisms and destroy them. These substances are called *antibodies* and *antitoxins*. The organisms are said to act as *antigens* to produce antibodies.

The antibodies and antitoxins produced, e.g. against the diphtheria organism, will have effect only against this organism and will have no effect against any other organism.

Antibodies do not persist indefinitely. Some last for many years, but others only for a few weeks or months.

Antibodies are a form of protein known as gamma globulin and are produced by lymphocytes and special plasma cells. These cells seem capable of producing millions of different antibodies to deal with all the different kinds of antigens that are encountered and just how this happens is a subject of much recent research. It appears that the thymus gland plays an important part in the development of immunity in the fetus, and that the lymph nodes and the spleen are a factory for the development of the lymphocytes in the adult.

Naturally acquired immunity

Natural immunity to a particular disease may be acquired in several different ways:

The individual has an actual attack of the disease. When the body is invaded by an infection, certain protective substances are produced by the lymphocytes to counteract and neutralise the invader. These protective substances are known as *antibodies*. These antibodies will protect against the particular infection for which they were formed, but not against other infections. If there is considerable antibody formation, the patient will be immune from further attacks of the same infection. However, not all infections give rise to antibody formation, so that immunity is not always acquired to further attacks of the same disease.

The individual is exposed to repeated infection in small doses, so that an actual attack of the disease does not occur. By repeated stimulation of the body's protective mechanisms by infections too small to cause an actual attack of the disease (*sub-clinical infection*) a complete development of antibodies can occur in the course of time. These can then resist a full dose of infection, which would normally set up an attack of the disease. This method of developing an immunity to a particular disease explains why some people are immune or resistant to a disease without ever having suffered from an actual attack.

Resistance to a disease is inherited. For example, an infant may be immune for a short period owing to the passage of the mother's protective substances into its circulation by way of the placenta or through the mother's milk.

In addition to the above, there is the natural immunity of animals to such diseases as syphilis and gonorrhoea. Again, certain animals may be immune to a disease whilst others are highly susceptible, e.g. sheep and cattle are very susceptible to the disease anthrax while dogs and rats are practically immune.

Artificially acquired immunity (active and passive)

Artificial immunity is the result of a deliberate and successful attempt, by one means or another, to make the body develop protective substances against disease. The history of the discovery of this process is of great interest and helps in understanding immunity.

In 1798 Jenner observed that people who suffered from the mild disease known as cowpox, caught from cattle, rarely suffered from the much more serious and often fatal disease known as smallpox. If they did contract smallpox the attack was usually mild. From this he inferred that the cowpox attack in some way conferred a resistance or immunity to smallpox in the person concerned. He also believed that probably the organism causing cowpox was almost identical with that causing smallpox, but of a milder nature.

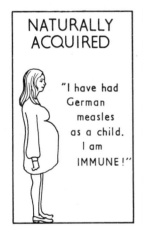

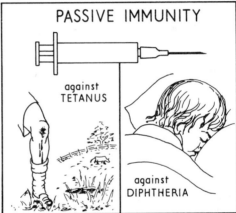

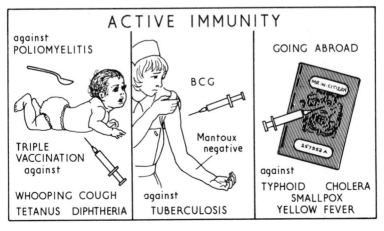

Fig. 3.8   Some types of immunity.

Jenner then proceeded to inoculate a boy with cowpox, and after the boy had overcome this mild complaint, demonstrated that he could not be infected with smallpox. This brilliant experiment of Jenner's has laid the whole foundation of vaccination.

The next advance in the artificial creation of immunity was due to Pasteur. In 1885 he discovered that certain bacteria could be rendered harmless by various means, so that they could be injected into human subjects with complete safety. Although these bacteria could no longer cause disease, they retained their capacity to stimulate the formation of antibodies. Thus infecting an individual with this modified type of organism created an immunity or resistance in the person without causing an attack of the disease. The means Pasteur adopted to modify the virulence or activity of an organism were heating the organism, adding an antiseptic, or passing it through an animal. Passage of an organism through an animal for some reason modifies it so that it is no longer capable of setting up active disease in man but can still create an immunity to infection by active organisms. The term *vaccine* is given to a suspension of modified avirulent organisms, and the procedure of inoculating is spoken of as vaccination or immunisation.

Instead of using modified avirulent organisms, the toxins produced by organisms, suitably modified, may be used as an alternative in order to create an immunity. Modified toxin as used in immunisation is known as *toxoid*.

In addition to the above-mentioned type of artificial immunity, which is called *active immunity*, there is still a further form, known as *passive immunity*. Passive immunity will be discussed later (see p. 65).

Clinical use of vaccination (immunisation) and serum treatment

Vaccination is the method frequently used to produce immunity to certain infectious diseases which can become widespread and serious. Thus to protect against typhoid fever dead typhoid bacilli are used to prepare a vaccine. When this vaccine is inoculated the body forms antibodies which afford protection against typhoid fever for over a year. In areas where typhoid fever is rampant inoculation must be repeated at intervals to renew antibody formation. This type of immunity is known as *active immunity* since it depends on the activity of the vaccinated person's own lymphocytes to produce the appropriate antibody.

DISEASES IN WHICH VACCINATION (ACTIVE IMMUNITY) IS OF VALUE

Smallpox
Diphtheria
Tuberculosis
Typhoid
Tetanus

Whooping-cough
Poliomyelitis
Rubella.

An individual who has recovered from an infection will have circulating in his blood the specific antibodies to the particular organism responsible for his illness. Thus a patient recovering from measles has abundant antibodies to measles circulating in his blood. This blood can now be withdrawn and the serum used to prevent measles in a child who has been exposed to this infection. This is known as *passive immunity* since the antibodies are not actively produced by the child who receives the serum.

DISEASES IN WHICH ANTITOXIN SERUM (PASSIVE IMMUNITY) CAN BE USED
Diphtheria
Tetanus
Measles.

In practice today actual convalescent serum is no longer used to prevent measles for fear of transmitting other infections. Instead the protein which contains the antibodies (gamma globulin) is isolated from the serum, purified and stored for future use.

In diphtheria the horse is used as the source of antitoxin serum. He is repeatedly inoculated with inactivated diphtheria bacilli until sufficient antitoxin is formed. The horse is then bled, the serum sterilised and kept for emergency use in severe diphtheria (p. 71).

ORGAN TRANSPLANTATION

As has been discussed (p. 43), the introduction of bacteria or other foreign material (known as the antigen) leads to the production of antibodies, mainly by the lymphocytes. These antibodies block the effect of the antigen. Any material introduced into the body acts as an antigen unless it is naturally part of the body, or at least so similar to the natural product as to be indistinguishable from it. For example, a transfusion of blood from another person will produce serious antibody reactions unless the blood is of a similar group. It is this problem of antibody reaction that makes so difficult the transplantation of organs. The surgeon may wish to transplant a kidney from someone who has just died from a road accident into a patient suffering from hopeless kidney disease. Technically this is not difficult in experienced hands but unless the kidney is from an identical twin, antibodies are formed which react with the transplanted kidney and prevent it from functioning. This process is known as rejection. Much research is being conducted on the best methods of preventing this rejection.

  (a) Steroids, such as prednisone, help to suppress the antigen–antibody reaction but have to be given in large doses.
  (b) Certain cytotoxic drugs, especially azathioprine, prevent the

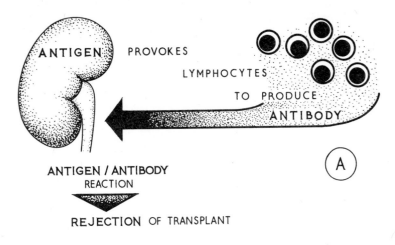

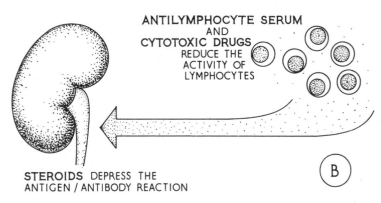

FIG. 3.9   Organ transplant. (A) Causes of rejection. (B) Prevention of rejection.

production of antibodies. They have toxic effects and have to be administered cautiously.

(c) Antilymphocytic serum may be given to suppress the lymphocytes which supply the antibodies. Human lymphocytes injected into a horse lead to the production of antibodies to these lymphocytes in the horse's serum. This now becomes the source of antilymphocytic serum. Thus in order to prevent the rejection of a transplanted organ, antilymphocytic serum is injected and treatment begun with prednisone and azathioprine.

With these precautions, transplanted organs may function well for a time and temporary success has been recorded with transplants of such organs as the kidney, liver, pancreas, lung and heart. Many problems remain to be solved before this operation can become routine. At present, the organ to be transplanted must be removed soon after the donor's death since no method is available for preserving it for more than a few hours without damage.

ANAPHYLAXIS, SERUM SICKNESS, HYPERSENSITIVENESS AND ALLERGY

All the above conditions are in some way allied to each other and the terms are often used in different senses by different people. This is especially so with the term *allergy*. To explain the above conditions, which are rather difficult to understand, it is best to describe how they are seen in clinical practice.

Anaphylaxis

In some people who have been given an injection of serum a second injection, if it is given more than 10 to 14 days after the first, may be followed by a very severe and often fatal reaction known as anaphylaxis. The essential features of the reaction are a spasm of smooth muscle and a dilatation of small capillaries. This leads to collapse, extreme difficulty in breathing, convulsions and, in some cases, death. These effects are supposed to be due to the action of a foreign protein in the first serum injection which produces an excess of sensitive antibodies which, on the second serum injection, cause this violent reaction. If the second injection is given before 10 days have elapsed, the anaphylactic reaction does not for some reason develop.

Anaphylaxis is very rare, and in the treatment the immediate injection of adrenaline (0·5 to 1 ml of 1 : 1000 dilution) is of great value. When injecting serum of any kind, adrenaline should always be readily available.

Serum sickness

About seven to 14 days after an injection of serum (especially of large amounts) the person may develop an urticarial reaction in the skin, joint pains, fever and enlarged glands. These symptoms occur after the first injection of serum. As in anaphylaxis, they are due to a sensitisation of the body against a foreign protein in the serum. Serum sickness, however, unlike anaphylaxis, is never fatal.

The antihistamine drugs (Phenergan, Benadryl, etc.) will often relieve symptoms, and adrenaline is also helpful by injection. Should these measures fail, cortisone or its allies are usually prescribed.

Hypersensitiveness

Anaphylaxis and serum sickness, just discussed, are of the nature of hypersensitive reactions, but these terms are usually reserved for sensitiveness following serum injections only. Many individuals, however, are sensitive to a great many different foreign proteins present in foods, dust, flowers, drugs, etc. When they come in contact with the offending substances by eating, inhaling or touching them, they develop certain characteristic reactions such as:

(a) Laboured wheezing breathing (asthma)
(b) Wheals, like bites on the skin (urticaria)
(c) Vomiting and diarrhoea
(d) Severe running from the nose and eyes (similar to hay fever)
(e) Fever.

These individuals are said to have an idiosyncrasy to the offending substance or to be 'allergic'. Certain diseases such as asthma, urticaria, hay fever and eczema are often due to a sensitiveness to a food, plant, or drug, etc., and are therefore called allergic·diseases.

CHEMOTHERAPY

Chemotherapy is the treatment of infections by substances which destroy or suppress bacteria.

The sulphonamides were the first group of chemical drugs to be used successfully in the treatment of common infections. They exert their effect by inhibiting the growth of invading bacteria, thus allowing the defensive mechanism of the body to overcome susceptible organisms. Unfortunately the sulphonamides are ineffective against many dangerous bacteria.

The discovery of penicillin represented a major victory in the fight against bacteria, and greatly increases the range of bacteria which can be overcome. Penicillin is not a chemical drug but is, in fact, the product of a living mould. It is called an *antibiotic* and destroys the germs directly. Several other potent antibiotics are now available. Streptomycin is the first agent to be effective against the tubercle bacillus, while chloramphenicol suppresses the typhoid group of bacteria. The tetracycline antibiotics have further extended the scope of chemotherapy. One great difficulty has arisen in the use of antibiotics; in some cases bacteria at first susceptible to a particular antibiotic later become resistant to it. For example, nowadays staphylococci grown from hospital dust are nearly always resistant to penicillin.

THE SULPHONAMIDES

The original sulphonamide drugs were often toxic, but they have gradually been replaced by much safer preparations. There are now many sulphonamides available, all with slightly different properties. Some act best in the kidneys, some in the bowel. Some are less powerful but can safely be given for long periods. Sulphonamides are less expensive than antibiotics and are usually given by mouth in tablet form.

1. Sulphadimidine and sulphadiazine

These sulphonamides are used for acute systemic infections, such as pneumonia, meningococcal septicaemia, streptococcal tonsillitis, and pyelitis. A large initial dose of 2 to 3 g is followed by a smaller dose varying from 1 to 1·5 g four to eight-hourly. In successful cases the temperature falls very quickly with obvious improvement in the patient's condition. Treatment should be sustained for several days but normally should not be continued for more than a week, especially if there is no effect, in view of the possibility of toxic effects after this time. Sulphadiazine is well absorbed into the cerebrospinal fluid and so is particularly useful in the treatment of meningococcal meningitis.

2. **Sulphafurazole and sulphamethizole**

These preparations are rapidly concentrated in the kidneys and are therefore valuable for treating renal infections. Prolonged treatment at a low dosage may be necessary.

3. **Sulphaguanidine and phthalylsulphathiazole**

These are poorly absorbed from the intestinal tract and so exert their effect locally in the bowel. For this reason they can be given in high dosage (e.g. 2 g four to six-hourly) in such infections of the intestinal tract as dysentery or enteritis. Usually the temperature falls and the diarrhoea ceases within a few days of treatment.

4. **Co-trimoxazole (septrin)**

This is a combination of trimethoprim with a sulphonamide sulphamethoxazole. Trimethoprim enhances the antibacterial action of sulphonamides and the combination is effective against a wide range of Gram-positive and Gram-negative bacteria. It is particularly valuable as first treatment for bronchopneumonia in the elderly and is widely used for chest and renal infections. It is normally prescribed in tablet form to be taken twice a day but is also available as an intravenous infusion for very ill patients. When given intravenously it has to be diluted and given by drip transfusion.

Toxic effects of sulphonamides

In some patients sulphonamides may cause nausea or even vomiting. Skin rashes may develop. Particularly following high dosage or prolonged treatment, *agranulocytosis* may rarely occur. In this condition, the number of white cells diminish and disposes the patient to other infections.

ANTIBIOTICS

Penicillin was first used in the treatment of infections in 1943 and since then an increasing number of antibiotics have become available. Some forms of bacteria are resistant to the action of penicillin from the start, while others become insensitive to its action after prolonged treatment. Hence there is a need for more effective antibiotics in these situations. The first step in the treatment of an infection is to isolate and to identify the causative organism. It can then be cultured and its sensitivity tested to various antibiotics. The appropriate bacteriological specimen (sputum, urine, throat swab, pus, blood culture, cerebrospinal fluid, etc.) is sent to the laboratory and the organism is cultured by incubation in a suitable medium (p. 39). On the culture plate are placed small discs of filter paper impregnated with the various antibiotics or sulphonamide. If the organism is sensitive to an antibiotic or sulphonamide preparation, it will not grow in the immediate vicinity of the disc impregnated with that antibiotic or sulphonamide preparation. On the other hand, if the organism is resistant to an antibiotic, growth of the organism will not be affected in the immediate vicinity of the disc. Unfortunately, these sensitivity tests take a few days to perform and if the patient is ill, it may not be wise to wait for the results to come through. Consequently, the physician will choose a chemotherapeutic agent on his estimate of the likely bacterial cause of the infection and on the severity of the illness. After a time, if it is evident that the patient is not responding to this initial treatment, the antibiotic can be changed in the light of the sensitivity tests.

Antibiotics may be divided into two types according to their action on bacteria. *Bacteriostatic* antibiotics inhibit the growth and multiplication of bacteria. *Bactericidal* antibiotics destroy bacteria in the process of multiplication. Thus tetracycline is bacteriostatic and penicillin is bactericidal. They should not be given together since the action of tetracycline in inhibiting multiplication of bacterial actually protects them from the effect of penicillin.

Some antibiotics (e.g. penicillin) are effective mainly against Gram-positive bacteria, and others (e.g. streptomycin) against Gram-negative bacilli. Hence in seriously ill patients where the infective organisms are not known, both antibiotics may be given together. It can be seen that a knowledge of the action of the antibiotic and of the type of bacterial infection will enable the physician to decide the treatment to be prescribed. In making his choice of antibiotic he will also be influenced by the cost of the drug (some antibiotics are very expensive), by its possible toxic effects and by knowledge of whether the patient is known to be sensitive to any particular preparations. For example, if a patient is known to be sensitive to penicillin and has had a reaction to it in the past, some alternative antibiotic must be chosen.

Penicillin

Penicillin acts by preventing the organisms from growing and also by actually destroying the organisms. Its action varies with different bacteria, being highly effective against some while having little or no effect against others.

Main uses of penicillin

Table IV gives the main diseases and their causative organisms for which penicillin is used.

TABLE IV

Diseases	Causative organisms
Septic infections (wounds, abscesses) Osteomyelitis Septicaemia	Streptococci and staphylococci
Acute tonsillitis Bacterial endocarditis Eye infections (conjunctivitis)	Streptococci
Pneumonia	Pneumococci, streptococci, staphylococci
Syphilis	*Treponema pallidum*
Gonorrhoea	Gonococci

Penicillin has little or no effect on such organisms as:
1. The enteric, dysentery and food poisoning group.
2. The *B. coli* group, which are frequently responsible for urinary tract infections (pyelitis, cystitis) and also for some cases of septic peritonitis.
3. The tubercle bacillus.
4. The whooping-cough bacillus.
5. Any of the viruses which are the causative organisms of so many acute infectious fevers (measles, poliomyelitis, chicken-pox, smallpox, etc.).

Doses and administration of penicillin
There are several preparations of penicillin in use, the following being those most widely used.

1. CRYSTALLINE BENZYLPENICILLIN
This is the ordinary soluble sodium (or potassium) salt which is usually referred to as 'penicillin'. This form of penicillin is very rapidly absorbed into the blood stream but is also quickly excreted by the kidneys. The larger the dose of penicillin given, the longer the therapeutic effect lasts, but up to a definite limit only. It is probable that even the largest doses are all excreted within eight hours. The dose of penicillin given depends both on the severity of the infection and the frequency of the injections. The tendency nowadays is to give very large doses of penicillin, at longer intervals.

For moderately severe systemic infections, 500,000 units of penicillin are normally given twelve-hourly; but in more serious infections, and particularly where it is known that the causative organism is not highly sensitive to penicillin, much higher doses can be employed.

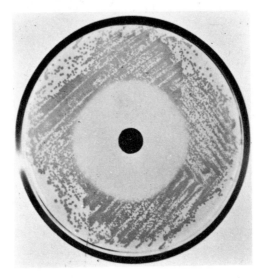

Fig. 3.10   Penicillin-sensitive staphylococci. The organisms have failed to grow in the immediate vicinity of the penicillin-impregnated paper disc.

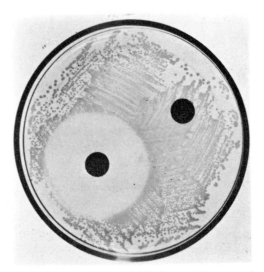

Fig. 3.11   Staphylococci resistant to penicillin, but sensitive to erythromycin. The paper disc on the right was impregnated with penicillin which failed to inhibit growth of the organisms, but around the erythromycin-impregnated disc on the left is a clear area where the organisms have failed to grow.

In addition to the above administration, crystalline penicillin is injected into the pleural cavity in cases of empyema.

2. PROCAINE BENZYLPENICILLIN (This preparation is usually referred to as procaine penicillin)

Combining procaine with crystalline soluble penicillin delays its absorption so that an effective blood concentration can be maintained for a much longer time. This means that less frequent injections can be given, usually at 12-hourly or 24-hourly intervals. Owing to its slow absorption, however, a high concentration of penicillin is not usually achieved with procaine penicillin and therefore severe systemic infections are usually treated, not with procaine penicillin, but with soluble crystalline penicillin.

Procaine penicillin is thus mainly used for treating localised infections or the less severe general systemic infections. The usual dose is 300,000 to 600,000 units at 12-hourly or 24-hourly intervals. For an immediate effect soluble crystalline penicillin (100,000 units) is often combined with procaine penicillin.

3. PHENOXYMETHYLPENICILLIN (PENICILLIN V)

This preparation of penicillin is fully effective when given by mouth, unlike most other forms of penicillin, which are largely destroyed by the acid gastric juice. Except for severe general infections, oral therapy with penicillin V is usually sufficient and obviates the need to give frequent intramuscular injections. This is of particular value when treating children.

Phenoxymethylpenicillin is given in 60 to 125 mg doses four-hourly to six-hourly. The last daily dose may be doubled to avoid waking the patient at night.

In recent years chemists have been able to work out the actual structure of the penicillin molecule, and so have been able to prepare new forms of penicillin in the laboratory. Many of these preparations are effective in the treatment of bacterial infections resistant to the action of penicillin itself.

Ampicillin

This is effective in overcoming a wide range of bacterial infections when given by mouth. It is available in 250 mg capsules and can be given every six hours, the dose depending on the type and severity of the infection. As its absorption from the bowel into the blood is variable, it should be given before meals. In severe infections, it can be given by intramuscular injection or by intravenous drip infusion. As with penicillin, it is liable to give rise to urticarial reactions.

Amoxycillin is similar to ampicillin but better absorbed.

Cloxacillin

Some bacteria produce an enzyme called *penicillinase* and this can inactivate the action of penicillin. Cloxacillin is not affected by penicillinase and so can be effective against this type of infection. It has to be given by intramuscular injection in doses of 250 mg every 6 hours.

Flucloxacillin is very similar to cloxacillin but can be given by mouth. One 250 mg capsule should be taken four times daily about an hour before taking food.

Tetracyclines

This group includes tetracycline, oxytetracycline and doxycline.

These antibiotics have a very wide range of activity—they are often referred to as 'broad-spectrum antibiotics'—being effective in streptococcal, staphylococcal, pneumococcal, meningococcal, gonococcal and *Bacillus coli* infections. In addition they are effective in rickettsial and certain virus infections.

Tetracycline and oxytetracycline are usually given by mouth in 250 mg doses six-hourly. Demethylchlortetracycline is more long acting so that 300 mg twice daily is usually sufficient. In those very severe infections where the patient, for whatever reason, cannot take oral therapy, tetracycline and oxytetracycline may be given by intravenous or intramuscular injection. Local irritation and pain are likely to occur, however, with parenteral therapy, so that as soon as possible oral therapy is started.

The tetracycline antibiotics are also used for local application in a 1 per cent ointment for bacterial skin diseases such as impetigo and sycosis.

Toxic effects

Nausea, vomiting and diarrhoea are not infrequently seen, particularly after intensive and prolonged therapy. Tetracycline causes the least gastrointestinal upset. With prolonged therapy, excessive growth of insensitive organisms, such as fungi and staphylococci, may occur in the bowel with resultant infection of the gastrointestinal tract. This infection may cause acute inflammation of the bowel (ileocolitis) with severe diarrhoea and fever and in some few cases has proved fatal.

Another adverse effect very likely to arise with prolonged therapy or with heavy dosage is vitamin deficiency, particularly of vitamins B and K. This is due to the alteration of the normal intestinal bacterial flora. When the tetracyclines are given for more than a few days, vitamin B complex should be given.

Chloramphenicol (chloromycetin)

Chloramphenicol is similar in its action to the tetracyclines but in addition it is the one antibiotic effective in the treatment of typhoid fever. Chloramphenicol is given in oral doses of 500 mg six-hourly.

The toxic effects of chloramphenicol are similar to those of the tetracyclines, whilst, in addition, chloramphenicol may give rise to the more serious danger of severe *aplastic anaemia*. Aplastic anaemia, which is often fatal, has most often occurred in children on prolonged and heavy dosage. The use of chloramphenicol is best restricted to the treatment of typhoid fever and to infections not responding to penicillin or the tetracyclines.

Erythromycin

Erythromycin is an antibiotic effective against staphylococci, streptococci and pneumococci. Its action is in many ways similar to that of penicillin. The chief use of erythromycin is in the treatment of staphylococcal infections resistant to penicillin and the other antibiotics. Staphylococci, probably more than any other organisms, are very likely to become resistant to penicillin or other antibiotics, and for these infections erythromycin has proved very valuable.

Erythromycin is given by mouth in tablets, in 200 to 300 mg doses six-hourly. No serious side effects have so far been noted and it is said that erythromycin does not materially alter the normal intestinal flora, with the result that it rarely causes gastrointestinal upset or vitamin deficiency.

Neomycin

Neomycin is an antibiotic with a very wide range of activity. It is never given by injection as it is too toxic, causing severe kidney damage and deafness.

Uses

1. Neomycin is mainly used for local application in bacterial skin infections such as impetigo, sycosis and infected eczema. Unlike penicillin, bacterial resistance to neomycin rarely develops.

2. In bacterial infections of the eye, neomycin in ointment form is often very effective.

3. Neomycin is not readily absorbed when given by mouth, so severe toxic effects are not likely to develop when it is given in this way. Neomycin is therefore used orally in the treatment of gastro-enteritis of infants.

4. Oral neomycin is also given before operations on the intestinal tract.

5. In severe cirrhosis of the liver, when the patient shows mental changes, neomycin is given to sterilise the bowel and reduce toxic absorption.

Lincomycin

Lincomycin is particularly effective against pyogenic (pus-forming) Gram-positive pathogen which are resistant to the action of penicillin. It is valuable in the treatment of bone infections (osteomyelitis) and can be given by mouth (500 mg every 8 hours) for mild infections or intramuscularly (600 mg twice daily) for severe cases.

Clindamycin is a similar preparation. It can be given by mouth (300 mg every 6 hours) and is used in the treatment of chronic wound infections not responding to penicillin.

Cephalosporine

This group of broad-spectrum antibiotics includes cephaloridin and cephaloxin. Cephaloxin is active against Gram-negative organisms such as *E. coli* and is used in the treatment of resistant urinary tract infections and bronchitis. It can be given by mouth (250 mg every 6 hours).

Gentamicin

· Gentamicin is a powerful antibiotic against many Gram-negative organisms, including those resistant to other antibiotics. It has to be given by injection but is liable to give rise to deafness and vertigo if the dose given is too high or too prolonged. This is particularly prone to occur where kidney function is impaired and the drug is not excreted in the urine. In any event it is advisable to monitor the dose given by measuring the level of gentamicin in the blood and discontinuing this treatment if the blood levels are likely to be toxic to the auditory nerve.

Streptomycin

Streptomycin was the first antibiotic to be successful in the treatment of tuberculosis and is still used in this way. However, many other drugs are now available in this field (see p. 182).

Streptomycin has to be given by intramuscular injection and is effective against many Gram-negative bacilli. As with gentamicin, it has a toxic effect on the auditory nerve and can cause vertigo, tinnitus (noises in the ear) and deafness.

Other antituberculous drugs are described in the treatment of pulmonary tuberculosis (see p. 175).

OTHER CHEMOTHERAPEUTIC AGENTS

Urinary tract antiseptics

Nitrofurantoin and nalidixic acid are two chemotherapeutic drugs excreted in the urine in an active form, and of value in the treatment of persistent urinary tract infections (see p. 379).

Antifungal agents

One of the disadvantages of antibiotic treatment of bacterial infections is that they allow infection by various fungi to flourish. Strangely enough, many antibiotics, themselves derived from fungi, are effective in the treatment of fungal infections.

NYSTATIN

Monilia albicans is a fungus which can affect the mouth (thrush), the bowel (moniliasis) and the vagina (monilial vaginitis). Nystatin is available for appropriate treatment in the form of a liquid suspension for the mouth, tablets for the intestinal infection and pessaries for vaginal infection. Nystatin is effective treatment and indeed can be given prophylactically to prevent fungal infection in patients on long-term antibiotic therapy.

AMPHOTERICIN B

This can be used for rare systemic fungal infections and has to be given by intravenous drip infusion.

GRISEOFULVIN

This oral antibiotic is effective in ringworm and other fungal infections of the skin, nails and hair. It has to be taken four times a day (250 mg) and, to be effective, treatment must be continued for many months.

Drugs acting on protozoa

Malaria. Effective drugs are available both for protection against malaria and for its treatment (see p. 84).

Amoebic dysentery. Drugs such as emetine and metronidazole (see p. 85) are successfully employed in the overcoming amoebiasis.

Anthelmintics

These are drugs used in the treatment of various worms (see p. 238).

4 Infectious Illnesses (Acute Infectious Fevers; Some Tropical Diseases; Venereal Diseases)

ACUTE INFECTIOUS FEVERS

Although the term acute infectious fever might be applied to any viral or bacterial infection, in practice it refers to a group of particular ailments easily spread from person to person, often occurring in epidemics and particularly common in babies and children. In the developed part of the world, these ailments no longer lead to the high death rate in children that used to occur. This is because:

(a) Improved standards of nutrition. Children today are better fed than they were and more able to resist infection as a result.

(b) Improved private and public hygiene, including a pure water supply; standards of cleanliness in the sale and provision of food; proper sanitation in homes, public places and places of work; and an efficient sewerage system and disposal of refuse. All these are factors which reduce the spread of infection.

(c) Protection of children by an organised programme of immunisation against common infections. Ailments such as diphtheria, smallpox and poliomyelitis, previously so deadly to small children, have almost been eradicated thanks to immunisation.

(d) The introduction of chemotherapy for the treatment of various complications occurring in these ailments.

Despite these evident successes, it would be unwise to be complacent. Ailments such as poliomyelitis and smallpox can be successfully prevented by immunisation, but treatment is largely ineffective should they be allowed to spread.

The term *acute infectious fever* is therefore usually reserved for those infections which tend to display the following characteristics:

1. The onset is acute with rise of temperature.
2. The disease is caused by a specific bacterium or virus.
3. It tends to run a definite course and often occurs in epidemic form.
4. It is very infectious.
5. In many cases one attack confers immunity from a second attack. (Common important exceptions to this do occur, however.)

Certain terms are frequently used in discussing the infectious fevers and are best explained at the outset.

Epidemic. When a large number of cases occur at the same time, to be followed by a period in which few or no cases occur.

Endemic. Where the disease is regularly found.

Sporadic. Where scattered cases only of the disease arise.

Pandemic. Where there is a worldwide distribution of the disease.

Isolation and period of isolation. Most cases of infectious disease are isolated to prevent the disease spreading to other people. The period of isolation required varies with the different diseases, but in any case generally lasts until the patient no longer harbours the infecting organisms. With some people, however, the organisms may persist indefinitely, even when they themselves have fully recovered from the illness. Such people are called *carriers*, because they carry virulent organisms capable of spreading disease to others. It should further be noted that these people can also carry virulent organisms without themselves ever having had an actual attack of the disease. This is because they have a natural resistance or immunity to the disease.

Incubation period. The incubation period is the length of time which elapses between the patient's becoming infected and the appearance of the first symptoms. The incubation period varies with the different diseases.

Quarantine. Quarantine is the restriction of the activities of people who have been in contact with a case of infectious disease until such time as it is known whether they have acquired the disease or not. The period of quarantine is just longer than the incubation period. In practice, strict quarantine of contacts is not usually enforced except in cases of such serious infectious diseases as smallpox or typhus. Known contacts of most other infectious diseases are nowadays simply kept under medical observation so that they can be isolated as soon as any symptoms develop. Strict quarantine of all known contacts involves too much disruption of everyday life, and in most cases close observation, with prompt isolation if necessary, is just as effective in controlling the incidence of infectious diseases.

Notifiable diseases. Certain diseases, usually the infectious diseases, have to be notified to the public health authorities. This is to enable the authorities to take all necessary measures to prevent spread of the disease. Some diseases are notifiable only at certain times, e.g. when they are especially prevalent or there is a large epidemic of the disease.

General features

Infectious fevers are ushered in by a rise in temperature, general malaise, headache, loss of appetite or vomiting, a dry mouth, a hot dry skin and a diminished output of concentrated urine. In rubella, a rash appears on the first day: in measles, the rash is not apparent until the fourth day of the illness. In adults, when the infection is severe, the onset may be ushered in with a rigor (see p. 305). In small babies, a convulsion or fit may occur.

In nursing patients with infectious illnesses, precautions must be taken not to spread the infection to others. The patient is best isolated in a separate room, particularly for enteric fevers. Disposable eating utensils and bedpans should be employed, but if these are not available care should be taken to ensure that the patient's utensils are marked and adequately sterilised after use. The nurse should use a gown kept outside the cubicle when attending the patient and should carefully wash her hands before leaving the room. Where the infection is respiratory, a facemask should be worn.

Most fevers occurring in children can be treated in the home but admission to hospital becomes necessary if the infection is severe or home conditions unsuitable.

Inoculation schedule

A regular programme of immunisation is recommended to protect children from particular infectious fevers.

A triple vaccine has been prepared against diphtheria, tetanus and whooping cough (pertussis) but a single injection of this triple vaccine does not offer sufficient protection. Three interval injections should be given in babyhood, the first at about 6 months, the second a month or two later and the third at about 1 year. Booster inoculations against diphtheria and tetanus can be given at 5 years old or on starting school, and again at age 10 to 12. A final dose can be given on leaving school.

At the same time as these injections are given, an oral poliomyelitis vaccine should be administered. Three drops can be absorbed onto a lump of sugar which is then eaten. This simple technique has prevented an ailment responsible for great suffering and disability.

Active immunisation against measles employs an attenuated virus and is effective for many years. It is usually given between the first and second birthday.

Rubella (German measles), as will be seen, can severely damage the foetus if the mother is infected during pregnancy. Hence it is wise to protect girls between the age of 11 and 14 by vaccinating them against rubella.

Protection against tuberculosis (see p. 179) can be given to boys and girls between the ages of 10 to 13 who are shown to be susceptible by the tuberculin test. Tuberculin-negative children are given an inoculation of B.C.G. (Bacille Calmette-Guérin).

The table that follows is a simplification. In practice, the times of inoculation need not be precise and will vary according to convenience and circumstances.

Vaccine		Recommended age (approximate only)
Diphtheria	⎫	6 months
Whooping cough	⎬ Triple combined	8 months
Tetanus	⎭	1 year
Poliomyelitis		
Diphtheria	⎫ Combined	5 years
Tetanus	⎭	11 years
Poliomyelitis		18 years
Measles		2 years
Rubella		12 years (girls)
B.C.G. (TB)		12 years (Tuberculin-negative)

MEASLES

CAUSE. Virus infection.

SPREAD. Spread is by direct contact through droplet infection from sneezing or coughing. It is very contagious, especially in the catarrhal stage before the rash appears.

INCUBATION PERIOD. Ten to 14 days.

INCIDENCE. The maximum incidence of the disease is between the ages of 8 months and 5 years. Attacks are commonest in winter and spring when widespread epidemics may occur.

Symptoms and signs

1. The onset is usually abrupt with the following catarrhal symptoms predominant:
   (a) Coryza
   (b) Conjunctivitis
   (c) Photophobia
   (d) Bronchitis.

With these symptoms the child gives a picture of running eyes and nose, coughing and sneezing. In some cases a laryngitis with hoarseness is present.

2. At this stage, before the rash appears, many cases will show the typical *Koplik's spots*. These are small white spots on the mucous membrane of the mouth beside the molar teeth. They often disappear when the rash comes out. Koplik's spots are seen only in measles.

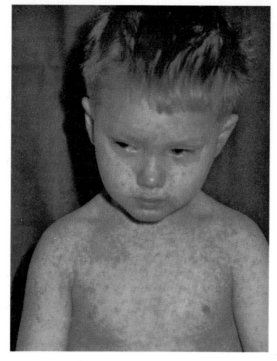

Fig. 4.1   Measles. Note the conjunctivitis.

3. The temperature rises on the first day, often to 100° to 103° F (37·8° to 39·4° C). It usually falls slightly on the third day, to rise again on the fourth day with the onset of the rash.

4. The rash appears on the fourth day of the illness. It is seen first on the forehead and behind the ears, and soon spreads all over the face and body. The rash is a dusky red macular eruption which gives a bloated, swollen appearance to the face.

5. The rash gradually fades and is gone in a week whilst the temperature falls slowly. The infection varies in severity from mild to seriously ill cases.

Complications

1. Bronchopneumonia is the most important complication of measles and is responsible for most of the deaths. It is especially frequent in young children.

2. Acute gastroenteritis. This is particularly liable to arise in infants and children under 2 years of age.

3. Conjunctivitis, blepharitis and corneal ulceration.
4. Otitis media and mastoiditis.
5. Stomatitis.
6. Inflammation of the brain and spinal cord (encephalomyelitis) is a rare complication of measles, as it is of many of the other infectious fevers.

Treatment

The patient is nursed in strict isolation in a well-ventilated room. The usual nursing care as outlined in the general treatment of any fever case with regard to diet, bowels, sleep, etc. is given.

In view of the danger of conjunctivitis, corneal ulceration and stomatitis, particular attention should be paid to the eyes and mouth. If the eyes are discharging they should be bathed in warm water. Direct sunlight on the eyes should be avoided.

A careful watch must be kept on the breathing as quickening of the respiratory rate may herald the onset of bronchopneumonia. Penicillin or other antibiotics will be given if there is any suspicion of pneumonia or other bacterial complication.

Pain in the ear, discharge from the ear or swelling behind the ear will denote an otitis media or mastoiditis, and one of the antibiotic drugs will be given to clear up the inflammation. In those cases which do not rapidly clear up, incising the drum of the ear (myringotomy) to provide proper drainage may be necessary.

The patient is kept in bed until the temperature has been normal for several days at least and until all signs in the chest have gone. This may take several weeks in moderately severe cases.

All the clothes, linen, utensils, etc. are disinfected at the end of the illness as with any infectious case.

Preventive treatment—immunisation

ACTIVE. A live attenuated measles vaccine is now available and offers effective protection. A vial contains the dried powder for a single dose and this is dissolved in water for injection. It may give rise to a temperature and should not be used in babies until 9 months old.

PASSIVE. A passive immunity to measles can be given by the injection of gamma globulin. Gamma globulin is that part of the serum protein which contains the antibodies, and is prepared from the serum of healthy adults who have had measles in the past.

If gamma globulin is given to contacts within five days of exposure to infection, an attack of measles can be completely prevented. If the gamma globulin is given between six and nine days after exposure, a modified mild attack of measles develops. In practice, full protection is usually given to infants under 2 years, where the danger of bronchopneumonia and gastroenteritis is greatest. Above the age of 2, unless the child is already ill with another disease, full immunisation is not usually carried out.

RUBELLA (German measles)

CAUSE. Virus infection.

SPREAD. By direct contact and droplet infection on coughing, sneezing, etc.

INCUBATION PERIOD. Fourteen to 19 days.

INCIDENCE. Adults as well as children are affected. The disease is most prevalent in spring and early summer.

Symptoms and signs

1. The onset is less acute than in measles and the patient is far less ill. There are the general symptoms of a mild infection, namely, malaise, headache, nasal catarrh and a slight temperature.

2. The rash appears on the first day of the illness. It begins on the face and spreads to the trunk and limbs. It is a discrete, pink, papular eruption, not usually as confluent and widespread as in measles. Koplik's spots do not occur.

3. The occipital and cervical lymph glands are characteristically enlarged.

Course and complications

The whole illness is usually mild and complications are very rare. If, however, rubella occurs in the first three months of pregnancy, in a certain number of cases it causes congenital deformities in the foetus, especially congenital heart disease. In view of this risk, it is desirable for girls to have had rubella while they were young and so to have developed immunity before marriage. A vaccine against rubella is available for girls between their 11th and 14th birthdays.

Treatment

Isolation is necessary (five to six days being sufficient) with the usual treatment for a mild fever case.

WHOOPING-COUGH (Pertussis)

CAUSE. An organism called the pertussis bacillus.

SPREAD. Usually by droplet infection in coughing; less commonly the disease is spread by contact with infected clothes or other articles (fomites).

INCUBATION PERIOD. Seven to 14 days.

INCIDENCE. The disease is most prevalent in spring and autumn. Children under the age of 5 are the usual sufferers, but adults may also be affected. Since the decline in the severity of scarlet fever and the reduction in the number of diphtheria cases through active immunisation, whooping-cough is nowadays the most serious acute specific fever in children.

Symptoms and signs

CATARRHAL OR PREPAROXYSMAL STAGE

This stage usually lasts about a week, during which time the child appears to be afflicted with a bad cold. Fever is often present, whilst the cough tends to be very persistent and may be associated with vomiting.

PAROXYSMAL STAGE

When this stage is reached there is no mistaking the nature of the illness. Paroxysmal attacks of severe coughing occur, the child going blue in the face and holding his breath. When it seems that the child must suffocate, a long, deep inspiration with a loud 'whoop' takes place.

Vomiting frequently occurs at the end of a paroxysm.

Thick sticky mucus is expectorated.

There may be as many as 20 or more of these bouts (which are especially frequent at night) in a severe attack leaving the child utterly exhausted.

COURSE. The paroxysmal stage usually lasts for three or more weeks, the bouts gradually becoming less severe. The younger the child the more severe the disease, so that most of the deaths occur in children under 1 year of age.

DIAGNOSIS. This is obvious in the paroxysmal stage. Before this stage, whooping-cough should be suspected in any child with a severe cold and cough associated with vomiting. A swab suitably curved for insertion into the post-nasal region is taken and then cultured on a special medium in the laboratory, when it will reveal the whooping-cough bacillus in a large percentage of cases.

Complications

Bronchopneumonia. This is the outstanding complication of whooping-cough and is responsible for most of the deaths among infants.

Bronchiectasis. Collapse of a part of the lung may occur in the acute stage owing to the thick mucus obstructing a bronchus. If the lung does not re-expand, the permanent collapse may give rise to bronchiectasis.

Gastroenteritis. In children under 2 whooping-cough often leads to gastroenteritis, particularly in the summer months when enteritis is prevalent.

Convulsions. Repeated convulsions are serious and may prove fatal.

Treatment

1. In mild cases, where the paroxysms are few and the child's general health is good, the patient should be kept in the fresh air as much as possible.

2. In the more severe cases, with frequent paroxysms and fever, the child is put to bed. A well-ventilated room is particularly important in the treatment of whooping-cough.

3. Diet is of special importance because of the frequent vomiting.

The child is best fed with small, frequent, light meals immediately after each bout of coughing. Skilled attention will be necessary to induce the child to take sufficient nourishment. This is especially so with infants. Routine bottle feeds may have to be abandoned and the infant fed whenever it will take its feeds.

4. To reduce the paroxysms of coughing, various drugs have been tried. Phenobarbitone, 30 mg twice a day (15 mg b.d. for infants), may be effective.

5. Convulsions are best treated with oxygen and by giving phenobarbitone, 60 mg immediately, followed by smaller doses afterwards. It is important that the sedatives should not be given in such quantities as to make the child too drowsy, as the cough reflex then becomes depressed with resultant retention of the thick bronchial mucus.

6. Penicillin is given at the first suspicion of pneumonia.

7. The tetracycline antibiotics are sometimes given in severe attacks as it is believed by some that these drugs reduce the number and severity of the paroxysms.

PREVENTIVE TREATMENT

An effective vaccine is available for active immunisation. The vaccine is usually combined with those against diphtheria and tetanus (triple vaccine) and three injections are recommended to give full protection. The first is given at about 6 months, the second at about 8 months, and the final injection at about 1 year. Very rarely, inoculation has been followed by encephalitis (brain damage). To offset this remote danger are the undoubted benefits of the inoculation in saving life from whooping cough and preventing long term complications to the lungs.

SCARLET FEVER

CAUSE. Haemolytic streptococcus.

SPREAD. Mainly by droplet infection. Less often, fomites (infected articles such as toys, books, etc.) may be responsible. Milk infected by a carrier may cause a widespread outbreak of the disease.

The organism generally enters the body through the throat and a streptococcal sore throat is an initial symptom of the disease. In puerperal women the infection may occur via the genital tract— *puerperal scarlet fever.*

INCUBATION PERIOD. Two to four days.

INCIDENCE. Primarily in children, especially during the winter.

Symptoms and signs

1. The onset is nearly always sudden, with fever, severe headache, vomiting and sore throat.

2. The pulse rate is very fast, more so than one would expect from the degree of fever.

3. The throat is very red, and exudate is usually present on both tonsils, often giving the appearance of a membrane.

4. The tongue is heavily furred and the red papillae seen through the fur gives the appearance referred to as the *strawberry tongue*. After a few days the tongue peels, becoming red and raw—*red strawberry tongue*.

5. *Rash.* The rash appears on the second day and has the following characteristics:

(a) It avoids the face, which is, however, flushed, except around the mouth. (This condition is the well-recognised *circumoral pallor*.)

(b) It appears first around the neck and chest and soon spreads rapidly all over the body.

(c) It is a bright red erythema which blanches on pressure.

(d) It fades in about a week, to be followed by the typical desquamation. Here the skin peels off, either in large scales or in a small form which produces 'pin holes' in the skin.

TYPES

Simple. This is the ordinary, relatively mild type with symptoms and signs as just described.

Toxic. Here severe toxaemia is present and many patients die. This form is now very rare in Great Britain but is still commonly seen in Eastern Europe.

Septic. In this type the septic complications are a predominant feature.

DIAGNOSIS

The diagnosis is usually made on the streptococcal sore throat accompanied by the erythematous rash. If the rash is so slight that it is missed, the occurrence of desquamation later on in the illness is suggestive of scarlet fever.

Dick test. This is a similar test to the Schick test used in diphtheria. Scarlatinal toxin is injected into the skin, and if the person is susceptible to scarlet fever a bright erythema develops in 12 hours and is gone in 24 hours. The test can be used up to the third day or so of the disease if the toxin is inserted into an area of skin where no rash is present.

Complications of scarlet fever

Scarlet fever can be accompanied by septic infections or may be followed by toxic or allergic disorders.

Septic. The septic complications are caused by the infection spreading to the surrounding tissues. They usually develop in the early stage of the disease, unlike the toxic complications which tend to arise in the second and third weeks. The main septic complications are:

(a) Septic cervical adenitis

(b) Otitis media, which may spread to cause mastoiditis

(c) Quinsy (peritonsillar abscess).

Toxic and allergic. The main complications in this group are:
(a) Acute myocarditis and endocarditis. The heart involvement in scarlet fever is closely related to that in acute rheumatic fever and is treated in the same way.
(b) Acute nephritis. This is identical with the ordinary form of acute nephritis described in Chapter 11.
(c) Arthritis.

Treatment

The patient is nursed in bed with the isolation procedure and nursing care usual in a fever case. In view of the mild form of the present-day scarlet fever, patients are not usually nursed in hospital where there is an added risk of cross-infection from other strains of haemolytic streptococci.

Penicillin is most valuable in the treatment of scarlet fever and considerably reduces the risk of complications.

Isolation for two weeks is usually sufficient except where there are any septic discharges which may contain the organisms.

ERYSIPELAS

CAUSE. Haemolytic streptococcus.

SPREAD. By direct contact, entry into the body usually being through a skin abrasion or wound.

INCIDENCE. Erysipelas was formerly a very common infection in hospitals and institutions, especially in surgical wards where infected wounds and abscesses spread the disease. Nowadays, however, with proper aseptic technique, and particularly with the introduction of the sulphonamides and the various antibiotics, the disease is much less common and can be quickly controlled.

Symptoms and signs

1. Erysipelas is most frequently seen in middle-aged and elderly people, and the presence of some debilitating disease or chronic alcoholism is particularly likely to give rise to the infection.
2. The onset is usually sudden, with fever, general constitutional upset and rigors.
3. The characteristic lesion is a bright red erythema of the skin which is swollen and tense with a clear-cut border. The most frequent site of this local lesion is the face, and it often spreads in a butterfly distribution over the nose and cheeks. Another common site is around the margin of a surgical wound.

Course and treatment

Before the use of sulphonamides and penicillin, erysipelas was a prevalent disease and often serious. Penicillin, however, usually clears up the infection in a few days and thereby also reduces the risk of the infection spreading. The general treatment consists of bed rest and the routine care for an acute fever case.

DIPHTHERIA

CAUSE. Infection with the diphtheria bacillus, of which there are several strains, the gravis strain being the most severe.

SPREAD. Mainly by droplet infection. Indirect spread (e.g. from sucking infected pencils) also often occurs.

INCUBATION PERIOD. Short—two to four days.

INCIDENCE. Children are chiefly affected, although diphtheria may also be seen in adults, especially during epidemics. Winter is the most usual season for diphtheria.

PATHOLOGY. The illness takes the form of a typical local lesion with a severe general toxaemia.

The local lesion is a membranous exudate which usually occurs in the throat, causing faucial diphtheria. Less often it is situated either in the nose (causing nasal diphtheria) or in the larynx (causing laryngeal diphtheria). Combined lesions may occur, in rarer cases, skin diphtheria may be present.

Although the organisms remain in the membrane, they produce a very powerful toxin which causes a general toxaemia. The toxin particularly attacks the heart muscle (myocardium), causing an acute myocarditis, and the nervous system, causing various forms of paralysis.

Diphtheria can affect primarily the fauces, the nose or the larynx.

Symptoms and signs

1. The onset may be insidious without obvious fever. But the pulse is rapid and there may be marked exhaustion and general malaise.

2. Examination of the throat reveals that the tonsils are covered by a greyish-white membrane. This membrane may extend over the soft palate and cannot be wiped off with a swab. The breath has a musty smell.

3. The tonsillar glands in the neck are enlarged, giving the neck a swollen appearance.

4. In nasal diphtheria, the membrane is confined to the nose, causing a blood-stained nasal discharge.

5. When the membrane involves the larynx, breathing becomes obstructed and the trachea may have to be opened surgically (tracheostomy) to allow the child to breathe.

6. Myocarditis may be caused by the toxins produced by the diphtheria bacilli. The pulse becomes very rapid, the blood pressure falls and death can follow.

7. Paralysis of the nerves and muscles may also be caused by the toxins, leading to difficulty in breathing and swallowing.

DIAGNOSIS

A throat swab is taken and sent to the laboratory for culture. This will reveal the presence of the diphtheria bacillus.

Treatment

Once the diagnosis of diphtheria is suspected, it is best to give treatment straight away without waiting for the result of the throat swab. This is because the diphtheria toxin can spread so rapidly. Diphtheria antitoxin is injected intramuscularly, usually in a dose of 24,000 units. In cases more severe or collapsed, a bigger dose may be given intravenously. In addition, penicillin should be administered to overcome the spread of the bacilli.

Prevention

Epidemics of diphtheria used to be a feature of town life and special fever hospitals were built to accommodate these and similar cases. Thanks to the success of the immunisation programme, the disease has almost been eradicated. Inoculation against diphtheria is combined with vaccines against whooping cough and tetanus (triple vaccine) and given to babies at approximately 6 months, at 8 months and again at 1 year. Booster doses may be given at 5, at 11 and at 18 years.

CHICKENPOX (Varicella)

CAUSE. Virus infection.

SPREAD. By droplet infection or by the hands and clothing of attendants.

INCUBATION PERIOD. Twelve to 21 days, usually 14.

INCIDENCE. The disease is very common, attacking all age groups, but especially children under 10. Chickenpox is most prevalent in autumn and winter.

Symptoms and signs

The onset is usually mild, the patient merely feeling 'off colour,' with a slight pyrexia. In children, quite often the first sign of the disease is the appearance of the rash.

The *rash* of chickenpox has the following characteristics:

(a) It appears first on the trunk, particularly the back, and then spreads to the face and limbs. The eruption is densest on the trunk and the upper parts of the limbs.

(b) Red papules appear first, which rapidly change to vesicles and pustules. Within a few days the pustules dry up and form scabs which quickly fall off.

(c) The rash appears in crops so that all types of lesion, papules, vesicles, pustules and crusts are seen together.

Complications

Chickenpox is nearly always a mild disease, severe toxic types being very rare. The most frequent complication is infection of the rash through scratching.

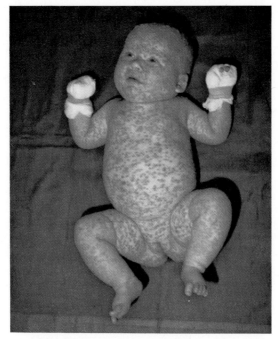

Fig. 4.2 Extensive chickenpox.

Diagnosis

The most important part in diagnosis is to distinguish a severe case of chickenpox from a mild case of smallpox. This differentiation usually rests on the order of appearance, the distribution and, in smallpox, the protracted development of the rash. The main points of difference are given under Smallpox.

Chickenpox may also be mistaken for various skin diseases like impetigo, urticaria and scabies.

Treatment

Treatment of chickenpox is mainly concerned with the prevention of secondary infection of the lesions. In children the finger nails should be cut short and, if itching is severe, gloves or splints should be applied. The itching may be alleviated by using a soothing lotion such as calamine with 1 per cent phenol. If the lesions are profuse, penicillin may be given to prevent secondary infection.

Isolation is necessary till all the crusts have separated.

SMALLPOX

CAUSE. Virus infection.

SPREAD. By direct contact and droplet infection through the

respiratory tract. Smallpox was the most infectious of all known infectious fevers.

INCIDENCE. Smallpox, which once threatened every family in the land, has at last been eradicated, and will never be seen again. This is thanks to a vigorous programme of vaccination by the World Health Organisation in countries where smallpox was endemic and also thanks to international agreement that all travellers to and from such countries had to be vaccinated.

Symptoms and signs

The rash of smallpox had similarities with chickenpox but the vesicles were more prolific on the face and the limbs than on the trunk. The vesicles were deeper and became purulent, leaving scars when they healed ('pockmarks'). There were serious constitutional manifestations with high fever, headache and prostration. It carried a high mortality rate.

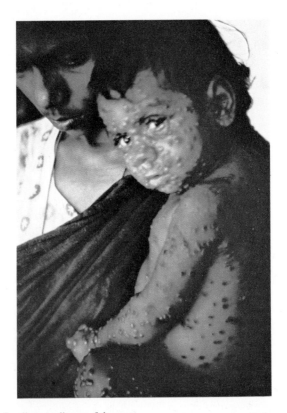

FIG. 4.3   Smallpox, a disease of the past.

Successful eradication of smallpox (vaccination)

It was in smallpox that the first brilliant instances of the prevention of disease by vaccination were obtained by Jenner. In vaccination against smallpox the vaccine used was a suspension of a virus which caused cowpox in cattle. The virus of cowpox (*vaccinia*) appears to be similar to the virus of smallpox except that its effect on human beings is much less virulent. Inoculating a person with a vaccine containing the virus of cowpox caused an attack of vaccinia and led to the formation of antibodies. As a result the person became immune to the much more serious disease, smallpox, and so prevented its spread.

MUMPS (Epidemic parotitis)

CAUSE. Virus infection.

SPREAD. By droplet infection through the respiratory tract.

INCUBATION PERIOD. Twelve to 28 days, usually 17 days.

INCIDENCE. Mumps is chiefly seen in children between the ages of 5 and 15 years and also in young adults. Epidemics occur mainly in schools and institutions.

Symptoms and signs

1. In some cases the first sign of the disease may be the swollen face. Usually, however, the initial symptoms of pyrexia, headache and sore throat arise a few days before the characteristic swelling of the parotid glands.

2. The enlarged parotid glands produce a swelling below the angle of the jaw and the skin over the glands becomes tense and shiny. One gland is usually enlarged for a short time before the other. There is often a complaint of pain on eating and it may be difficult to open the mouth.

3. The enlargement of the glands usually subsides within seven to ten days. The temperature falls when the glands begin to subside, which is generally within a few days.

Complications

Orchitis, or inflammation of the testis, is a well-recognised complication which is most frequently seen in older children and adults. With the onset of orchitis, fever returns, with pain and swelling of the testis.

Rarer complications of mumps include mastitis (inflammation of the breast), oophoritis (inflammation of the ovary), pancreatitis and encephalitis.

Treatment

There is no specific treatment for mumps. Children are nursed in bed till the temperature has subsided and are kept away from school until all the swelling has gone. Adults, however, in view of the likelihood of complications, are usually kept in bed for a longer period until all the parotid swelling has subsided. Aspirin or codeine may

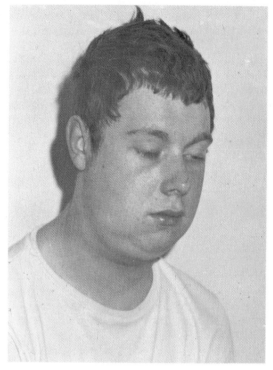

FIG. 4.4 Mumps, showing swelling of the right parotid gland.

be needed to relieve pain. If chewing is difficult, a soft diet is given and fluid can be sucked through a straw.

If orchitis develops, cortisone or allied steroid often brings about rapid relief of the swelling and pain and is therefore usually prescribed.

INFLUENZA

CAUSE. Virus infection of which there are several different strains.

SPREAD. By droplet infection. Influenza is a highly infectious disease.

INCUBATION PERIOD. Short, one to three days.

INCIDENCE. Influenza occurs throughout the world in widespread epidemics, which vary considerably both in their clinical picture and fatality rates. Pandemics (world-wide epidemics), with a very high mortality rate, also occasionally occur—the last in 1918 when millions died of the disease. In more localised outbreaks influenza is fairly mild.

Symptoms and signs

1. The onset is usually sudden, with symptoms similar to those

of the common cold or an acute bronchitis. The symptoms tend to vary, however, with different epidemics.

2. The general constitutional upset is more severe than one would expect with an ordinary cold. Headache, chills and lethargy are common.

3. A cough, sneezing, running eyes and nose, and laryngitis are usual symptoms.

4. Nausea, vomiting and abdominal pains are a feature of some outbreaks.

Complications

Bronchopneumonia is the most important complication and is responsible for most of the deaths. The pneumonia is usually caused by secondary infection with such organisms as the influenzal bacilli, streptococci and staphylococci. Elderly people are more prone to develop pneumonia.

Treatment

All patients are best nursed in bed with the usual nursing care for a fever case. Isolation is not often possible owing to the rapidity of development of the disease and the difficulty of early diagnosis.

There is no specific treatment for influenza. Aspirin or codeine is useful for the headache. Penicillin or other antibiotics are usually given for the treatment of the secondary infections.

As the immunity to influenza lasts for a short period only, recurrent attacks are usual.

Prevention

Vaccines are available against some strains of influenza. They offer partial immunity for some months and are of limited value when there is an epidemic.

GLANDULAR FEVER (Infectious mononucleosis)

CAUSE. Virus infection.

INCUBATION PERIOD. Five to 10 days.

INCIDENCE. Chiefly in children and young adults of either sex. It occurs both sporadically and in epidemics.

Symptoms and signs

1. The onset is usually gradual with general malaise, tiredness, loss of appetite and rise of temperature.

2. In some cases there is a sore throat, which may be covered with exudate. A measles type of rash may develop.

3. The lymph glands become enlarged, usually after a few weeks. The cervical glands are particularly enlarged but axillary and inguinal glands are also affected. The spleen enlarges.

4. Blood examination reveals an increased number of white cells (leucocytosis), and especially the monocytes—hence the name

mononucleosis. There are also unusual forms of lymphocytes which the pathologist can recognise as typical of this virus infection.

5. The diagnosis can be confirmed by an agglutination test called the Paul-Bunnell test, though this is not always positive.

Course and treatment

Patients should be kept in bed while the temperature is raised. Unfortunately many patients continue to feel unwell and tired for several weeks or even months, with occasional fever. There is no specific remedy.

TYPHOID FEVER

CAUSE. Bacillus typhosus (*Salmonella typhosa*).

SPREAD AND INCIDENCE. Typhoid fever is spread mainly through the contamination of water, milk, or food with sewage. Human carriers excrete the organisms in the faeces or urine, and if proper hygiene and sanitation are lacking, contamination of water or food results. For this reason typhoid fever is particularly likely to arise in armies during times of war and also in areas where adequate sanitation is lacking.

INCUBATION PERIOD. Usually 10 to 14 days.

PATHOLOGY. The bacilli enter the blood stream from the bowel and cause septicaemia with fever. They settle mainly in the small intestine where they cause inflammation and ultimately ulcers occur. Bacteria may also invade the gall bladder and even the bones, sometimes leading to abscesses. The heart may be affected by bacterial toxins.

Symptoms and signs

1. The onset is gradual with headaches, gradually rising fever and marked malaise. The pulse may be slow in relation to the temperature.

2. The abdomen may be distended and tender. Constipation is often present in the early stage.

3. Usually after a week, diarrhoea supervenes with frequent watery motions ('pea soup' stools), sometimes streaked with blood. The patient at this stage has a high temperature and is dehydrated and exhausted. He may lapse into a comatose confused state.

4. A rash usually appears on the abdomen, consisting of small round red areas ('rose spots').

5. Complications are common in the untreated case. Haemorrhage from the bowel, intestinal perforation, bronchopneumonia and heart failure can lead to a fatal termination.

DIAGNOSIS

1. *Blood culture.* The bacilli circulate in the blood stream during the first week. In suspected cases, several blood specimens should be sent to the laboratory for culture and identification of the typhoid bacilli if they are present.

2. *Widal reaction.* Antibodies to typhoid bacilli develop in the blood

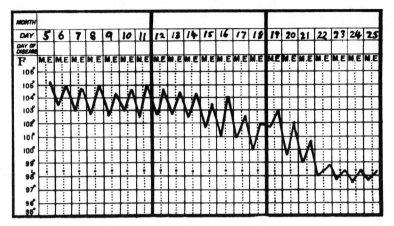

FIG. 4.5   Temperature chart from a case of uncomplicated typhoid fever, not treated with chloramphenicol. The temperature became normal on the 23rd day.

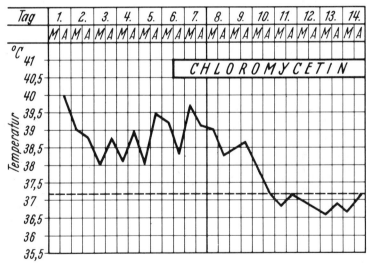

FIG. 4.6   Temperature chart from a case of typhoid fever showing the response to chloramphenicol.

and are present in appreciable amounts after the first week of the infection. These antibodies can be measured by the Widal reaction and confirm the diagnosis if they have increased over the first week. There is a difficulty. Antibodies are induced in any person who has been vaccinated against typhoid and this fact has to be borne in mind in interpreting the result.

3. *Faeces.* Specimens are sent to the laboratory for isolation of the organisms.

Treatment

Typhoid cases must be nursed in isolation and disposable eating utensils, urinals and bedpans are advisable. Suitable disinfectants should be added to excreta, and the nurse should wear gloves and a gown when attending to the patient.

Chloramphenicol is a very effective antibiotic in the treatment of typhoid fever and is given by mouth in capsule form 0·5 g every 6 hours for a week or more. Because prolonged treatment with chloramphenicol may give rise to agranulocytosis (absence of white cells), other treatments have been tried. These include ampicillin and co-trimoxazole (see pp. 51 and 55).

CARRIERS

Some people harbour typhoid bacilli in the bowel or in the gall-bladder without any detriment to their own health. However, they may be a great danger to others and, particularly if they are

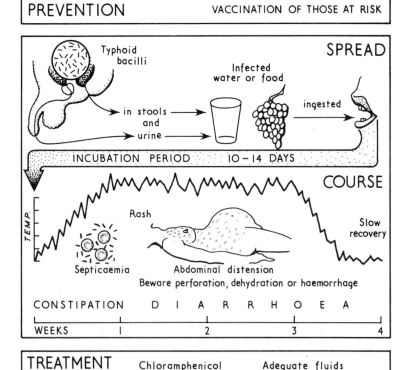

FIG. 4.7   Typhoid fever.

employed in handling food, can cause an outbreak of typhoid fever. Treatment with an antibiotic is often effective in clearing the infection, but sometimes a cholecystectomy (removal of gallbladder) is necessary. Carriers should be warned of the danger they can bring to others if strict personal hygiene is not observed; indeed, carriers are forbidden by law from handling food on sale to the public.

PREVENTION

An active immunity to typhoid fever can be created by means of the highly effective vaccine available. It is necessary, however, to revaccinate once a year if an effective immunity is to be maintained. Vaccination against typhoid is usually practised in any circumstances wherein the sanitation and hygiene are such that they cannot be relied upon to prevent the disease arising. For troops during war and for people who, because of travel, may be exposed to contaminated food or water, typhoid vaccination is essential.

PARATYPHOID FEVERS

Paratyphoid fevers are caused by infection with the paratyphoid bacilli, referred to as A, B and C. These bacilli are very like the typhoid bacillus in their action. Paratyphoid fevers and typhoid fever are often grouped together under the heading of *enteric fever*. Typhoid fever, which formerly was much the commonest type of enteric fever seen in Great Britain, is now less common; on the other hand, paratyphoid B infection is now more prevalent.

Paratyphoid infection tends, on the whole, to be much less severe and toxic than typhoid, but the general symptoms and the treatment are all very similar. For this reason all that has been said about typhoid applies to paratyphoid fever. The exact diagnosis of the specific organism causing the enteric fever is made on bacteriological examination.

BACILLARY DYSENTERY

CAUSE. Dysentery bacilli, of which there are several types including Sonne, Flexner and Shiga.

SPREAD. The method of spread of the disease is similar to that of enteric fever. The bacilli are excreted in the faeces, and through defective sanitation and bad hygiene, food and water can then become contaminated. Flies, too, frequently cause contamination of food and are a prevalent mode of spread of the disease.

INCIDENCE. Although dysentery is commonest in tropical countries it is becoming more frequent in Great Britain, especially in camps, nurseries and large institutions subject to overcrowding. Sonne infections in children are commonly seen in this country. Flexner dysentery, which usually occurs in adults, is less common in Great

Britain but is more severe. The most virulent infections are caused by the Shiga bacilli but these are rarely seen outside the tropics.

PATHOLOGY. There is an acute inflammation of the large intestine with ulceration in severe cases.

Symptoms and signs

In *Sonne* dysentery in children the disease is usually mild, with few constitutional symptoms and only slight fever. The pre-dominating signs are diarrhoea, with the passage of blood and mucus in the stools. The number of stools passed in the day rarely exceeds five or six. Slight abdominal colic is usually present.

In *Flexner* infections, toxaemia is more marked, with headache, loss of appetite, thrist and lassitude all present. Severe abdominal colic with the rapid onset of urgent diarrhoea are the main symptoms. As many as 15 to 20 stools a day may be passed. The typical dysenteric stool is small and consists entirely of blood and mucus or muco-pus, with no faecal matter present. In severe cases shreds of mucous membrane are present.

Shiga infections are usually accompanied by profound prostration and dehydration.

DIAGNOSIS. Laboratory examination of the stools or of a rectal swab is carried out in all cases and usually reveals the causative organism.

Treatment

The usual nursing care and isolation precautions outlined under typhoid fever are necessary. The form of dysentery usually seen in Great Britain (Sonne) is highly infectious, and when dealing with the disease in children it is most important that different nurses should attend to the feeding and to the changing. Destructible napkins should be used.

In the acute stage a fluid diet is given, but as soon as the stools become more solid, additions to the diet are quickly made in the form of soft, bland, low-residue foods. For severe cases, where de-hydration is present, intravenous fluids may be necessary.

Ampicillin usually leads to a rapid improvement but occasionally the bacteria are resistant to it and an alternative antibiotic will be needed.

The patient is considered infectious until successive bacteriological examination of the stools are negative.

FOOD POISONING

CAUSE. Food poisoning is caused by the contamination of food with bacteria, or with the toxins of bacteria. The most common causes of food poisoning are the Salmonella group of bacilli and the toxins produced by the Staphylococcus.

The rare form of food poisoning known as *botulism* is caused by the improper canning of foods.

SPREAD. Food poisoning may arise through contamination of food due to lack of proper hygiene on the part of people who, while harbouring the organisms in their faeces, are engaged in handling food. Animals such as rats and mice may also infect food. Such foods as reheated pies, cooked meats and duck eggs are especially liable to contamination by Salmonella organisms, whilst cakes, custards and ham are most frequently infected by staphylococcal toxin.

Symptoms and signs

Food poisoning due to staphylococcal toxin causes a severe acute gastroenteritis with vomiting, abdominal colic and diarrhoea. These symptoms usually start within a few hours of the eating of the offending food. Usually all the people who eat the food are similarly affected.

Food poisoning caused by the Salmonella bacilli produces a similar picture of an acute gastroenteritis. The onset, however, is not so rapid as in staphylococcal poisoning, as it takes 6 to 24 hours to develop, and the symptoms may persist for a longer period—over several days.

In botulism the symptoms usually develop about 24 hours after the poisoned canned food was eaten. The predominating symptoms are various forms of paralysis; in most cases the outcome is fatal.

DIAGNOSIS

The diagnosis of food poisoning is usually easily made when vomiting, abdominal pain and diarrhoea occur in several people after they have eaten the same food. Dysentery, which also causes abdominal colic and diarrhoea, is differentiated from food poisoning by the absence of vomiting and also by the presence of blood in the stools, which is rarely seen in food poisoning.

Treatment

Most patients with food poisoning recover fairly rapidly with rest in bed and a fluid diet. If abdominal colic and diarrhoea are severe, a kaolin and opium mixture may be given.

In staphylococcal cases which do not quickly clear up, the antibiotics, erythromycin or terramycin, may be used with some effect. In Salmonella food poisoning there is no specific therapy, but chloramphenicol or the tetracycline antibiotics may be of value in some cases.

Preventive treatment is most important and entails the proper handling and storage of all foods. Full hygienic measures must be employed in all kitchens, and care taken to see that flies, rats and mice cannot get at the food. In addition, all people handling food must be free from any infection.

SOME TROPICAL DISEASES

With the spread of international airway travel, diseases previously found only in tropical or subtropical areas are now appearing in Britain as well.

MALARIA

Malaria is the commonest disease in tropical countries and is responsible for much ill health and many deaths each year.

It is caused by a parasite of the genus *Plasmodium*. The parasite undergoes a complicated life cycle, with division and cyst formation. Part of this life cycle takes place in the blood cells and liver of man, and part in the stomach and salivary glands of the anopheles mosquito. When the infected anopheles mosquito bites a man, the parasite is introduced into his blood stream and causes malaria. At the same time, when the mosquito sucks infected blood from a man with malaria the parasite completes the other part of the cycle in the mosquito.

There are four different types of plasmodia, the two commoner types giving rise to benign and malignant varieties of the malaria. Tertian malaria is characterised by recurrent bouts of high fever occurring every third day. This fever is accompanied by severe rigors, profuse sweating, prostrating headaches, and vomiting. The attack then subsides, and the temperature becomes normal for a few days until the next attack.

In malignant tertian malaria, the parasite can invade the brain, leading to convulsions, coma and death.

Treatment

In areas where malaria is rife, suppressive therapy to protect against an attack of malaria may be given. From the 17th century until modern times Cinchona bark or quinine has been the traditional remedy, but this has now been largely replaced by more effective drugs. Chloroquine at present is the drug of choice for an acute attack.

For those entering an area where malaria may be present, it is most important to take preventive tablet treatment, not only while in the area but also for four weeks after returning home. Proguanil (Paludrine) 100 mg daily is usually advised in this respect.

PREVENTION

1. Measures must be taken to prevent the breeding of anopheles mosquitoes by drainage of stagnant waters or spreading the surface with oil.

2. Protective measures must be observed by people against mosquito bites such as sleeping under nets and wearing protective clothing.

3. Insistence that visitors to malarial areas take preventive tablets before, during and after their visit.

AMOEBIASIS

Amoebiasis is caused by a parasite called *Entamoeba histolytica* and is spread from contaminated vegetables and water. The parasite invades the colon and is carried by the portal vein to the liver.

Amoebic dysentery

Characterised by abdominal discomfort and frequent loose stools containing blood and mucus. The condition can become chronic with loss of weight, malaise and intermittent episodes of diarrhoea.

A fresh specimen of stool is examined under the microscope and the diagnosis can be made by identifying the entamoeba.

Amoebic liver abscess

The liver becomes enlarged and tender, with abscess formation which may rupture into the chest.

Treatment

Metronidazole is effective treatment for amoebic dysentery and should be given by mouth, 800 mg eight-hourly for 5 days. It is also effective for amoebic hepatitis but when abscess formation has occurred, surgical drainage may be necessary.

CHOLERA

Cholera can be an extremely severe and sometimes fatal disease seen in the tropics. It is caused by a bacillus called the *Vibrio comma*. Infection is spread through contamination of water in particular, and also of food. The disease occurs in large epidemics and the main features are an intense diarrhoea with watery stools containing shreds of mucous membrane from the intestinal wall—the typical 'rice-water' stools of cholera. In addition, a rapid and severe dehydration sets in as a result of the loss of fluid from the body. The eyes become sunken, the skin pinched and dry, whilst severe cramps arise in the muscles owing to the dehydration and loss of salt.

The treatment of cholera lies in the urgent relief of the usual intense dehydration by the use of intravenous fluids. Tetracycline given by mouth reduces the number of stools and the loss of fluid. A vaccine is available for those at risk and is effective for up to six months. Two doses are given at an interval of a week and booster doses are needed every six months for those living in endemic areas.

TYPHUS FEVER

Included in the term *typhus fever* are many different forms, all of which are caused by a group of organisms called Rickettsiae. These organisms are found in rats and other rodents, and are conveyed to man through the bites of lice, fleas, ticks and mites. The various forms of typhus are seen in different parts of the world under the names of tropical scrub typhus, Rocky Mountain spotted fever (America, Canada), Q fever (Australia, America) and epidemic typhus (Eastern Europe, Asia). The severity of the different forms varies in different outbreaks from a mild to a highly fatal disease.

The characteristics of most forms consist of a sudden abrupt high fever, severe toxaemia and a purpuric rash. The fever usually runs a course of two to three weeks. The forms of typhus which are spread by lice and rat fleas are especially prone to occur in overcrowded camps and institutions where there is a lack of proper hygiene.

In typhus fever general nursing care is most important in order to maintain the patient's resistance. The strictest measures are necessary to prevent the nurse herself and the other patients being bitten by any lice or fleas. Thorough delousing of all patients is necessary. The specific treatment of typhus consists of the administration of one of the tetracycline antibiotics or chloramphenicol, which have a rapid effect in most cases.

PLAGUE

Plague is a highly infectious and often fatal disease seen in tropical areas. It often occurs in widespread epidemics. It is caused by a bacillus which is found in rats and the infection can be conveyed to man by the bite of the rat flea. Two main forms are seen, the *bubonic* where the lymph glands become enlarged, and the *pneumonic* where the principal feature is a severe bronchopneumonia. In both types severe prostration and toxaemia are present and the death rate is high.

In preventing the spread of infection the suppression of rats and their eradication from ships (which can carry infected rats from one area to another) is most important. The treatment of an individual attack consists of the routine nursing care of a severe infectious fever and the administration of streptomycin, which is effective in plague.

LEPROSY

Leprosy which in former years was world-wide in distribution is nowadays mainly confined to Asia and certain parts of the Americas. The causative agent is a bacillus which is generally found in the nasal secretions. It is a chronic disease of which the main effects are on the skin and nerves. The face especially becomes thickened and nodular. In advanced cases destruction of the bones of the nose and face develops and blindness is also common. Affection of the nerves causes loss of sensation leading to trophic ulcers.

Most cases are segregated in special leper colonies so as to prevent spread of the disease. Drugs such as dapsone or thiambutosine are usually effective, but treatment must be maintained for many months.

RABIES (Hydrophobia)

Rabies is a virus infection which occurs in dogs and is transmitted to man by the bite of an infected dog. It is not seen in Great Britain owing to the strict quarantine enforced on dogs brought into the country. Dogs infected with the virus go mad and die. In man the chief symptoms are severe spasms of the muscles, especially of the throat, and swallowing or even the sight of food or water sets up these spasms: hence the name hydrophobia—fear of water. Death occurs through exhaustion and dehydration.

People bitten by a dog which might be rabid must be given anti-rabies vaccine without delay, since this offers complete protection.

TETANUS (Lockjaw)

Tetanus is caused by bacteria which usually gain entrance to the body through wounds, especially deep penetrating stab wounds, e.g. from nails. The bacillus is most commonly present in soil and manure, and wounds so infected are particularly dangerous. The main symptoms are severe muscular spasms which usually start in the jaw muscles, causing difficulty in opening the mouth—lockjaw. The spasms then rapidly spread to other muscles so that the severe muscle spasms become generalised. Death results from exhaustion.

The widespread use of preventive inoculation with tetanus toxoid (combined with vaccines against diphtheria and whooping cough) to babies of two months has reduced enormously the incidence of the disease in Europe. Where there is a possibility of tetanus in any wound, injured children and adults should receive 1 ml tetanus toxoid if they have been properly immunised within the previous 10 years. Otherwise they should be given ATS (antitetanus serum), and this must be followed after six weeks by a course of three injections of toxoid to avoid the need for future injections of ATS. Repeated injections of ATS lose their effect and frequently give rise to serum sickness. In treatment, sedation and curare to control the severe spasms are used, combined with large doses of tetanus antitoxin. In severe cases a tracheostomy may be necessary as a temporary expedient to ensure a clear airway.

BRUCELLOSIS (Undulant fever)

Brucellosis, formerly known as undulant fever, is primarily an animal disease which is caused by infection with the Brucella organisms, of which there are several types. The organisms are present in infected cows, pigs and goats, and the infection is carried to man through handling or ingestion of contaminated milk, cheese, meat, or pork. Farm workers and packing house employees are frequently affected.

The chief symptoms are a prolonged fever, often with few constitutional signs. Severe sweating and joint pains are a feature of many cases. The spleen is usually enlarged. The diagnosis is confirmed by finding the organisms in the blood (by means of a blood culture) or, more often, by an agglutination reaction similar to the Widal reaction of typhoid.

The specific treatment is the administration of one of the tetracycline antibiotics. Relapses are, however, commonly seen.

VENEREAL DISEASES

Diseases transmitted during sexual intercourse are known as *venereal diseases*.

SYPHILIS

Syphilis is a widespread disease throughout the world and is caused by the spirochaete *Treponema pallidum*. It is transmitted during sexual intercourse with an infected person. If untreated it can become chronic and cause constitutional disorders many years after the original infection.

The signs and symptoms can be described in three stages:

1. *The primary stage.* A firm, painless ulcer, called a chancre, appears on the penis in the male or the labia in the female. The chancre may bleed easily and gives rise to painful enlargement of the inguinal lymph glands. Occasionally this primary sore appears on the lips, the breasts or the fingers. It usually occurs about a month after the infected intercourse and takes a few weeks to heal. Unless treated it is followed by

2. *The secondary stage*, usually a few weeks after the chancre. There may be generalised enlargement of the lymph glands, general malaise, mild fever and a skin rash. The rash usually appears on the trunk, it is ham-coloured and does not itch.

3. *The tertiary stage.* Some years after the original infection, serious constitutional effects may occur, including (a) involvement of the aorta which may lead to aortic aneurysm and aortic regurgitation (see p. 127), (b) involvement of the nervous system leading to tabes dorsalis and general paralysis of the insane (p. 314).

Congenital syphilis

Syphilis may be transmitted to the foetus by an infected mother. If the baby is born alive, it may develop disorders of growth, of the eyes or of the nervous system.

Diagnosis

In the primary stage, a scraping from the chancre may reveal the spirochaete when examined under the microscope.

Reliable blood tests are available to establish the diagnosis. The older tests (Wasserman and Kahn) are not specific for syphilis and although positive in syphilis may also be positive in other ailments. More specific tests should be performed if the WR (Wasserman reaction) is positive, such as the TPI (*Treponoma pallidum* immobilisation test).

Treatment

Penicillin given daily for 10 days by intromuscular injection is successful treatment both to cure the disease in the primary and secondary stages and to arrest the damage and promote healing in the tertiary stage. Careful supervision and follow-up is necessary until the blood tests show that the infection has been safely overcome.

NON-SPECIFIC URETHRITIS

This is commonest in young men and is due to a non-gonococcal infection of the urethra, perhaps in some cases to an unidentified virus. The symptoms are those of frequency of micturition, burning discomfort on passing water and a mucopurulent urethral discharge. These features are sometimes associated with conjunctivitis and acute arthritis: this condition is then known as Reiter's syndrome.

Although the symptoms subside after a few weeks, they frequently recur and the joints can become chronically inflamed.

Tetracycline is often prescribed but the response is not consistent.

GONORRHOEA

Gonorrhoea is due to infection by the gonococcus, which is an organism causing an acute, purulent inflammation. It is a widespread disease, especially common in time of war, as is all venereal disease.

Gonorrhoeal infection in the adult results from sexual intercourse with an infected person and gives rise both to acute and to chronic disorders.

Acute

The main lesions in acute gonorrhoea are as follows:

(a) Acute inflammation of the urethra (acute urethritis) in the male and of the cervix of the uterus in the female. This inflammation causes a thick, purulent, yellow discharge often combined with painful micturition, and is the predominating sign of gonorrhoea.

(b) The inflammation often spreads to neighbouring organs, causing prostatitis and epididymo-orchitis in the male, and salpingitis and oophoritis in the female. The latter leads to pelvic peritonitis.

(c) Blood-stream infection develops in some cases, resulting in:
  (i) Septicaemia, with the organisms growing in the blood. This may be associated with an infective bacterial endocarditis and also a meningitis.
  (ii) Acute arthritis ('gonococcal rheumatism').
  (iii) Inflammation of the eyes. Iritis and conjunctivitis are common.

Chronic

In the late stages the common results of gonorrhoea are a urethral stricture and chronic prostatitis with prostatic abscess in the male, and in the female, chronic salpingitis with sterility.

Gonococcal ophthalmia of infants

The gonococcus may set up an acute inflammation of the eyes in an infant as a result of contamination during its birth in cases where the mother suffers from acute gonorrhoea.

Severe conjunctivitis, iritis and corneal ulceration can result and lead to blindness. The presenting sign is a discharge from the eyes of a newborn infant. This may, however, be caused by organisms other than the gonococcus, but in all cases swabs from the eyes are taken to establish the causative organism.

Treatment of gonorrhoea

PROPHYLACTIC

Formerly penicillin or sulphacetamide (Albucid) drops were usually instilled into the eyes of the newborn infant to prevent ophthalmia. Nowadays, however, antenatal care, by detecting cases of active gonorrhoea, is the most important item in the prevention of gonococcal ophthalmia of infants.

CURATIVE

Practically all acute cases of gonorrhoea will respond to one or two injections of procaine penicillin. In the chronic stages of gonorrhoea, penicillin, in larger doses for a longer period, is also very effective.

In the chronic stages, if a urethral stricture is present, dilatation with bougies is performed.

For infants with ophthalmia, penicillin is also the best treatment. If only one eye is affected the good eye must be protected by a shield (Buller's shield) and the infant should lie on the affected side.

The importance of proper isolation in all cases of active acute gonorrhoea must be stressed. Any discharge present contains the gonococci, therefore the greatest care must be taken in handling all dressings or soiled linen.

All cases of discharge from the eyes in newborn infants must be treated with the strictest isolation procedure. Infection can spread with the utmost rapidity to other infants unless the greatest care is taken. It should be remembered that eye discharges are seen in infants which are caused by other organisms than the gonococcus, e.g. by streptococci or staphylococci. These cases are also extremely infectious and must be treated with strict isolation technique to prevent spread of infection.

5 Diseases of the Circulatory System

The heart is a muscular pump which propels the blood throughout the body and the arteries are the pipelines by means of which fresh blood is carried to all organs and tissues. Used blood is returned to the heart in the veins. The blood in the arteries has been oxygenated in the lungs and supplies the tissues with oxygen necessary for metabolism. Arterial blood is bright red because of its oxygen content. The blood in the veins contains carbon dioxide, the waste product of metabolism, and venous blood is darker in colour than arterial blood because of the lack of oxygen in it.

THE CIRCULATION

The right ventricle drives venous blood through the lungs to be oxygenated. The left ventricle propels fresh oxygenated blood through the body. This continuous process is known as the circulation.

1. The left ventricle drives fresh oxygenated blood through the aortic valve, into the aorta and thence in the arteries to all parts of the body.
2. Arterial blood supplies oxygen to the tissues in exchange for carbon dioxide and is then returned by the veins to the right atrium.
3. Venous blood from the right atrium passes through the tricuspid valve into the right ventricle.
4. The right ventricle drives the venous blood through the pulmonary valve into the pulmonary arteries and so through the lungs.
5. Blood having been oxygenated by the lungs is carried by the pulmonary veins to the left atrium.
6. Oxygenated blood from the left atrium passes through the mitral valve to the left ventricle.

The heart cycle is divided into two periods—systole and diastole. The systolic period is when the heart is contracting to propel the blood into the lungs and out into the arterial circulation. The right

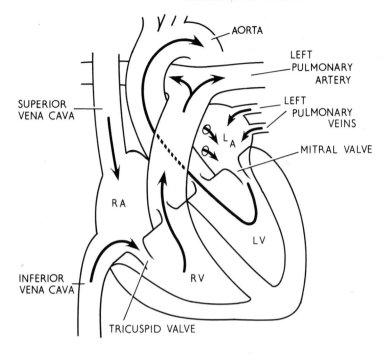

FIG. 5.1 Diagram of the circulation. (RA, right atrium; LA, left atrium; RV, right ventricle; LV, left ventricle.)

and left ventricles contract at the same time. As can be readily understood, the pulmonary and aortic valves are open during systole to allow the blood to pass through. The atrioventricular (auriculo-ventricular) valves (mitral and tricuspid), however, are closed. This is to prevent blood being forced back into the atria (auricles) when the ventricles are contracting. When the ventricles cease to contract the period of rest or diastole begins. At this stage the pulmonary and aortic valves close to prevent wasteful regurgitation of blood back into the ventricles. On the other hand, the atrioventricular valves, which were closed during systole, now open to refill the empty ventricles in time for the next systole of the heart. The function of the valves is therefore to prevent a wasteful backward flow of blood.

CONDUCTION SYSTEM

The heart normally beats at a regular rate, usually between 70 and 80 times a minute. There is a specialised conducting mechanism in the heart which is responsible for the proper initiation and conduction of the heart impulse. The cardiac impulse normally starts in the upper part of the right atrial, in what is called the *sino-atrial node*, or

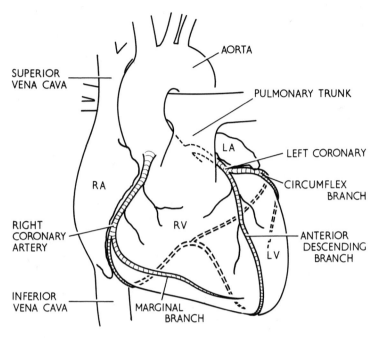

FIG. 5.2 The coronary arteries.

pacemaker, of the heart. The impulse quickly fans out over both atria causing them to contract. The impulse now passes to a second area of specialised tissue known as the *atrio-ventricular node*, which lies close to the septum between the atria. From here the impulse passes to the ventricles by a special pathway in the intraventricular septum called the *bundle of His*. The latter divides up into two branches, right and left, to carry the impulse to both ventricles. The contraction of the ventricles is therefore normally controlled by an impulse which arises in the atria, thus causing the atria and ventricles to beat at the same rate and in a regular fashion. When the conducting pathway is diseased, so that the passage of the impulse is interfered with, the atria and ventricles may, however, cease to beat at the same rate. In extreme cases, where disease in the conducting pathway may completely block the passage of all impulses from the atria to the ventricles, the latter start to beat on their own accord and at their own rate. It should be noted that this ventricular rate is not around 70 to 80 beats a minute but is approximately 40 beats a minute.

The pacemaker of the heart, the sino-atrial node, is under the influence of two nerves—the vagus, which slows, and the sympathetic, which quickens the heart rate.

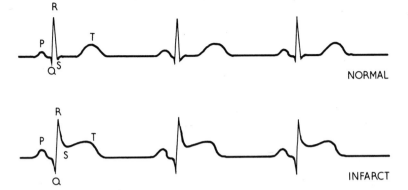

Fig. 5.3   Electrocardiogram tracings in the normal heart and after a myocardial infarct.

Electrocardiogram

The spread of the heart contraction, first from the sino-atrial node to the atrio-ventricular node and then through the bundle of His to the ventricles, is associated with a change in electrical voltage.

The electrocardiogram is an instrument which records the electrical changes produced during the contraction and relaxation of the heart muscle as it beats. Electrodes (known as leads) are attached to the limbs and chest of the patient and the electrical changes are amplified and recorded on a moving paper to yield a permanent tracing.

A normal tracing shows characteristic waves, given letters to identify them. The first wave is called the P wave and is caused by atrial contraction. This is followed by the QRS complex produced by contraction of the ventricles. Finally, the T wave is formed as the ventricle relaxes.

Clearly, important information as to the heart's action can be gleaned from study of the electrocardiogram.

IRREGULAR HEART ACTION

Types of irregular heart action

The following are the more common forms of irregular heart action:

1. Sinus arrhythmia
2. Extrasystoles
3. Atrial fibrillation
4. Heart block
5. Paroxysmal tachycardia
6. Atrial flutter
7. Ventricular fibrillation.

SINUS ARRHYTHMIA

Sinus arrhythmia is a very common condition wherein there is an increase in the rate of the heart on inspiration, with a corresponding slowing of the heart rate on expiration. It is most frequently seen in young children. It is of no significance and is not a sign of heart disease.

EXTRASYSTOLES

Extrasystoles (ectopic beats) are one or more extra or premature beats which occur before the next normal beat is due. After the premature beat there is usually a long pause in the heart action. This premature or extra beat may be so weak that the impulse does not travel to the pulse at the wrist so that there is a missed beat. If the ectopic beats are very numerous the patient may complain of palpitations due to the irregular heart action.

CAUSES

The causes of extrasystoles may be conveniently divided into two groups, important and unimportant.

1. *Important.* Here the extrasystoles are of significance and there is usually heart disease present.

(a) In myocardial infarction, the onset of ectopic beats may presage more dangerous and prolonged irregularities, particularly ventricular fibrillation. Hence the presence of these extrasystoles may require appropriate treatment p. 114).

(b) Thyrotoxicosis, by its effect on the heart, commonly causes numerous extrasystoles as well as atrial fibrillation.

(c) Digitalis poisoning. Overdosage with digoxin often produces an extrasystole after every other heart beat so that a characteristic coupling of the pulse rhythm occurs—pulsus bigeminus. The presence of this irregularity calls for a reduction in the dose of the drug.

2. *Unimportant.* Extrasystoles are often present without any evidence of heart damage and no significance need then be attached to them. Extrasystoles are common in those who smoke excessively.

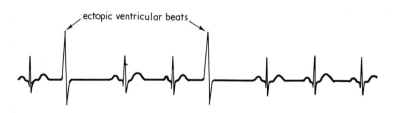

Fig. 5.4   Ectopic ventricular beats.

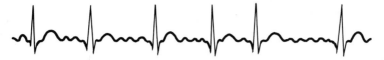

Fig. 5.5   Atrial fibrillation. Note absence of regular P waves.

ATRIAL FIBRILLATION

Atrial fibrillation is the most important type of irregular heart action and after extrasystoles it is also the most common. Atrial fibrillation is usually associated with heart disease.

Instead of the normal orderly contraction of the atria which follows when the cardiac impulse starts in the sino-atrial node, the atria undergo a very rapid twitching called fibrillation. There is no proper contraction of the atria. The ventricles are continuously stimulated by these rapid twitchings but respond only to the stronger impulses. The result is that the ventricles contract in a most irregular fashion both as regards the rate and force.

Causes
   1. Rheumatic heart disease, usually associated with mitral stenosis, is the commonest cause before the age of 50.
   2. Thyrotoxicosis, when the atrial fibrillation may recur in paroxysmal attacks or may be permanent.
   3. Coronary arteriosclerosis and hypertension in later life.
   Atrial fibrillation may be caused by any form of heart disease, but the above are the most frequent causes.

Symptoms and signs
   The diagnostic clinical sign is the complete irregularity of the heart's action in both the rate and the force. The rate in untreated cases is often 120 to 160 beats a minute. There is in most cases a difference between the rate as counted by the pulse at the wrist and that counted directly over the heart with a stethoscope, which is known as a 'pulse deficit'. The pulse deficit may be as much as 20 beats a minute. The pulse deficit is caused by some heart beats being too weak to be transmitted to the pulse at the wrist.
   As most cases of atrial fibrillation are associated with heart disease, signs of the latter are usually present. Very often the onset of atrial fibrillation precipitates congestive heart failure.

Treatment
DIGOXIN
   Unless due to thyrotoxicosis, the specific drug for the treatment of atrial fibrillation is digitalis. The most commonly used preparation of digitalis is digoxin and this is available in two strengths: 0·25 mg tablets are usually prescribed for adults but a weaker 0·0625 mg tablet is available for children or the elderly. Ampoules of 0·5 mg digoxin are also available for intravenous use.

Digoxin delays conduction from the atrium to the ventricle, thus reducing the number of impulses reaching the ventricle. Slowing of the heart rate results and the action of the ventricles becomes stronger and more efficient.

In patients not already taking digoxin and where the heart rate is very rapid, the initial dose of digoxin may be given intravenously, usually 0·5 mg. In less urgent cases, digoxin is given as tablets by mouth, often at an initial dose of 0·5 mg and then 0·25 mg six hourly until the heart rate has slowed.

Once the heart rate is controlled at a suitable rate, digoxin may be given at a daily dose of 0·25 mg or less each day. Where there is doubt as to the most effective dose, the level of digoxin can be measured in the blood. If the dose of digoxin is too high, toxic effects may follow. Particularly in patients who have been taking digoxin regularly for some years, it is easy to forget the potential poisonous effects of digoxin and to ascribe the symptoms to some other cause. The results of digoxin overdosage include:

1. Loss of appetite, nausea and vomiting.
2. Marked slowing of the heart rate with a pulse rate of less than 50.
3. Numerous ectopic ventricular beats sometimes with pulsus bigeminus in which every normal beat is followed by an ectopic beat.

ELECTRIC CARDIOVERSION

The cardioverter is an apparatus which passes an electric current through the heart and successfully restores sinus rhythm in the majority of cases of atrial fibrillation. In patients with enlargement of the heart or where the fibrillation has been present for a long time, the rhythm usually relapses into fibrillation again after treatment. This being so, the treatment is usually reserved for patients where the atrial fibrillation is of recent origin and where the heart is not enlarged. Cardioversion is performed under short-term anaesthesia so that the patient is not frightened by the procedure. When sinus rhythm has been restored, drugs such as quinidine or disopyramide may be prescribed daily to prevent relapse.

ANTICOAGULATION

When the heart is enlarged and the atrium is not contracting properly because it is fibrillating, blood clots may form on the wall of the atrium (mural thrombi). Slowing the heart either by digoxin or by cardioversion can lead to a dislodgement of the clot forming an embolus which may reach and obstruct the cerebral circulation. To avoid the possibility of this disaster, anticoagulant therapy with warfarin or heparin is sometimes used.

THYROTOXICOSIS

When atrial fibrillation is due to thyrotoxicosis (page 441), treatment of the thyroid disorder usually leads to restoration of sinus rhythm. If it does not, quinidine may be administered or cardioversion can be applied.

HEART BLOCK

Disease affecting the conducting mechanism of the heart may interfere with the proper conduction of the cardiac impulse, so that blocking of the beats may occur. There are very many different types of heart block but it is sufficient for the nurse to know the main types. In *incomplete* heart block, isolated impulses fail to reach the ventricles from the atria; consequently the ventricles fail to contract, with the result that a beat is missed or dropped. The rhythm of the heart rate in incomplete heart block is usually irregular. In *complete* heart block no impulses reach the ventricles from the atria and the ventricles beat at their own independent rate, usually about 40 beats a minute. The rhythm of the heart in complete block is regular.

Stokes-Adams syndrome

In Stokes-Adams syndrome the ventricles fail to contract for a period as the result of a severe degree of heart block. In most of these patients coronary arteriosclerosis is the cause of the heart block. In severe cases the patient falls unconscious and a convulsion or fit may occur, usually with cyanosis. If the heart fails to beat within two minutes the patient dies; less severe attacks usually cause a feeling of faintness and giddiness with a transient 'black-out'.

Treatment

In many cases isoprenaline, 30 mg three times a day, is useful as it tends to quicken the heart rate. Prednisone is sometimes helpful in early cases. In severe attacks, if the patient is unconscious, adrenaline (1 ml) may have to be injected direct into the heart.

Where attacks are frequent and severe despite this treatment, an artificial pace-maker may be used. This is a small electrical device, placed in the heart and motivated by a battery. The pace-maker provides rhythmic stimulation directly to the heart and so prevents dangerous failures of contraction.

PAROXYSMAL TACHYCARDIA

Paroxysmal tachycardia is a common irregularity of the heart but is not often seen by the nurse, as most of these patients do not require in-patient hospital treatment. Paroxysmal tachycardia is not usually associated with any other evidence of heart disease.

Symptoms and signs

1. Sudden onset of extreme tachycardia so that the heart beats about 180 to 200 times a minute and never less than 160.

2. Rhythm of the heart is absolutely regular.

3. The attack may last from several minutes to several hours, or even in severe cases for days. During the attack the patient may complain of palpitations and/or dyspnoea.

4. The attack passes off as suddenly as it occurs.

Treatment

Stimulation of the vagus nerve in an effort to slow the heart rate may occasionally stop an attack. This may be induced reflexly by firm pressure over the carotid artery in the upper part of the neck or by painful pressure over the eyeballs.

If the rapid heart rate can be shown to start in the atrium, intravenous digoxin or verapamil is usually successful in slowing the heart to its normal rate. If the tachycardia originates in the ventricle (as shown on the electrocardiogram), drugs such as lignocaine or practolol should be given intravenously. If all these measures fail to restore normal rhythm, cardioversion may be necessary. The patient is given a short anaesthetic and a direct electric current shock is applied to the chest. This usually is effective in controlling the heart rate.

ATRIAL FLUTTER

Atrial flutter is due to the same causes as atrial fibrillation and has a similar type of action except that the heart is often regular instead of irregular. The treatment is the same as for atrial fibrillation.

HYPERTENSION (High blood pressure)

The blood pressure is measured with a sphygmomanometer (see p. 7) and depends on two main factors. First, the strength of the contraction of the heart, known as the cardiac output. Second, the peripheral resistance to the blood flow, which is determined by the calibre of the smaller arteries; the more constricted the arterioles, the greater the peripheral resistance. The blood pressure rises when the cardiac output increases or when there is vasoconstriction of the peripheral arterioles.

As we get older, the arteries become thicker and less elastic, a condition known as arteriosclerosis. This leads to an increase in blood pressure and explains why the blood pressure tends to be higher in older people. Thus a blood pressure of 170/90 might be regarded as normal for a man of 70 but would certainly be abnormal for someone aged 20. Consequently, in defining what is meant by the term hypertension, the age of the patient is an important factor. More important than the definition of hypertension is an understanding of the dangers of an elevated blood pressure and what level of blood pressure is likely to be harmful. It is not always necessary to recommend treatment merely because the blood pressure is above a certain level. In this respect, the diastolic pressure may be of more significance than the systolic pressure. The systolic pressure, produced when the heart contracts, is more susceptible to changes induced by exercise and emotion, and more liable to fall when the subject is at rest. The diastolic pressure, the pressure maintained when the heart relaxes between beats, is more dependent on the state of the arteries and less likely to be affected by extraneous events: it is more constant

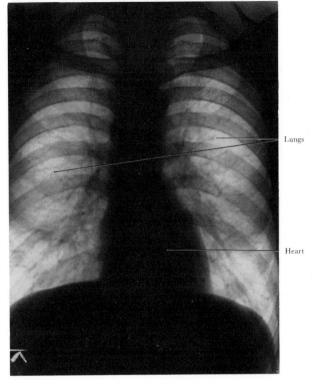

Lungs

Heart

FIG. 5.6   X-ray showing the shape and size of the normal heart and also the X-ray appearance of the normal lungs.

than the systolic pressure. Below the age of 50, the diastolic pressure is normally less than 85.

Causes of hypertension

In the majority of patients with high blood pressure, no obvious cause can be found. This type of hypertension is known as *essential hypertension.*

Some forms of kidney disease lead to high blood pressure, particularly chronic nephritis or pyelonephritis (see p. 371). Consequently, particularly in young people, the presence of hypertension will lead to investigation of the kidneys and their function. Hypertension itself can cause damage to the kidneys so that sometimes it is difficult to know which came first, the high blood pressure or the kidney ailment.

Certain endocrine disorders can cause hypertension. Phaeochromocytoma (see p. 451) is a tumour of the adrenal medulla which produces large amounts of adrenalin: this causes vasoconstriction and a rise in blood pressure. In Cushing's syndrome (see p. 450)

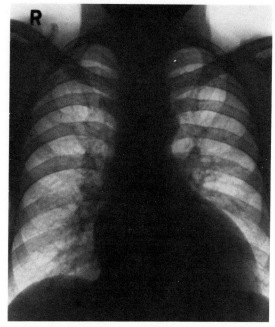

FIG. 5.7 X-ray showing a markedly enlarged heart due to hypertension.

excess cortisone causes retention of salt and fluid, leading to hypertension.

Hence although in most cases of hypertension no other abnormalities can be found, sometimes investigation is indicated to exclude possible causes.

Pathology

The effects of the increased pressure in the arteries are numerous and in most cases serious.

1. The left ventricle of the heart enlarges and hypertrophies to counteract the extra pressure in the arteries. Eventually, if the strain becomes too severe the heart cannot cope and heart failure sets in.

2. The renal arteries, owing to increased pressure, become thickened and narrowed, which leads to a diminished blood supply to the kidneys. This causes in turn a loss of function and may lead to chronic renal failure (uraemia).

3. The raised pressure commonly causes rupture of certain arteries, especially the cerebral arteries. This results in cerebral haemorrhage (apoplexy or stroke).

4. The continuous raised pressure often aggravates or predisposes to sclerotic changes in the arteries with the result that angina pectoris, coronary thrombosis and cerebral thrombosis are all frequently seen in association with hypertension.

Symptoms

Hypertension is often present for many years—perhaps 10 or 15—during which time it causes few symptoms. Headache, giddiness, ringing in the ears and epistaxis are symptoms which only occur when the blood pressure is very high. Eventually, however, owing to the persistently increased pressure against which the heart has to work, heart failure develops. Even mild exertion leads to breathlessness, and attacks of cardiac asthma may supervene (see Left Heart Failure). In addition, the patients may complain of anginal pain resulting from coronary arteriosclerosis, since hypertension predisposes to the occurrence of coronary arteriosclerosis. For the same reason, coronary thrombosis is common in hypertensive people, whilst another frequent result of hypertension is apoplexy caused by a cerebral haemorrhage.

In severe cases of hypertension attacks known as *hypertensive encephalopathy* may arise. Severe headaches, vomiting, convulsions and paralysis are usually present. These attacks are also particularly frequent in the form of hypertension called *malignant hypertension*. Here, in contrast to the prolonged course of the more usual type of essential hypertension (often called benign essential hypertension to contrast it with the malignant form), the whole tempo of the disease is much more rapid and death takes place within a few years of the onset. The kidneys are especially affected in malignant hypertension and renal failure (uraemia) is a frequent feature. Malignant hypertension also tends to affect much younger people than the benign form.

Treatment

Effective drug treatment is now available for lowering the blood pressure but this treatment is generally reserved for the more severe grades of hypertension. Mild hypertension often does not require any treatment and it may be wiser not to mention to the patient that the blood pressure is raised, since this knowledge can cause un-necessary uneasiness.

When it is necessary to treat blood pressure to avoid the risks of future heart strain, the co-operation of the patient must be sought. He should reduce weight if he is obese, he should give up cigarette smoking and he should learn to lead a more restful existence.

Many drugs are now available for the treatment of hypertension but there is a good deal of variation in individual response. Quite often a combination of drugs are more effective than a single one. The hypotensive drugs most frequently used at present include:

(a) Propranolol (Inderal). This is one of many drugs which block the constricting effect of adrenaline on blood vessels. They are known as beta-blockers and are effective not only in reducing the blood pressure but also in slowing the heart rate and relieving angina (see p. 108).

(b) Bethanidine (Esbatal) 10 mg daily as an initial dose, gradually increased until the blood pressure is controlled. It acts by

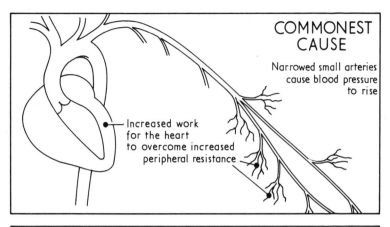

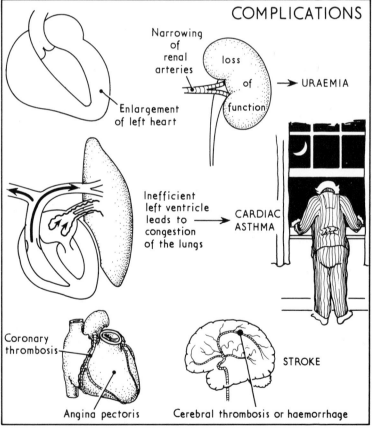

FIG. 5.8 Hypertension.

relieving sympathetic nerve constriction of blood vessels and can lead to a dangerous fall in blood pressure after exercise. Debrisoquine (Declinax) is another useful drug of this type and the dose can be increased from an initial 10 mg̊ daily until the blood pressure is controlled.

(c) Methyldopa (Aldomet) lowers the blood pressure by preventing the formation of adrenalin. The effective dose varies from 0·5 to 4 g daily and is most useful for patients with moderate hypertension.

(d) Rauwolfia and its alkaloid reserpine (Serpasil) are milder hypotensive agents with a sedative effect. If given for too long a time, severe mental depression and trembling of the hands may result.

The action of these hypotensive drugs is greatly enhanced when the oral diuretic chlorothiazide (Saluric), or one of its derivatives, is given at the same time.

During the initial period of stabilisation on hypotensive drugs, care must be taken to increase the dose only gradually, since the blood pressure may fall suddenly. If the patient is in the ward, the blood pressure must be recorded daily.

CORONARY ARTERY DISEASE

Coronary artery disease has become the major cause of death in middle and old age in the Western world.

The coronary arteries are the first arteries to come off the ascending aorta and they carry fresh oxygenated blood to supply the entire myocardium. The left coronary artery divides into two branches, the anterior descending and the circumflex. These branches supply the left ventricle. The right coronary artery supplies blood to the right ventricle (Fig. 5.2).

In coronary artery disease, thickening and narrowing of the coronary vessels occurs so that the blood supply to the heart muscle is diminished. This process, known as arteriosclerosis, begins in early middle age and usually shows gradual progression with the years. Most men and women over the age of 50 show some arteriosclerosis of the coronary arteries, though there are great individual variations. When the coronaries became very narrowed, the blood flow in them may become sluggish and a thrombosis or clot may form in one branch. This *coronary thrombosis* deprives part of the heart muscle of its blood supply: the myocardium involved cannot survive and this is known as a *myocardial infarction*.

Factors disposing to coronary artery disease

The increasing frequency of coronary thrombosis as a cause of death in the developed countries has led to an intensive search into all the factors which could explain this increase.

1. Diet. One of the features of arteriosclerosis is the deposition of fatty plaques on the inner lining (intima) of the coronary arteries.

These deposits are formed from the products of fat in the blood and in particular, cholesterol. Cholesterol is partly derived from the animal fats in our food, particularly meat, fat, butter, eggs, milk and cream. Cholesterol also is formed if we take large quantities of sugar. Hence, if we have a high intake of animal fats and sugar, an excess of cholesterol forms in the blood and leads to fatty deposits on the lining of the coronary arteries. Some people have a familial tendency to form high levels of blood cholesterol even though their diet is not to blame.

2. Cigarette smoking disposes to coronary thrombosis and the risk for smokers of dying from coronary disease is about double that of non-smokers.

3. Lack of exercise. There is a tendency today for many people to go to and from work by bus, to sit at a desk during the day and to sit in a chair watching television in the evenings. This sedentary existence leads to a sluggish circulation and disposes to coronary artery disease.

4. Obesity. Fat people are more prone to heart disease than those who are thin.

5. The stress and strain of modern life disposes to coronary thrombosis. Electrocardiographic tracings of motorists taken while driving revealed abnormal changes when the motorist gets caught in a traffic jam or other stressful situations.

6. In women over 40, the contraceptive pill may be a factor disposing to coronary disease.

7. Patients with hypertension and

8. Those with diabetes are more liable to coronary artery disease.

ANGINA PECTORIS

This is a clinical syndrome produced by a reduction in the blood supply to the muscle of the heart. When a muscle has to work with a deficient oxygen supply a severe cramping pain occurs. This pain, due to oxygen deficiency, is common to all muscles: an example can readily be provided by applying a blood-pressure cuff to the arm and opening and shutting the hand several times. This, after a time, brings on severe pain in the hand which is due to the lack of oxygen caused by cutting off the blood supply by the blood-pressure cuff.

In angina the pain is characteristically felt across the upper part of the chest, and it most frequently radiates down the left arm. It may also radiate into the right arm, into the neck, or, more rarely, into the upper abdomen. It is of a dull, gripping nature. It results from exertion, the patient usually stating that he notices it when he goes up an incline or climbs stairs. The pain is relieved by rest. The patient usually stops and after a minute or so the pain passes off. It is only in very advanced cases that the pain comes on at rest.

Causes of angina

The majority of cases are due to arteriosclerosis of the coronary

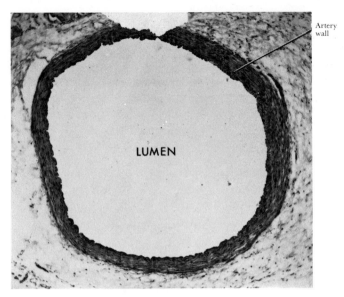

Artery
wall

LUMEN

FIG. 5.9 Photomicrograph of a normal coronary artery showing the width of the lumen of the artery in relation to the thickness of the walls.

arteries, which become too narrowed to provide an adequate blood supply to the heart muscle. High blood pressure is another factor in producing angina, since this leads to enlargement of the heart and greater oxygen requirements. Other less common causes of angina are aortic aneurysm (which narrows the openings of the coronary arteries), severe anaemia (the blood carries less oxygen) and aortic stenosis (the pressure falls in the coronary arteries).

Treatment of angina

There is no medical treatment which cures angina but much can be done to relieve the pain and to prevent extra strain on the damaged heart. The patient is warned to avoid exertion which will bring on the pain, though it is important that the patient should lead as normal and active a life as possible. Regular moderate exercise is to be encouraged. In patients of an anxious temperament where emotional upsets cause angina, sedative drugs such as small doses of diazepam are useful. Diet is also of importance in angina. Obesity, if present, throws an added strain on the heart, and therefore a low calorie diet is given to reduce the patient's weight to normal or slightly below normal. Individual meals must always be light, because a heavy meal increases the work of the heart to an appreciable extent; indeed, anginal pain may be noticed after a heavy meal, the patients imagining they suffer from 'indigestion'.

Thickened
wall

Thrombus
in lumen

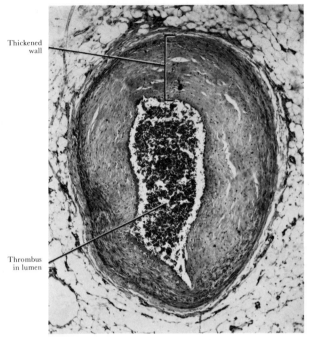

Fig. 5.10 Photomicrograph of an arteriosclerotic coronary artery showing the marked thickening of the wall which results in diminished blood supply to the heart. In addition, in this case, a thrombus has formed in the coronary artery blocking the circulation.

Cigarette smoking increases the risks of angina, perhaps because nicotine causes constriction of the coronary arteries. Although it is not easy for habitual smokers to give up cigarettes, angina patients must be urged to do so. If the blood pressure is raised, treatment should be given to reduce it.

Several drugs, apart from the sedatives already mentioned, are used in the treatment of angina, all of which act by producing a dilatation of the coronary arteries and thus improving the blood supply to the heart. Amyl nitrite is in the form of a capsule, which the patient crushes, then inhaling the drug. Glyceryl trinitrate (trinitrin) (0·5 mg) is in the form of a tablet, which can be chewed or allowed to dissolve under the tongue, and is very effective in relieving an attack of angina. When angina is more frequent and persistent, use of the beta-blocker drugs often provides relief of symptoms. These drugs protect the coronary arteries from the effect of adrenaline: they lower the blood pressure and slow the heart rate. There are many varieties of beta-blocker drugs. Propranolol or oxprenolol 40 mg or more three times a day are two in common use and are often successful in reducing the frequency and severity of these incapacitating and worrying anginal symptoms.

Sometimes angina is unrelieved by any medical treatment and becomes persistent even at rest. The patient's activities and enjoyment of life are seriously curtailed. In such cases the possibility of surgery must be considered. The first step is to perform coronary arteriography, a procedure in which radio-opaque fluid (which shows up on X-ray) is injected directly into the coronary arteries. A catheter is inserted into the brachial artery and then eased into the aorta until the tip is inserted first into the left and then into the right coronary artery. The radio-opaque fluid is injected through the catheter and a series of X-rays taken outlining the coronary arteries. These reveal where the narrowings and obstructions occur in the coronary arteries and allow the surgeon to decide whether operation is feasible. The operation consists of bypassing the obstructed vessel, using a length of saphenous vein taken from the leg. One end is inserted into the aorta and the other into the coronary artery beyond the obstruction. The results of this operation relieve the symptoms in the majority of angina patients and enable them to lead a fuller life.

CORONARY THROMBOSIS (Myocardial infarction)

In patients with narrowed thickened coronary arteries there is always the danger of clot formation (coronary thrombosis) completely blocking one of the branches of the coronary tree. If a major branch is suddenly occluded, the heart will be unable to maintain its action and sudden death occurs. If only a small branch is blocked, the region of heart muscle supplied by it becomes necrotic and dead: this area is known as an *infarction*. After a time, the dead heart muscle is absorbed and replaced by a fibrous scar. If the scar is not a large one, it may interfere very little or not at all with the action of the heart. If it is a large one, however, the force of the heart beat may be seriously impaired and congestive heart failure may follow (see p. 134).

Symptoms and signs

A coronary thrombosis may occur out of the blue in someone who has always thought himself to be in good health. Indeed, coronary thrombosis is a common cause of unexpected sudden death. In other patients a coronary thrombosis is the culmination of months or even years of angina.

The onset of coronary thrombosis may occur at any time, while moving about or while at rest, during the day or in bed at night. The patient experiences pain in the chest which may spread into the neck or into the left arm. The pain may be no more than a dull ache, often mistaken for indigestion, or it may be of great and unbearable severity. It lasts much longer than an attack of angina

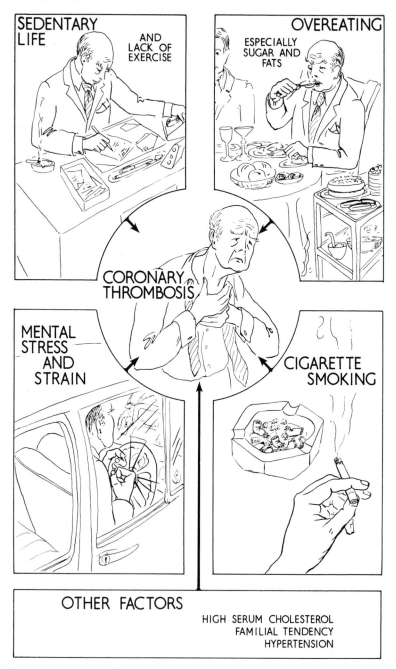

Fig. 5.11   Factors disposing to coronary thrombosis.

and usually persists for several hours. It may be associated with burping of wind or with vomiting.

In a severe case, the patient may be in severe pain, restless and sweating. There may be signs of shock with a rapid pulse of poor volume, a low blood pressure and the patient cold and clammy.

The course of the progress of a myocardial infarction can be treacherous. Although the signs and symptoms may be mild at the start, the thrombosis can spread leading to increased pain, irregularity of the heart action and collapse.

Diagnosis

1. The site of the pain, its persistence over several hours and other associated features usually make the diagnosis clear on clinical grounds.

2. Changes occur in the electrocardiogram which confirm that a myocardial infarction has occurred (Fig. 5.3).

3. The infarcted myocardium releases enzymes from the breaking-down muscle fibres and these can be detected and measured in the blood. Some of these enzymes are known as transaminases and are elevated in the blood after the first day of the infarction, remaining raised for several days.

4. The white count is increased since the polymorphs are mobilised to help absorb the damaged muscle.

Course and complications

Many patients who develop a coronary thrombosis die within a few hours of onset and before they can be taken to hospital. In others, the pain is not severe and the course is uneventful. Various complications are liable, particularly in the first few days.

ARRHYTHMIAS

Irregularity of heart rhythm is common and may vary from occasional extra beats to total irregularity of the atrial and ventricular beats. Ventricular fibrillation is the state in which the ventricles contract rapidly and irregularly and unless controlled leads to a fatal outcome.

THROMBOSIS AND EMBOLI

Patients lying immobile with a low blood pressure are particularly liable to form a clot (thrombosis) in the deep veins in the legs or in the heart itself over the infarcted area. Part of the thrombotic clot may become detached from the vein into the blood stream and cause a pulmonary embolus in the lung: or from the heart into the cerebral circulation, giving rise to a stroke.

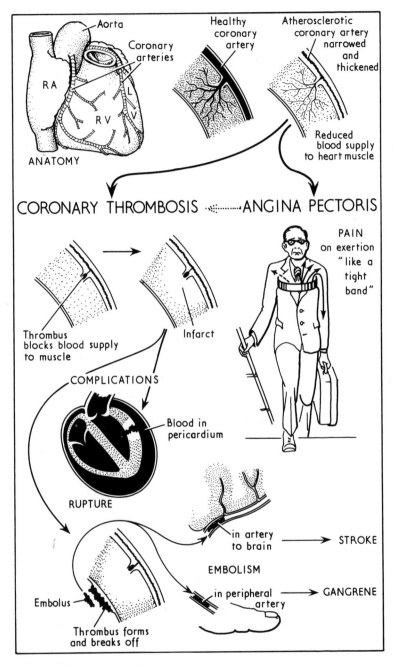

Fig. 5.12   Coronary artery disease.

HEART FAILURE

The patient goes into shock with cold extremities, a low blood pressure, rapid or irregular pulse and breathlessness. The outlook is grave.

Treatment

1. Relief of pain. Where this is persistent, diamorphine (5 to 10 mg subcutaneously) should be given at regular intervals. Diamorphine is preferable to morphine since it is much less liable to cause nausea or vomiting. If nausea is troublesome, an antihistamine such as cyclizine can be given as well. In milder cases, pentazocine 30 mg can be given subcutaneously.

2. Patients should be nursed in a posture comfortable to themselves. If there is evidence of cardiac dyspnoea (left ventricular failure—see p. 132), the patient is best propped up in bed or allowed to sit up in a high arm chair. Where there is evidence of shock and a low blood pressure, the patient is kept flat with the foot of the bed elevated.

3. Apart from cases in shock, patients should be allowed to feed themselves and to use a bedside commode, although the nurse may help with washing and shaving according to the general state of the patient.

4. In severe cases, oxygen may be administered through a disposable face mask in the hope of improving the oxygen supply to the myocardium.

5. Treatment of arrhythmias. Especially over the first 48 hours, all but the mildest of cases should be monitored for the early detection of irregularity of rhythm. The patient is supervised on the oscilloscope which displays a constant electrocardiograph on a bedside screen. This takes the place of constant pulse taking but requires regular supervision just the same.

When ectopic ventricular beats begin to occur, lignocaine is the treatment of choice. It is best administered in an intravenous infusion, perhaps with an initial dose of 100 mg and then at a dose level of about 2 mg every minute.

With atrial fibrillation, digoxin is administered, usually intravenously initially and then by mouth.

If these measures are not successful, other drugs such as procaine amide, phenytoin or bretylium may all be tried to slow the dangerously rapid heart beat.

If ventricular fibrillation occurs and fails to respond to drug treatment, electric cardioversion must be applied. A strong electric current is passed through the chest and is usually successful in restoring normal rhythm though sometimes the fibrillation recurs after a time.

6. Anticoagulants are sometimes used in severe cases where a venous thrombosis in the legs is suspected. Heparin is given sub-

cutaneously for the first 48 hours and then warfarin thereafter: these drugs help prevent emboli. However, the best way to avoid phlebo-thrombosis is to mobilise the patient as soon as possible.

SUBSEQUENT MANAGEMENT

In an uncomplicated case with no pain after the onset, a regular pulse and a good blood pressure, there is no advantage in keeping the patient confined to bed after the first few days. It is good for his morale if he is told from the start that he has had a coronary thrombosis, that he will make a complete recovery, that he will be able to go home in two weeks (or thereabouts) and that he will be able to lead a full life.

In more severe cases, advice will have to be modified by the degree of myocardial damage. Arrhythmias such as atrial fibrillation may persist, angina pectoris may occur and there may be evidence of left ventricular failure. Patients with these disabilities may not be well enough to continue with a job demanding a good deal of physical effort.

A coronary thrombosis imposes a severe strain on the patient's confidence and morale. He may feel afraid to be active lest he precipitate another attack and well-meaning advice to take it easy can reinforce these fears. In fact there is no evidence that ordinary activity disposes to coronary thrombosis: indeed the contrary is more likely to be the case. Regular moderate exercise is to be encouraged and the patient should be advised to lead as normal a life as possible.

As far as diet is concerned, obese patients must reduce weight. Sugar should be omitted entirely and carbohydrates eaten sparingly. As there is evidence that a diet containing a high proportion of saturated fats (dairy produce such as butter, eggs, meat, fat and cheese) increases the cholesterol in the blood and may predispose to atherosclerosis, some physicians prescribe a restricted diet in this respect. Certain unsaturated fats (vegetable oils such as corn oil) do not cause elevation of cholesterol and commercial products containing these fats can replace dairy products in the diet. To offset the dubious advantages, thought must be given to the expense, inconvenience and unpalatability of this sort of diet.

Cigarette smoking is known to dispose to coronary thrombosis and patients should be discouraged from this unhealthy habit.

Coronary care units. Some hospitals have special units of four to six beds specially for the care of the more severe coronary cases. These are sometimes part of an Intensive Treatment Unit where other emergencies are also treated. These units allow round-the-clock supervision and apparatus is at hand to keep the airway clear, to administer oxygen, to provide resuscitation and to treat cardiac arrhythmia. Most importantly, by means of a central series of oscilloscopes, one nurse can supervise the cardiac rhythm in several patients simultaneously. However, it is neither feasible nor necessarily

TABLE V

	Administration	Rapidity of action	Danger	Antidote	Clinical use	Control	Average dose
Heparin	By intravenous injection every 4 to 6 hours, or intramuscularly every 8 to 12 hours	Immediate	Haemorrhage	Immediately neutralised by intravenous injection of 5 ml of protamine sulphate	Best given at onset of attack of thrombosis till phenindione or other drugs take effect		Depends on the clotting time. Usually 5000 units every 4 to 6 hours intravenously, or 12,500 units every 12 hours intramuscularly
Phenindione (or Warfarin)	By mouth in single or divided doses	Takes effect in 24 to 36 hours	Haemorrhage, especially haematuria	Vitamin K₁, 5 to 20 mg orally or intravenously, repeated if necessary. Takes 2 to 6 hours to act. Blood transfusions essential with severe haemorrhage	Better than heparin for long-term treatment, as it can be given by mouth	Prothrombin estimations (a form of clotting time) essential	Depends on the prothrombin time. Maintenance dose about 12.5 to 50 mg daily for phenindione and 3 to 10 mg daily for warfarin

desirable for all patients with coronary thrombosis to be treated in special units, since adequate supervision and treatment can be undertaken in a general ward.

Cardiac resuscitation

Occasionally, after an attack of coronary thrombosis, during an operation or after a severe electric shock the heart stops beating. Providing not more than a few moments are allowed to elapse, in some cases the heart beat can be restarted. If cardiac resuscitation is to be effective action must be prompt and efficient. The patient must be laid supine on the floor and external cardiac massage commenced. Two hands are placed on the sternum and strong rhythmical pressure exerted at the rate of 60 to 80 per minute. At the same time another operator performs mouth-to-mouth artificial respiration. The head of the patient is extended and the nose held (see Fig. 5.13). After a deep inhalation the mouth is placed on the patient's mouth and the breath is blown out forcibly into the patient's lungs. If it is available, a Brook airway should be used for this purpose, since it is less unpleasant and more effective than direct

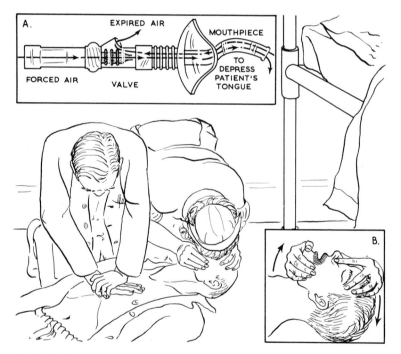

FIG. 5.13 Cardiac resuscitation: first-aid treatment. (A) Brook airway. (B) Position of patient's head and nurse's hands. Shaded area to be covered by nurse's mouth if airway not available.

mouth-to-mouth. This airway contains a valve which allows the operator to blow into the patient's lungs, but any expired air from the patient is diverted to a side outlet. These methods are first-aid treatments and are designed to keep the patient alive until more effective remedies are made available. A cardiac resuscitation team is sometimes formed for such emergencies and will contain an anaesthetist as well as a physician. Special apparatus, including an oscilloscope, a defibrillator and intubators, are kept in readiness with the necessary drugs.

When the heart starts beating again in response to first-aid treatment, the rhythm is often irregular. The patient must be monitored by the oscilloscope which displays a continuous electro-cardiogram on a screen. Appropriate drugs (such as adrenalin, atropine, digoxin, lignocaine and practolol) can be given intra-venously to restore sinus rhythm. Fibrillation of the ventricles is very much more serious than atrial fibrillation and electric shocks must be administered to restore normal ventricular action through electrodes placed on the chest from the defibrillator.

Intubation is performed by the anaesthetist by inserting a tube into the larynx. This makes sure the airway is kept patent and mucus can be sucked out. Ventilation can be assisted and oxygen ad-ministered by pressure from a bag attached to the tube.

Severe acidosis occurs during cardiac arrest and this must be over-come by the intravenous injection of sodium bicarbonate.

It can be seen that to be successful cardiac resuscitation requires skill, time and organisation, as well as expensive apparatus. Never-theless, many lives have been saved by these methods and by the devotion and speedy action of nurses and doctors.

Prevention of coronary thrombosis

Advice as to care of the health can do much to avoid the dangers of developing this common disorder in middle age.

1. Diet. Particularly in those with a family history of coronary disease and in those known to have a high cholesterol in the blood, a diet should be recommended with a low sugar and animal fat content. Sugar and cream should be avoided entirely, butter replaced by a vegetable margarine and eggs restricted to no more than five a week. Cooking fats such as lard should be replaced by corn oil since this helps to reduce the blood cholesterol.

2. The weight must be kept down to a level appropriate to the height and age, and obesity must be avoided.

3. Regular exercise should be taken suitable for the age and fitness of the patient.

4. Cigarette smoking should be discontinued entirely.

5. Treatment should be given for diabetes and hypertension where these are present.

PULMONARY HEART DISEASE

The right ventricle has to propel blood through the pulmonary circulation. When this circulation is impeded by lung damage, a strain is imposed on the work of the heart.

Pulmonary embolism

A pulmonary embolus most commonly arises from a blood clot detached from a thrombosis of a deep vein in the leg or the pelvis (Fig. 5.28).

A massive pulmonary embolus causes sudden tightness in the chest and breathlessness: this can be followed by collapse and death.

Smaller emboli may cause very little symptoms at the time but may be associated with increasing breathlessness and haemoptysis.

The diagnosis can be confirmed by finding evidence of phlebo-thrombosis in the legs or pelvis and by the chest X-ray which shows shadows typical of pulmonary infarction. The electrocardiogram may also show characteristic changes.

It should be remembered that women taking the contraceptive pill are particularly prone to develop venous thromboses in the legs and pulmonary emboli may follow.

Once the diagnosis has been confirmed, anticoagulant treatment should be maintained for several months.

Cor pulmonale

This is the name given to the form of heart failure occurring in patients with chronic bronchitis and emphysema (see p. 161). These patients become very cyanosed because the heart failure exacerbates the already impaired pulmonary function. Oedema and ascites usually are present and although these may respond in part to diuretics, the ultimate outlook depends on the state of the lungs.

RHEUMATIC HEART DISEASE

Rheumatic heart disease is an important cause of heart disease in young and middle-aged people. Rheumatic heart disease occurs in two main forms—acute and chronic.

Acute rheumatic heart disease

Rheumatic heart disease is usually caused by rheumatic fever, but occasionally it also occurs in chorea. Chorea is described under Diseases of the Nervous System, and it appears to be related to rheumatic fever in that both complaints are due to streptococcal infection.

Rheumatic fever usually follows a streptococcal sore throat after a lapse of seven to 21 days. One attack gives no immunity; in fact there is a definite susceptibility to recurrences. Most cases occur in young children and the disease is unusual after the age of 25. The younger the patient and the more frequent the attacks, the greater the liability that permanent heart damage will result.

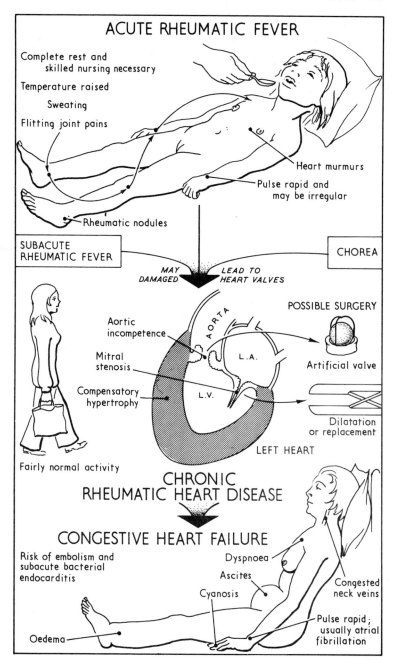

Fig. 5.14 The course of rheumatic heart disease.

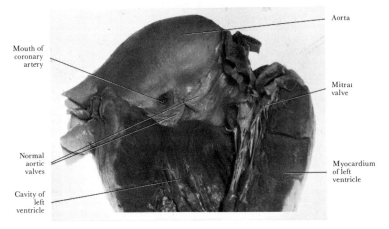

Aorta

Mouth of
coronary
artery

Mitral
valve

Normal
aortic
valves

Myocardium
of left
ventricle

Cavity of
left
ventricle

FIG. 5.15   Normal aortic valves.

PATHOLOGY. Rheumatic fever is a general infection which can permanently damage the valves of the heart; the myocardium and pericardium may also be affected. The joints are swollen in the acute stage of the illness but the effect is temporary. Hence the old adage, 'Rheumatic fever licks the joints but bites the heart'.

Rheumatic endocarditis. Endocarditis is an inflammation of the endocardium of the heart, affecting particularly the valves of the heart. Endocarditis (valvular disease of the heart), as we shall see later, has many causes, but rheumatic endocarditis is the commonest form in young and middle-aged people.

Characteristic lesions called vegetations occur on the valves as a result of the endocarditis. Vegetations are small clots (thrombi) which look like a row of beads on the valves. These vegetations are composed of fibrin, red cells and platelets, and in contrast to the vegetations which form in bacterial endocarditis, comparatively rarely break off to travel in the circulation and cause embolism. The valves themselves become swollen and distorted owing to the inflammation. As a result, the normal heart sounds are altered when heard through the stethoscope, and a blowing murmur can be detected.

Rheumatic myocarditis and pericarditis. In the acute stage of rheumatic heart disease the heart muscle (myocardium) is affected and acute myocarditis is present. Acute myocarditis is of particular importance because death in the acute stage of rheumatic heart disease is usually due to failure of the heart muscle. The unduly rapid and occasionally irregular pulse seen in rheumatic fever is a most important sign of an underlying acute myocarditis.

Inflammation of the pericardium (pericarditis) occurs generally in the more severe cases of acute rheumatic fever. The pericarditis may be dry or wet (pericardial effusion). A large pericardial effusion

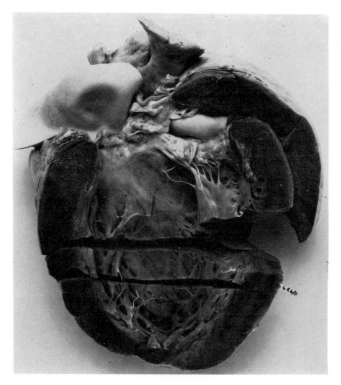

Fig. 5.16   Heart with rheumatic endocarditis.

may press on the heart causing severe embarrassment to an already damaged heart (p. 173).

Symptoms and signs of acute rheumatic fever

1. The onset is often preceded, as mentioned earlier, by a sore throat seven to 21 days beforehand.

2. There is general malaise with a high temperature and heavy sweating. The profuse perspiration may cause a sweat rash.

3. The involvement of the joints is very characteristic and the diagnosis of acute rheumatic fever is often made on the joint lesions alone. Pains occur over the affected joints, the typical feature being their flitting nature so that different joints are affected at different times. There is swelling and tenderness of the affected joints but seldom to any severe degree. The joints never suppurate as in cases of septic arthritis.

4. The main signs of heart involvement are the very rapid pulse rate and the presence of heart murmurs. The pulse rate is faster than one would expect from the degree of fever, and the rhythm may be irregular. Any irregularity of the pulse must be carefully

noted by the nurse as it may be one of the few signs of heart damage.

5. *Rheumatic nodules*. These are small fibrous nodules which occur around the joints and tendons, usually behind the elbows, on the back of the scalp, or ankles. They are tender and painful and their presence usually denotes a severe attack affecting the heart.

Treatment of acute rheumatic fever

NURSING

In the acute stage the patient is kept at rest in bed, although it requires both kindness and explanation to persuade young patients to lie quietly. Help will be needed with washing and personal hygiene but independence should be restored as soon as the medical condition allows. Children easily get bored and despondent when they have nothing to do: parents and family should be encouraged to visit and the limitations of the position explained to them.

If the joints are unduly swollen and painful, wrapping in warm cotton-wool is often most useful to relieve the pains. The affected joints should be protected from the weight of the bed-clothes by bed-cradles.

During the acute stage of the fever light diet only will be needed which will be increased as the acute symptoms subside.

DRUGS

There is no specific cure as yet for acute rheumatic fever although *sodium salicylate* or *calcium aspirin* dramatically relieves the joint pains and lowers the temperature. Salicylates have little or no effect on the heart lesions. Calcium aspirin is usually given in doses of 1 g every four hours. Toxic symptoms may occur from the large doses of salicylates used, but no real harm results as these toxic symptoms rapidly subside when the drug is reduced. Buzzing in the ears (tinnitus), deafness, nausea and vomiting are the usual toxic symptoms noticed.

In severe cases of rheumatic fever accompanied by carditis *cortisone* or *prednisolone* may be prescribed. These steroids are sometimes more effective than salicylates in suppressing pain and fever, but it is still undecided whether damage to the heart valves can be prevented.

A course of penicillin injections is often given at the start of treatment to destroy any streptococci still in the throat. It is important in children to give penicillin by mouth for up to five years after a severe attack of rheumatic fever to prevent further attacks and further damage to the heart.

CONVALESCENCE

Complete rest in bed is enforced until the active stage of the disease is over. This is usually revealed by the return of the pulse rate to normal and a fall in the *sedimentation rate* (p. 333). When the pulse rate and the sedimentation rate have been settled, the patient is allowed to sit out of bed.

Chronic rheumatic valvular disease

Chronic rheumatic valvular disease follows the acute stage but many years may elapse before the effects are noticed. Most cases of chronic rheumatic heart disease therefore have a history of rheumatic fever, or chorea, in childhood. In some cases, however, there is no history of the acute stage of the disease, and in these patients it is presumed that the symptoms in the acute stage were so mild that they escaped notice.

PATHOLOGY. In chronic rheumatic heart disease it is the valves that are particularly damaged, chronic inflammation causing thickening, distortion and loss of the normal elasticity. As a result the valves cannot function properly.

Two main effects follow this chronic inflammatory change:

1. The valves may adhere together, causing a narrowing of the valve opening and obstruction to the flow of blood. This is usually known as stenosis of the valve.
2. Because of the loss of elasticity and distortion of the valve the latter may not close properly, so that a leakage or regurgitation of blood results. This is known as incompetence of the valve.

Chronic rheumatic valvular disease may affect all the valves of the heart but those most commonly damaged are the mitral and aortic valves. *Mitral stenosis* and *aortic incompetence* are the conditions which most commonly arise, although mitral incompetence and aortic stenosis also occur. Quite often mitral stenosis and aortic incompetence develop in the same patient.

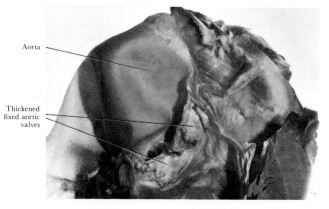

Aorta

Thickened
fixed aortic
valves

FIG. 5.17   Chronic rheumatic endocarditis involving aortic valves.

Symptoms, course and treatment

Until heart failure results from the added strain on the heart, chronic rheumatic valvular disease may cause few symptoms. Valvular lesions are easily diagnosed, however, if the heart is listened to with a stethoscope, whereupon the characteristic murmurs are heard. Indeed, the first indication of a valvular heart lesion may appear during the course of some routine examination, e.g. for military service or insurance purposes, the patient having previously been unaware of any disease. Enlargement of the heart may also be found owing to the compensatory muscular hypertrophy which takes place to overcome the strain on the heart. In mild cases the patient may suffer little disability and live to an advanced age, but with severe lesions heart failure develops, with death following a few years later.

During the prolonged period when there are no symptoms (the condition having perhaps been discovered only through some routine examination), the patient is advised to avoid any undue exertion which might tax the heart too much and so precipitate heart failure.

The operation of *mitral valvotomy* is often carried out in the treatment of mitral stenosis. The tightly stenosed valve is cut and dilated, thus relieving the obstruction at the valve and the engorgement in the lungs. Young patients with progressive and severe dyspnoea are particularly suitable for operative treatment. This usually leads to an immediate easement of breathing and a marked improvement in exercise tolerance. Valvotomy has also been performed with good immediate results in patients with aortic stenosis. Where the mitral valve has shrunken with resultant regurgitation, the whole valve can be replaced by an artificial plastic valve, usually of the ball and socket variety.

Complications of chronic rheumatic valvular disease

Heart failure. Heart failure is the eventual outcome of most cases of rheumatic valvular disease (p. 114). In those cases where there is a mitral stenosis, irregular heart action in the form of atrial fibrillation is usually present (p. 97).

Embolism. In cases of mitral stenosis, particularly if they are accompanied by atrial fibrillation, a clot (thrombus) may form in the enlarged left atrium of the heart. This clot often becomes dislodged with the result that it travels in the circulation, finally most frequently lodging in a cerebral artery, so causing cerebral embolism (one form of apoplexy); the embolus also frequently lodges in a peripheral artery of a leg, giving rise to peripheral embolism and its resultant gangrene of the leg. *Pulmonary* embolism may also arise in rheumatic valvular heart disease when heart failure develops. Here the embolus usually comes from thrombosed veins in the legs or pelvis as a result of the sluggish venous circulation which is a feature of heart failure.

Subacute bacterial endocarditis

This disease is nearly always caused by one organism, the non-haemolytic streptococcus called *Streptococcus viridans*. It is important to note that this organism never attacks perfectly normal valves— only those already diseased, usually from rheumatic endocarditis or some congenital lesions. The organisms settle on the valves and cause large vegetations much bigger than those seen in acute rheumatic endocarditis. The vegetations are very easily dislodged into the blood stream to cause the emboli typical of this form of endocarditis.

Streptococcus viridans is commonly found in the mouth and the teeth, and bacterial endocarditis frequently occurs after a dental extraction or other dental treatment, which releases the bacteria into the blood stream.

Symptoms and signs

1. The illness often begins with prolonged pyrexia of obscure origin until other signs develop to make the diagnosis clear. The fever is not usually high but can be accompanied by rigors and sweating. These signs are in fact those of a septicaemia, caused by the *Streptococcus viridans* being actually present in the blood stream.

2. The disease is a serious one and the patient is ill and anaemic from the toxaemia.

3. At some period, signs of embolism from the dislodged vegetations appear in most cases. The exact signs depend, of course, on the organs affected by the emboli. The following are the sites most commonly involved:

(a) Brain. Paralysis in the form of a hemiplegia (paralysis of one

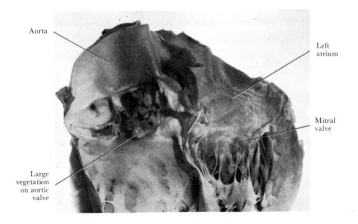

FIG. 5.18   Bacterial endocarditis involving aortic valves.

side of the body) usually occurs, the patient lapsing into coma for a temporary period.

(b) Kidneys. Emboli lodging in the kidneys cause pain in the loins with blood in the urine (haematuria).

(c) Skin. Multiple small emboli are common in the skin, producing petechial spots or larger purpuric haemorrhages. These petechial haemorrhages are especially common in the nails (splinter haemorrhages).

4. In addition to the above there are always murmurs to be heard when the heart is examined by the doctor with a stethoscope. These murmurs are due to the changes in the valves.

DIAGNOSIS

The diagnosis is often difficult in the early stages when the only sign may be continuing fever. Aids to diagnosis are:

1. A history of recent dental treatment or of previous rheumatic heart disease.

2. The presence of a heart murmur.

3. A positive blood culture. To obtain this a small amount of blood (2 ml) is withdrawn from a vein under strict asepsis to prevent contamination. The blood is put into a blood culture bottle, which contains a special medium (usually glucose broth) to aid the growth of bacteria. The broth is kept in gentle heat and after a few days the bacteria, if present, will multiply and form a surface scum. This bacterial growth can be identified under the microscope. Several blood cultures are often necessary before the bacteria are isolated.

Treatment of subacute bacterial endocarditis

Penicillin is usually the drug of choice. Large doses are needed, perhaps twelve million units a day in divided doses. If the temperature remains raised and the response is poor, then even greater doses may be given, perhaps with the addition of another antibiotic such as streptomycin. Other antibiotics may have to be used if the blood culture shows a growth of bacteria not sensitive to penicillin. Whatever drug or combination of drugs is used, treatment has to be continued for a prolonged period—about six weeks.

Preventive measures

Patients known to have valvular disease (such as mitral stenosis or aortic regurgitation) must always have penicillin injections before and after any dental treatment. This will prevent bacteria entering the blood and settling on the valves. Patients who have had bacterial endocarditis should have infected teeth removed to prevent further attacks.

Summary of the course of rheumatic heart disease

The usual history is the onset in childhood of acute rheumatic fever, or chorea, which is allied to rheumatic fever. During the attack of acute rheumatic fever or chorea the heart is often damaged. The acute heart lesions may completely clear up when the acute rheumatic fever is over. In many cases, however, after the acute rheumatic fever is over and when to all intents and purposes the child appears to be quite fit, the acute rheumatic endocarditis continues to smoulder, and after a lapse of many years becomes chronic. This chronic endocarditis gives rise to valvular heart disease (usually mitral stenosis or aortic incompetence, or both) in early adult life. At first little disability occurs, the heart compensating for the added strain by myocardial hypertrophy. Gradually, however, signs of failure of the heart develop, causing in the early stages shortness of breath on moderate or severe exertion only. Later, however, marked dyspnoea, cyanosis and oedema occur. Whether or not heart failure will develop early, i.e. within a few years of the initial attack of rheumatic fever, depends on the severity of the damage to the heart. In milder cases heart failure may not occur till middle age or even later still.

In addition to heart failure, embolism (either arterial or pulmonary) and subacute bacterial endocarditis may complicate chronic rheumatic valvular heart disease.

SYPHILITIC HEART DISEASE

Syphilis causes a chronic inflammation of the tissues and organs which results in fibrosis or scarring. The ascending aorta is commonly affected and this produces a marked weakening of the arterial wall. The high pressure on the aorta causes the weakened wall to stretch and eventually gross dilatation results. These changes in the ascending aorta may affect the heart in the following ways:

1. The marked dilatation of the aorta, which is known as *aneurysm* of the aorta, usually stretches the aortic valve opening and thus produces an aortic incompetence.

2. The syphilitic fibrosis commonly affects the mouths of the coronary arteries (which originate in the first part of the aorta) and so obstructs the flow of blood through these arteries. This, as will be seen when angina pectoris is discussed, may have a serious effect on the heart. Sudden death is a well-recognised feature of syphilitic angina.

Diagnosis

The presence of aortic incompetence in a middle-aged or elderly person with no evidence of rheumatic heart disease should be suspected as being due to syphilis. The presence of aneurysm is detected by X-ray examination, when the dilated aorta is seen. In many cases of syphilitic heart disease the specific blood tests (Wassermann and TPI) are positive.

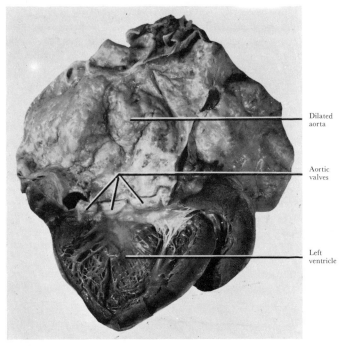

Dilated
aorta

Aortic
valves

Left
ventricle

FIG. 5.19 Advanced syphilitic aneurysm of the first part of the aorta with the characteristic gross dilatation of the aorta. The aortic valve cusps are thickened and separated from each other, causing aortic incompetence.

Treatment

In the early stages, before the onset of heart failure, anti-syphilitic treatment with penicillin is usually given. When failure occurs this is treated in the usual way. The treatment of syphilitic heart disease is, on the whole, very unsatisfactory.

THYROTOXIC HEART DISEASE

Thyrotoxicosis is due to overactivity of the thyroid gland, and is very liable to affect the heart. There is usually a persistent tachycardia and very often an irregular heart action of the type known as *atrial fibrillation*. The pronounced tachycardia is caused by a marked increase in the general metabolism produced by the over-activity of the thyroid gland. Increased metabolism means increased work for the body, and this calls for more oxygen. To supply this the output of the heart has to be increased, and this is brought about by the heart beating faster, i.e. tachycardia. If the thyrotoxicosis is allowed to go untreated, permanent damage with congestive heart failure very often develops.

Diagnosis and treatment

This will be more fully discussed under Diseases of the Endocrine Glands. The patient may be given one of the antithyroid drugs such as carbimazole (Neo-mercazole), or else operation to remove part of the thyroid is undertaken. Radioactive iodine is also used in selective cases. Any congestive heart failure or atrial fibrillation present is treated on the usual lines.

CONGENITAL HEART DISEASE

By this is meant an imperfect development of the heart during foetal life leading to various deformities. The cause of such deformities is usually unknown, but sometimes when the mother contracts rubella during the first few months of pregnancy, the foetal heart is affected in this way. There are many types of abnormalities and some are so severe that they are incompatible with life, the child either being born dead or dying soon after birth. Less severe deformity of the heart may be compatible with a short period of life; in milder cases still, the normal span of life may be only slightly reduced. The common types of defect which are met with are as follows.

Abnormal opening in the septum separating the atria or ventricles —called *atrial septal defect* or *ventricular septal defect.*

Patent ductus arteriosus. The ductus arteriosus is a normal communication present between the pulmonary artery and aorta which, during foetal life, 'shunts' the blood so that it bypasses the lungs which are not expanded. Soon after birth this opening normally closes to allow all the venous blood to go through the lungs, but in some cases it remains open, so causing signs of congenital heart disease.

Pulmonary stenosis. The pulmonary valve may be blocked so that it obstructs the blood going to the lungs from the right ventricle. This is commonly associated with other defects such as a patent septum between the ventricles, and is in these cases given the name of *Fallot's tetralogy.*

Coarctation of the aorta. In this form of congenital lesion there is a marked narrowing of the arch of the aorta so that the flow of blood into the lower parts of the body through the normal channels is inadequate. The intercostal and other arteries become much bigger and join up with arteries in the lower part of the body so as to carry sufficient blood into the lower limbs. The dilated intercostal arteries may be seen on the chest. Coarctation of the aorta causes a severe hypertension in the upper limbs but not the lower.

Symptoms and signs common to many congenital heart lesions

There are several symptoms and signs which lead one to suspect the presence of a congenital heart lesion.

Age of patient. In infancy or early childhood a heart lesion is probably congenital because other causes of heart disease do not occur or are very rare at this age. Stunted growth and evidence of mental retardation are often associated with severe congenital heart disease.

Cyanosis. This is especially marked around the lips, ears and fingers. Cyanosis maybe due to the mixing of the arterial and venous blood as the result of an abnormal connection between the right and left sides of the heart. If the venous blood flows into the left side, there will be an abnormal amount of unoxygenated blood in the arterial system, which causes cyanosis. Cyanosis may also be caused by a poor circulation in the lungs so that there is insufficient oxygen uptake from the lungs. Cyanosis is so marked a feature of many types of congenital heart disease that the term *blue baby* is often used to describe these patients.

Clubbing of the fingers. The ends of the fingers and even the toes are often enlarged and may look like 'drum-sticks'. The cause of this clubbing is unknown. It is also seen in some chronic respiratory diseases.

DIAGNOSIS

The diagnosis of congenital heart disease is made on the presence of severe cyanosis, clubbing of the fingers, dyspnoea and characteristic heart murmurs in an infant or young child. To diagnose the exact *type* of congenital lesion present is, however, except with the commoner types, more difficult. The marked advance in recent years of surgical treatment of congenital heart disease has, however, made such exact diagnosis of increasing importance in order to establish whether or not the lesion is of a type amenable to surgical treatment (not all types are).

To help in the diagnosis, specialised X-ray examinations are often carried out after injecting an opaque dye into a vein. The dye outlines the heart and its various chambers, and any abnormality may thus be visualised. This form of X-ray examination is called *angiocardiography*.

A cardiac catheter can be inserted in a vein in the arm and gently pushed into the superior vena cava, into the right atrium and even into the ventricle. The pressures can be recorded and other valuable information obtained. Cardiac catheterisation is of particular value in diagnosing congenital heart disease, but is also used in valvular disease of the heart.

Complications

In many types of congenital heart disease one of the commonest complications is bacterial endocarditis. This is very common in patent ductus arteriosus where infection occurs in the connection between the pulmonary artery and the aorta. It is also likely to complicate coarctation of the aorta.

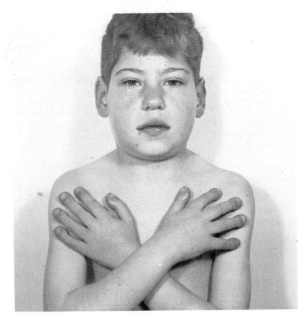

FIG. 5.20   Congenital heart disease. Note the cyanosis and clubbed fingers.

Treatment of congenital heart disease

In the past very little could be done for congenital heart disease, but now, owing to important advances in surgery and anaesthesia, the condition can be improved and often cured.

Surgery has produced the most dramatic results in cases of patent ductus arteriosus. The duct is ligatured, thus removing any abnormal strain and also preventing the development of bacterial endocarditis. Bacterial endocarditis which has already supervened on congenital heart disease is treated with penicillin or other antibiotics (p. 127).

In patients with Fallot's tetralogy an anastomosis between the pulmonary artery above the level of the stenosis and one of the main arteries, like the subclavian, is made. This allows a more adequate flow of blood into the lungs and effectively relieves the cyanosis.

In severe cases of pulmonary stenosis with no septal defects a *valvotomy* may be performed to widen the stenosed pulmonary valve and thus allow a free flow of blood into the lungs.

In cases of coarctation of the aorta, successful removal of the obstructed part of the aorta has been carried out, while cases of atrial septal defect can be successfully repaired.

The aims of surgery in the treatment of congenital heart disease are to relieve cyanosis and to improve the child's well-being.

CHRONIC HEART FAILURE

We have so far discussed the common causes of chronic heart disease and we have seen that many heart diseases cause symptoms only when failure of the heart develops. Before this stage the diagnosis of many forms of heart disease depends on the presence of signs which definitely indicate that the heart is not normal. Such signs include heart murmurs, irregular heart action and an enlarged heart. X-ray examination usually confirms or establishes the presence of an enlarged heart which, in nearly all cases, means that the heart is permanently damaged. Lastly, an electrocardiogram may show evidence of a diseased myocardium, particularly if it has been caused by coronary artery disease.

Chronic heart failure is usually the result of long-standing chronic heart disease which eventually affects the heart by severe strain over a long period. The heart usually enlarges and the muscle hypertrophies to overcome the added strain. This allows the heart for a time to act more efficiently. The stage is reached, however, when the enlargement and hypertrophy of the heart result in a severe weakening of the myocardium, and at this time heart failure develops.

If the strain on the heart is on the left side only, as commonly occurs in some heart diseases, then the left side of the heart may fail while the right side may continue to function normally. This stage is called *left ventricular failure*. Ultimately, however, failure of the left side of the heart throws a burden on the right side and this in turn fails, whereupon right heart failure, or as it is more often termed, *congestive heart failure*, arises.

Left ventricular failure

Here, as noted above, the strain is on the left ventricle. This commonly occurs in:
(a) Hypertension
(b) Aortic valvular disease
(c) Coronary artery disease.

Symptoms and signs

These are caused by failure of the left ventricle to pump the blood from the left side of the heart into the arterial system, with the result that as the right side of the heart continues to function properly, blood accumulates in the lungs causing severe congestion. We have then a condition wherein the right side of the heart continues to pump blood into overloaded and congested lungs.

The cardinal symptom is dyspnoea, which occurs on any moderate exertion. It may also come on, however, at night, waking the patient up from sleep gasping for breath, so that he has to sit up in bed, and often goes to an open window for more air. Gradually the attack passes off. These attacks are called paroxysmal nocturnal dyspnoea, or *cardiac asthma*. The signs present depend on the cause of the left heart failure and may include a raised blood pressure, or signs of aortic valvular disease, such as murmurs. In addition, the pulse is usually rapid and may be irregular in rhythm. In most cases of left heart failure the left ventricle of the heart is enlarged. It should be noted that the signs of gross congestion in the venous system and the oedema, which are both so prominent in congestive (right-sided) heart failure, are absent at this stage.

Treatment

For the attacks of cardiac asthma, morphine (15 mg) administered intravenously is of great value and usually relieves the attack fairly quickly. Aminophylline (250 mg given intravenously) is also effective in relieving the dyspnoea and a diuretic such as frusemide helps to clear oedema from the lungs. Oxygen may be administered.

In the long term, diuretics such as frusemide or bendrofluazide should be taken regularly. If the blood pressure is raised, hypotensive treatment is also indicated. Digoxin may be taken for atrial fibrillation.

Congestive heart failure

When the right ventricle fails to function properly, the right atrium becomes distended and this leads to stasis of the venous system.

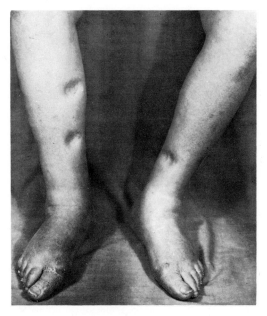

FIG. 5.21   Pitting oedema of the legs in a case of congestive heart failure.

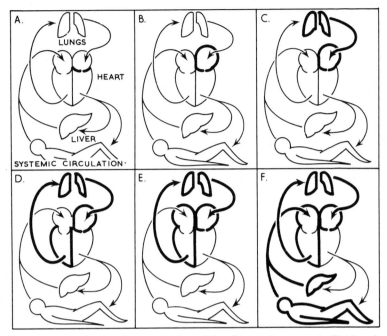

FIG. 5.22   Development of congestive heart failure due to mitral ~~stenosis~~. Thickened narrowed mitral valve (A) leads to enlargement of left atrium (B). Lungs become engorged (C) and so the right ventricle enlarges (D) to meet the extra work. When the right ventricle tires, the right atrium cannot empty fully and becomes distended (E). The whole venous system is now engorged, leading to an enlarged liver and generalised oedema (F).

The superior and inferior vena cavae cannot empty properly. The veins in the neck are distended, the liver becomes engorged, the legs become oedematous. This condition is known as congestive heart failure.

CAUSES. Any cause of heart disease may give rise to congestive heart failure. Some of these diseases may first cause left heart failure, whilst in others the right side of the heart is affected from the start. For instance, in chronic chest diseases, especially chronic bronchitis and emphysema, congestive (right-sided) failure develops without going first through the stages of left heart failure.

Symptoms and signs

1. *Dyspnoea*. Breathlessness is the cardinal symptom of congestive heart failure as it is of left heart failure. In congestive failure, however, the degree of dyspnoea is much more severe and usually occurs even on mild exertion, such as walking up an incline, climbing a flight of stairs, or walking fast on the flat. In very severe cases the patient may even be breathless lying in bed. Here the peculiar type of breathing known as Cheyne-Stokes respirations may be present;

the respirations wax and wane so that there are periods of deep, gasping respirations followed by periods of very quiet breathing. Cheyne-Stokes breathing denotes an advanced degree of failure.

2. *Cyanosis*. This is due to the stagnation of the blood in the venous system, and also to the severe congestion in the lungs causing imperfect oxygenation of the blood.

3. *The pulse*. In congestive failure the pulse is usually rapid and may be regular or irregular. The commonest type of irregularity of the pulse met with is atrial fibrillation.

4. The veins in the neck are distended and stand out owing to the venous congestion.

5. The congested lungs, in addition to producing the cardinal symptom of dyspnoea, also cause a cough and often haemoptysis. The latter is, however, never very severe.

6. The kidneys are also congested and this leads to a diminished output of urine (*oliguria*). The urine is usually highly concentrated, dark in colour, and contains albumin.

7. Congestion of the stomach and the intestines produces symptoms of dyspepsia, such as nausea, heartburn and vomiting.

8. *Oedema*. Oedema means the presence of fluid in the tissues. In congestive heart failure the fluid accumulates owing to the increased pressure in the venous circulation which forces fluid from the veins into the tissues. As the pressure in the venous circulation is greatest in the lower part of the body, oedema is usually first noticed around the ankles when the patient is up and about. In the later stages the fluid increases so that the legs become grossly swollen.

If the patient is in bed the oedema is usually most marked around the sacrum, producing the well-known sacral cushion or pad. This is because while the patient is in bed the sacral area becomes the lowest part of the body and the fluid sinks into this area.

The fluid may also accumulate in the different cavities of the body, such as the pleural cavity, producing what is known as a hydrothorax, and in the peritoneal cavity causing *ascites*.

In contrast to the oedema which is present in kidney disease— renal oedema—the face is never affected. This is because, as mentioned above, cardiac oedema is due to the increased pressure in the veins which causes the fluid by the force of gravity to settle in the lowest parts of the body.

Increased venous pressure is thus an important factor in the causation of cardiac oedema. In addition, there is the question of salt retention. In cardiac failure the kidneys fail to excrete salt properly and this retention of salt in turn causes retention of water.

Treatment of congestive heart failure

NURSING

The patient is comfortably propped up in bed. Patients with heart failure are unable to lie flat as this increases the congestion of the

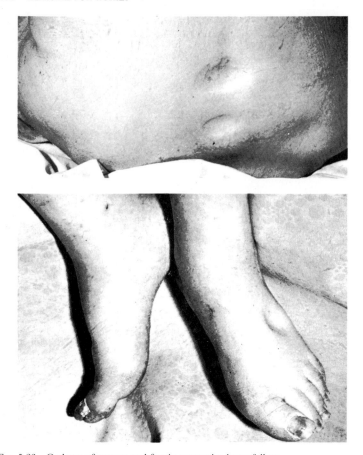

FIG. 5.23   Oedema of sacrum and feet in congestive heart failure.

lungs and so increases the dyspnoea. A bed-table on which the patient can lean is very useful. In many cases, however, the patient prefers to sit up in a chair so as to avoid the slipping down which may occur bed. In addition, special beds known as cardiac beds, to keep the patient well propped up in a sitting position, are available.

DIET

The diet must be light and easily digestible so as to avoid over-loading the already congested gastrointestinal system. Restriction of salt is advisable in congestive failure since the kidneys fail to excrete salt properly, which is therefore retained in the body. Retention of salt causes retention of water.

BOWELS

An aperient may be necessary to keep the bowels open and so prevent constipation and abdominal distension, with their added strain on the heart. The use of a commode at the bedside often causes less strain to patients than a bed-pan.

OXYGEN

Oxygen is needed to improve the oxygen content of the blood and thereby relieve the cyanosis. It also, for the same reason, relieves the dyspnoea. The B.L.B. mask, the disposable plastic mask and the Venturi facemask are all convenient and useful methods of administering oxygen, the last named having a flow meter to adjust the concentration of oxygen. It is most important that no open flame should come in contact with the oxygen owing to the risk of fire. For this reason smoking must be stopped and the patient warned about this danger.

DIURETICS

These compounds cause an increased output of salt and fluid by the kidneys and so relieve the oedema and circulatory congestion. They probably act by enhancing sodium excretion from the kidney tubules and this carries fluid with it. Potassium may also be lost and has to be replaced. Several diuretics are now available.

1. Chlorothiazide and its derivatives. This group includes bendrofluazide and frusemide (Lasix). Intravenous preparations are available for urgent effect but usually they are given as tablets, preferably in the morning to avoid nocturnal diuresis which might keep the patient awake. Where the oedema and congestion are severe, bendrofluazide 5 mg or frusemide 40 mg can be given each morning until the condition has subsided. Thereafter a maintenance dose one or two mornings a week helps to keep the patient free from oedema. Potassium supplements such as potassium chloride or potassium effervescent tablets should be given as a routine when prolonged therapy is necessary. Fresh fruit juice should be encouraged since this is a good source of potassium.

Chlorothiazide compounds have effects other than diuresis. They help to bring down the blood pressure and are often prescribed with more powerful hypotensive agents in the treatment of hypertension. They enhance the effect of digitalis so that in patients taking digoxin the dose of digoxin may have to be reduced to avoid toxic effects. They also cause a rise in blood uric acid and in blood sugar so that prolonged usage of these diuretics may precipitate gout or lead to diabetes.

2. Ethacrynic acid (Edecrin) is an extremely powerful diuretic which can be given orally or intravenously to relieve acute pulmonary congestion. It causes severe potassium depletion and is best used under hospital supervision.

3. Spironolactone (Aldactone) antagonises the hormone aldosterone and so causes loss of sodium and fluid from the kidneys. It is expensive and hence is reserved for cases not responding to chlorothiazide.

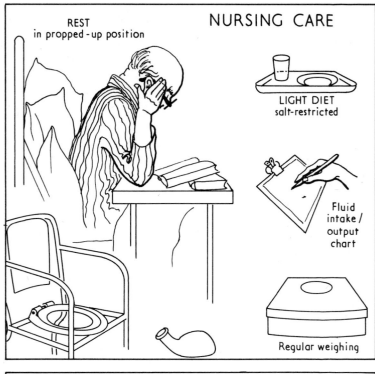

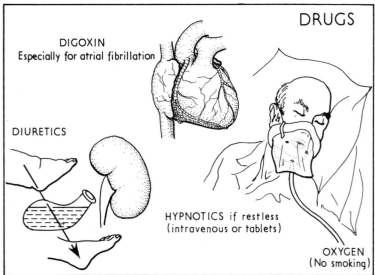

Fig. 5.24   Treatment of congestive heart failure.

A useful means of telling when the patient is responding to diuretic therapy or, on the other hand, beginning to develop oedema is regular weighing. As soon as they are fit, patients with heart failure should be weighed once or twice weekly.

DIGOXIN

This drug is of great benefit in the treatment of congestive failure. As has been noted, digitalis is the specific drug used in controlling atrial fibrillation, and the most dramatic results are obtained in those cases of congestive failure accompanied by atrial fibrillation. Digoxin is, however, also of value in those cases of failure not associated with atrial fibrillation.

SEDATIVES

Diamorphine is often given to ensure a good night's sleep and thus much needed rest. Most patients with heart failure before coming under treatment have probably lacked sleep for some time. Diamorphine in 5 mg doses is usually necessary for the first few nights, after which milder hypnotics such as nitrazepam will probably be sufficient. It is essential to see that the patient does fall asleep. In congestive failure due to chronic bronchitis and emphysema, morphine is best avoided owing to its depressant action on the cough reflex.

CONVALESCENCE

When the oedema has subsided and the congestion in the lungs improved, a gradual return to a limited activity is started. With the treatment outlined above, the patient may be able to get about again and even do light work. However, it is unfortunately likely that the patient will relapse, as in most cases the heart disease causing the failure cannot be cured.

PERICARDITIS

The pericardium is the outer covering of the heart and contains serous fluid which allows smooth movement when the heart contracts.

Pericarditis (inflammation of the pericardium) can be due to infection as a separate illness or it can be associated with rheumatic fever, systemic lupus erythematosis (see p. 471) or myocardial infarction.

1. Benign pericarditis is due to a virus infection. It is manifested by fever, malaise, breathlessness and chest pain. There may be an increase of pericardial fluid (pericardial effusion) which makes the heart shadow on X-ray appear very large. The disorder usually subsides without special treatment other than bed rest.

2. Infective pericarditis may be due to any bacterial infection including tuberculosis. It is associated with high fever, restlessness and dyspnoea. It responds to appropriate chemotherapy.

3. Pericarditis sometimes follows myocardial infarction, giving rise

to a rise in temperature and chest pain during the stage of recovery from the infarct. It is due to a non-infective inflammation and responds to steroid therapy.

4. Constrictive pericarditis. The pericardium becomes thickened and impairs the action of the heart beat by encasing it too tightly. This leads to breathlessness and congestion of the veins. Surgical removal of the constricting pericardium may become necessary.

DISEASES OF THE BLOOD VESSELS
A. THE ARTERIES

With increasing age, the arteries become thicker and less elastic, a condition known as arteriosclerosis. Arteries can be blocked by thrombosis or embolism and these disorders will now be described.

ARTERIOSCLEROSIS

Cause

Arteriosclerosis is a very common condition most frequently found in middle-aged and elderly people. The exact cause of arteriosclerosis is unknown, but certain factors do appear to play an important role in the causation of the disease.

1. There is a strong hereditary basis.

2. Certain diseases predispose to this lesion, e.g. diabetes is very often associated with arteriosclerosis.

3. High blood pressure (hypertension). This very common disease is distinct from arteriosclerosis, but there is some evidence that its presence aggravates or predisposes to the development of arteriosclerosis. Both conditions, however, may occur independently of each other.

4. The possible part played by the fat content of the diet in the causation of arteriosclerosis is now being investigated. It is believed that an excessive consumption of animal (saturated) fats (bacon, butter, cream, fat of meat) and a low intake of vegetable (unsaturated) fats may predispose to arteriosclerosis.

Pathology

Arteriosclerosis is known as a degenerative disease and causes thickening and narrowing of the arteries owing to changes in the inner wall of the vessels. Localised deposits of fatty material appear on the inner surface of the arteries, forming large patches known as atheromatous plaques. These plaques narrow the smaller arteries and so they cause deficient blood supply to organs and tissues. Atheromatous plaques are also very liable to break down and form ulcers. Thrombosis may then develop as a result of the roughening and ulceration of the inner coat of the arteries. Lastly, arteriosclerotic changes which commonly affect the aorta may spread down to the aortic valve to cause an incompetence or stenosis of the valve.

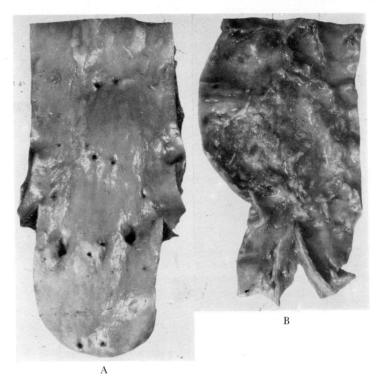

B

A

Fig. 5.25 (A) Photograph showing part of the normal smooth wall of the aorta. (B) Arteriosclerosis of the aorta showing the thickened, roughened and ulcerated wall. It is easy to see how clots can form on such damaged arterial surfaces.

Symptoms and signs

The symptoms and signs caused by arteriosclerosis are due to:

1. The narrowing of small arteries which reduces the blood supply to the various organs and tissues.

2. The thrombosis which is liable to occur in the diseased arteries.

In many arteries arteriosclerosis may have little effect, but in the following sites arteriosclerosis produces well-recognised diseases:

(a) In the *coronary* arteries where it causes:
(i) Angina pectoris.
(ii) Coronary thrombosis.
(b) In the *cerebral* arteries where it causes cerebral thrombosis (one form of 'stroke').
(c) In the *leg* arteries where it causes:
(i) Intermittent claudication, i.e. severe pain in the legs on exertion owing to the diminished blood flow through narrowed arteries.
(ii) Peripheral thrombosis with gangrene of the limb.

(d) In the *aortic valve* where it causes aortic incompetence or stenosis.

Treatment
Since the cause of arteriosclerosis is obscure there is no known method of preventing its occurrence. It may be that certain fats (especially animal fats) predispose to arteriosclerosis, and diets have been devised which employ substitutes, such as corn oil, instead of animal fats. Lack of exercise, obesity, cigarette smoking and nervous strain are all factors which seem to be associated with the early development of arteriosclerosis, and patients should be advised accordingly. Similarly the early recognition and treatment of diabetes is important in reducing the dangers of arteriosclerosis.

SYPHILITIC ARTERIAL DISEASE
Syphilis may set up a chronic inflammation in any artery. In most cases the result of syphilitic inflammation in the arteries is scarring and weakening of the vessel wall. The pressure in the arteries acting on the weakened walls eventually produces a marked dilatation of the artery known as an *aneurysm*. Syphilis is a common cause of aneurysm of the aorta. The most frequent sites for syphilitic aneurysm are the ascending aorta and the arch of the aorta.

Aneurysm of the aorta may result in so large a dilatation that pressure may be exerted on other structures in the chest. The aneurysm may press on the trachea, causing a troublesome cough; on the oesophagus, leading to difficulty in swallowing; or on the ribs with painful erosions of the bones. Syphilitic aneurysms cause breathlessness and angina.

Diagnosis
In most cases of aneurysm the diagnosis can be confirmed by X-ray examination in which the dilated artery may be seen. In addition, the specific blood tests for syphilis (Wassermann and TPI tests) may be positive.

Treatment
In advanced cases of aneurysm only palliative treatment is possible. In those cases which have been diagnosed early, anti-syphilitic treatment (penicillin) is given.

THROMBOSIS AND EMBOLISM

Arterial thrombosis
Thrombosis is clotting in a blood vessel. Apart from certain special arterial cases thrombosis is usually seen in the veins. The circulation in the arteries is normally too rapid for a clot to occur, but in the veins a sluggish circulation is not uncommon. However, when there is severe disease of an artery, particularly arteriosclerosis

(atherosclerosis), thrombosis does occur; it is also found as a result of injury to an artery.

The main types of arterial thrombosis are:

   (a) Coronary thrombosis in arteriosclerotic coronary arteries.
   (b) Cerebral thrombosis in arteriosclerotic or, less often, syphilitic cerebral arteries.
   (c) Thrombosis in arteriosclerotic arteries of the lower limbs.

Coronary and cerebral thrombosis have already been fully described elsewhere; there remains for discussion thrombosis in peripheral limb arteries.

In advanced cases of arteriosclerosis with gross narrowing of the arteries due to atheromatous plaques and also roughening of the inner wall, thrombosis may supervene and completely obstruct the already partially blocked vessel. The signs and symptoms that follow will depend on the sizes of the artery which is obstructed and whether other small blood vessels (the collateral circulation) can supply the area.

In a mild case, pain in the calves develops on walking any

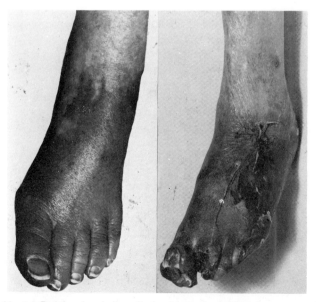

FIG. 5.26   (A) Peripheral embolism. Early changes in the foot due to an embolus lodging in the popliteal artery. The foot is mottled blue and dead cold, and the patient is unable to move it. The onset is marked by extreme pain. In this case the arterial embolus was dislodged from the heart, the patient having had a coronary thrombosis 12 days before. (B) A later stage of arterial embolism of the leg showing advanced gangrene. The foot is black and necrotic.

distance, a condition known as *intermittent claudication*. Examination shows that the foot pulses cannot be felt and the feet feel cold. Usually these symptoms improve with time, partly because the collateral circulation improves and partly because the patient learns to avoid exertion which brings on the pain.

When a major blood vessel is obstructed by a thrombus, gangrene may result. The foot becomes pulseless, cold and discoloured. Infection with gas gangrene may follow and endanger life.

An arteriogram is an X-ray of the artery after a dye has been injected and will show where the artery has been occluded. Sometimes a surgical operation can be undertaken to bypass the blocked area. A vein is removed and inserted into the artery above and below the obstructing thrombus to allow the blood to flow freely again. Unfortunately in many cases this repair operation is not possible and the leg has to be amputated.

Arterial embolism

Embolism in the arterial circulation is usually due to a clot becoming detached from the left side of the heart and travelling in the circulation, finally to lodge in an artery. There are three conditions which frequently give rise to a clot in the left side of the heart and so may cause arterial embolism:

(a) In *mitral stenosis* with atrial fibrillation a clot (thrombus) may form in the left atrium.

(b) In *coronary thrombosis* a clot may form on the endocardium of the heart over the damaged muscle (mural or wall thrombus, see p. 109).

(c) In *subacute bacterial endocarditis* the large vegetations on the valves are easily and repeatedly dislodged to travel in the circulation. These small emboli may then lodge in the skin, kidneys, brain, etc. (p. 126).

In the cases of (a) and (b) the embolus most frequently lodges in an artery in the brain, leg, kidney, or mesentery. In the brain it causes cerebral embolism with its consequential paralysis, usually

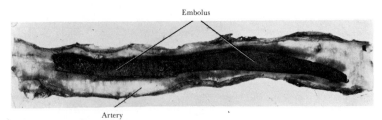

Embolus

Artery

Fig. 5.27   Excised portion of the femoral artery showing a part of an embolus which completely blocked the circulation to the leg.

in the form of a hemiplegia. In a peripheral artery of the leg it completely cuts off the blood supply causing severe pain in the leg, which becomes white, cold, paralysed and later gangrenous. The changes brought about by arterial thrombosis and embolism are essentially the same except that in embolism the changes are much more dramatic and usually more complete owing to the sudden onset. Sometimes surgical intervention can remove the clot from within the artery (*embolectomy*).

Thrombo-angiitis obliterans (Buerger's disease)

Thrombo-angiitis obliterans, although not as common as the arterial diseases already described, is not rare. For some unknown reason it rarely affects women. The exact cause is unknown and the only factor of established importance is that smoking appears to play a part. The underlying cause of the symptoms is the deficient blood supply to the affected limbs which is the result of the marked narrowing of the diseased arteries. The lower limbs are most commonly affected, the patient experiencing pain in the calves on exertion (intermittent claudication) which disappears with rest. (This pain is similar in type to that of angina pectoris, which is also due to deficient blood supply—ischaemia.) In the later stages gangrene sets in, usually starting in the toes. Gangrene is often precipitated by exposure to cold or to injury.

The treatment of thrombo-angiitis obliterans is unsatisfactory as there is no specific cure. The patient must take great care to avoid both the slightest injury to the feet and exposure to cold. Scrupulous attention to keeping the feet dry, warm and clean is essential. The nails must be trimmed with extreme care to avoid the slightest cut. If the patient is confined to bed special care must be taken to avoid pressure sores.

Regular leg exercises (Buerger's exercises) should be performed to improve the collateral circulation. The patient lies on a couch and the legs are supported 45 degrees above the horizontal until the feet blanch, usually after a few minutes. The legs are then lowered over the side until the feet flush pink. After a rest in the horizontal position the cycle is then repeated.

The operation of lumbar sympathectomy to cut the constricting sympathetic nerves is of value in early cases. When gangrene occurs a high amputation is usually necessary.

For the relief of pain sedatives such as codeine or aspirin are needed. Morphine or other habit-forming drugs must not be given. The patient must give up smoking.

Raynaud's disease

In contrast to thrombo-angiitis obliterans, Raynaud's disease is usually seen in women and very rarely in men. Furthermore, it

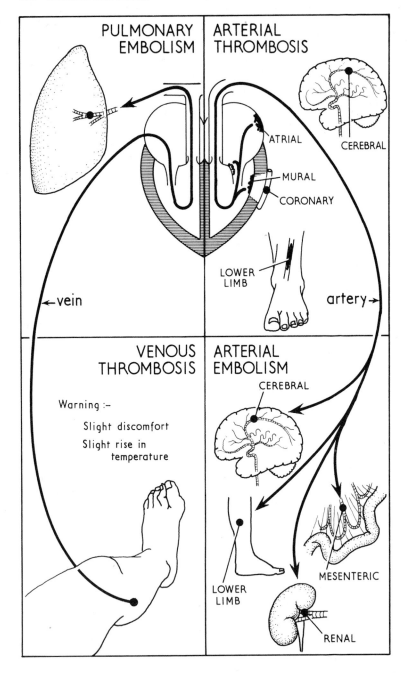

Fig. 5.28 Thrombosis and embolism.

usually affects the fingers and seldom the feet, whereas the effect of thrombo-angiitis obliterans is precisely the opposite. Raynaud's disease is due to spasm of the arteries of the fingers and hands, causing deficient circulation. The hands first go blue and then dead white and feel numb. Exposure to cold is the usual cause of these symptoms. In severe cases gangrene may develop, but it is not as common a complication as in thrombo-angiitis obliterans.

In the treatment of Raynaud's disease protection from cold is most important. In severe cases sympathectomy may result in marked improvement. Vasodilator drugs such as Priscol are said to relieve constriction of the arteries but in practice do not seem to be very effective.

B. THE VEINS

PHLEBITIS

Phlebitis, or inflammation of a vein, is a very common condition, especially in the lower limbs. Apart from the cases in which it occurs of its own accord for no obvious reason, phlebitis also frequently arises during prolonged serious infections such as typhoid fever, as a result of injury to a vein (such as may occur during an operation), and during the puerperium.

If a superficial vein is affected it produces localised swelling, redness and pain. In the case of a deep-seated vein, marked oedema or swelling of the affected area and pain are the most prominent features. The chief danger in a deep venous phlebitis is the likelihood of a clot forming in the inflamed vein, whereupon the condition of *thrombophlebitis* arises. If this happens, i.e. if a thrombus forms in cases of phlebitis, there is a risk that the clot may become dislodged, travel through the venous system, and lodge in the lungs, so causing pulmonary embolism.

VENOUS THROMBOSIS

Thrombosis frequently complicates a phlebitis but it may also arise of its own accord. Any condition that produces a slowing of the venous circulation creates a predisposition to the formation of a clot in the veins. Such slowing of the venous circulation is frequently seen in patients who are confined to bed for a long time, particularly if they do not move about in bed. It is for this reason that venous thrombosis often develops in patients after *major operations*, especially in elderly people who are more reluctant to alter their position in bed.

It has been confirmed that women taking the contraceptive pill have an increased liability to deep-vein thrombosis, probably because the pill contains oestrogens which disturb the normal clotting mechanism. The risk of hospital admission for venous thrombosis or pulmonary embolism is about nine times greater in women using oral contraceptives than in those who do not. To offset this, it should be added that pregnancy is another common cause of venous thrombosis.

Congestive heart failure, because of the resultant slowing of the venous circulation, also predisposes to venous thrombosis.

In many cases of venous thrombosis, especially where there is no evidence of phlebitis, the symptoms and signs may be so slight that the first indication of the condition may be the occurrence of pulmonary embolism, the clot having become detached and travelled to the lungs. In the post-operative cases the thrombus most commonly forms in the deep calf or pelvic veins. As a result the patient may notice a sense of heaviness or slight pain in the calf, whilst slight swelling may be present. It is important to realise that the pain and swelling may be minimal even though a potentially dangerous thrombosis is present. Due weight should therefore be given to these slight signs. In these patients a low-grade fever is also often present; after operation the presence of a slightly raised temperature for no obvious reason should arouse suspicion of a deep venous thrombosis.

Treatment of phlebitis and thrombosis

In the case of a superficial phlebitis the danger of pulmonary embolism is so very rare that it is unnecessary to put all patients to bed. In mild cases a supportive elastic dressing may be all that is required. In the cases of deep venous thrombosis where there is a very definite danger of embolism, complete rest to the affected limb is essential; a splint or sandbags are the most useful means of immobilising the limb, and a bed-cradle to take the weight of the clothes off the affected limb is also advisable.

In post-operative patients, where the risk of embolism is great, anticoagulant drugs may be given to lessen the clotting power of the blood, thus, by preventing the further spread of the thrombosis, reducing the risk of embolism. Heparin, warfarin and phenindione are the most useful anticoagulant drugs for this purpose.

When deep vein thrombosis leads to repeated attacks of emboli, surgical intervention must be considered. X-rays of the veins after injections of dye (venogram) will reveal where the thrombus lies and the surgeon may either remove the clot or tie off the vein above it to prevent further emboli.

Preventive treatment in those conditions likely to cause a venous thrombosis is most important. Early movement of the lower limbs combined with massage, to prevent undue slowing of the circulation, is most important. Elderly patients, who are especially reluctant to move about in bed, must be urged to undertake active movements. After major operations the patients must be encouraged to move their legs and not lie fixed in one position. Early ambulation after operation also reduces the risk of thrombosis and embolism.

SPECIAL CARDIAC INVESTIGATIONS

There are now many tests available which give detailed information of the heart's function and structure. Some of these require special instruments and techniques involving a specialist cardiac team.

1. *Phonocardiography*
This is a method of recording visually heart sounds and murmurs so that the physician can analyse and interpret them at leisure. Microphones are applied to the chest and the sounds are reproduced on a photographic recorder. An electrocardiogram is taken at the same time so that the relation of the murmur to systole and diastole can be determined.

2. *Echocardiography*
The heart contractions and the movement of the valves can be determined by photographing reflected sound waves. Using an ultrasound beam, the operator can take a recording of the pericardium, the walls of the ventricles and the valves. This technique can be used in the diagnosis of pericardial effusion, abnormalities of the ventricles or of mitral or aortic valve disease, as well as other similar conditions.

3. *Cardiac catheterisation*
The cardiac catheter is introduced into a vein in the arm or leg to investigate the right ventricle; or into an artery for investigation of the left ventricle. The catheter is manipulated into position under X-ray monitor and provides information as to the pressure in the atria, the ventricle and the main vessels. This information is vital to the surgeon before making a decision whether or not to operate in congenital heart disease or on the valves.

4. *Angiocardiography*
A special catheter is introduced into the heart, either through a vein or an artery and fluid is introduced which shows up on X-ray. This is recorded either on a ciné film or on multiple X-ray plates and enables a precise diagnosis to be made of many structural abnormalities, some congenital, some acquired.

5. *Coronary arteriography* (see p. 109).

In this procedure the tip of the catheter is placed in the origins of the right and the left coronary arteries and enables the surgeon to see if the coronary arteries are obstructed and suitable for surgery.

6 Diseases of the Respiratory System

The respiratory system can be described in two parts. The upper respiratory tract consists of the nose, air sinuses, pharynx and larynx. The lower respiratory tract comprises the trachea, bronchi and lungs. During breathing, air enters from the nose and mouth through the larynx and trachea and thence to the two main bronchi. The bronchi divide into smaller bronchioles and these open into the pulmonary alveoli.

The alveoli are large air sacs lined by thin flat cells and surrounded by capillary networks derived from the pulmonary arteries. It is in these alveoli that the interchange of gases takes place. The blood in the capillary network gives off carbon dioxide and exchanges it for the oxygen in the air freshly breathed into the alveoli. With each inspiration fresh oxygen is brought into the alveoli and with each expiration carbon dioxide is exhaled. In this way the blood circulating through the lungs replenishes its oxygen supply in exchange for its waste carbon dioxide.

THE MECHANISM OF RESPIRATION

Air is drawn into the lungs by the act of inspiration. During inspiration the chest cavity is inflated by contractions of the respiratory muscles attached to the bony cage of the chest, which pull out the ribs. The diaphragm descends during the act of inspiration, and this further helps to enlarge the chest cavity and so inflate the lungs. The lungs, in expanding, suck in air through the respiratory passages into each and every alveolus, and so allow the oxygen to be taken up and the waste product, carbon dioxide, to be given off. At the end of the inspiration the intercostal muscles and the diaphragm relax and allow the chest wall to fall back, thereby deflating the lungs. In addition, the elasticity of the lungs themselves, by exerting a pull on the chest wall, also plays an important role in expelling the air. This expulsion of air from the lungs is known as expiration.

CONTROL OF RESPIRATION

Respiration is controlled through the respiratory centre in the medulla of the spinal cord, which, through its influence on the nerves supplying the respiratory muscles and the diaphragm, can increase or decrease the act of respiration. Diseases which involve the respiratory centre may thus affect the rate of respiration. Furthermore, for the normal control of respiration the amount of carbon dioxide in the blood is most important. Even a slight increase in the amount of carbon dioxide stimulates the respiratory centre to increase the rate and depth of the respirations. A marked reduction in the oxygen content of the blood also stimulates the respirations.

INVESTIGATION OF CHEST DISEASES

1. A chest X-ray (radiograph) is undoubtedly the single most important investigation in every patient suspected of a chest disorder. It provides essential information not only of the lungs but also of the heart, the aorta, the pulmonary vessels and the hilar glands.

A tomograph is an X-ray focused on a selective plane of the lungs and helps to identify smaller shadows more accurately.

A bronchogram is an X-ray taken after an opaque fluid has been instilled into the trachea, so outlining with clarity the bronchi and the bronchioles.

2. Bronchoscopy. The bronchoscope is an illuminated tube which when passed into the bronchus allows the operator to inspect the

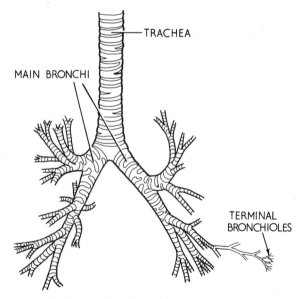

Fig. 6.1   Trachea, main bronchi and bronchioles.

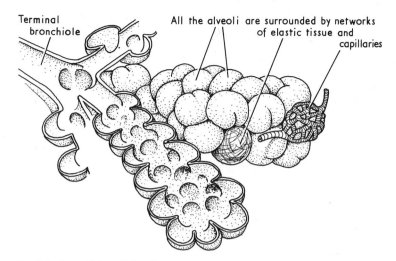

Terminal bronchiole

All the alveoli are surrounded by networks of elastic tissue and capillaries

FIG. 6.2   Bronchiole and alveoli.

lining of the bronchus and to take a biopsy or cutting of any suspicious area for examination under the microscope. Its main value is in the diagnosis of lung cancer. With the invention of a flexible bronchoscope, the smaller bronchi have become accessible to inspection and a biopsy can be taken under direct vision.

3. Pleural and lung biopsy. A special needle may be used to obtain a biopsy of pleura or lung, by penetrating through the chest wall.

4. Tests of lung function. Various simple tests are available to test the functional capacity of the lungs and are valuable in assessing the results of treatment to see if there is a measurable improvement. A spirometer is an apparatus for measuring the amount of air breathed into it. The patient is asked to take in as deep a breath as possible and then to blow it out into the spirometer as fully and quickly as possible. This gives the forced vital capacity (FVC). The volume expired in 1 second is known as the forced expiratory volume (FEV_1). Normally, about three quarters of the vital capacity can be blown out in one second. Expressed in symbols, this can be written as FEV/FVC = 75 per cent.

In ailments such as asthma or bronchitis, the air passages are obstructed and expiration is delayed. Hence the FEV/FVC ratio may only be 40 per cent. These disorders are therefore called *obstructive airway diseases*.

In chest ailments where the whole chest movement is restricted both FEV and FVC are greatly reduced but the ratio may remain normal. These disorders are known as *restrictive airway diseases*.

5. Blood gas analysis. The efficiency of the alveoli in ventilating the blood can be measured by estimating how much oxygen and how

much carbon dioxide is present in arterial blood. Normally the pressure of oxygen in arterial blood is 100 mm of mercury (expressed as $Po_2 = 100$ mmHg) while the pressure of CO_2 is 40 mm of mercury ($Pco_2 = 40$ mmHg).

In patients with chronic chest disease, there may be retention of CO_2 and inadequate oxygen. Pco_2 may rise above 100 mmHg, and this degree of carbon dioxide retention will lead to cyanosis and mental confusion. Since the arterial oxygen falls correspondingly, it may seem reasonable to give the patient pure oxygen to breathe: but this may do more harm than good. The only stimulus to increased respiration to drive off excess CO_2 is from the respiratory centre, and this is activated when the oxygen pressure is low. Hence oxygen should be given at a low concentration (28 per cent) by a special mask so that the Po_2 does not exceed 50 mmHg. If the oxygen content rises above this, the stimulus to breathe is diminished and more carbon dioxide is retained.

COMMON SYMPTOMS OF RESPIRATORY DISORDERS

Cough

A cough is an explosive expiration against a closed glottis. It is a reflex action produced by stimulation of nerve endings in the membranes lining the air passages. These nerve endings are sensitive to foreign particles inhaled from the air and to collections of mucus formed as a result of infection. Consequently, coughing is a response to these stimuli and helps to clear the air passages of unwanted material.

In many mild disorders of the respiratory tract and in the early stages of infection or of bronchial carcinoma, no mucus has formed and the cough is dry and *unproductive*, so called because no sputum or phlegm is produced. In nervous people, a dry cough can persist long after the original infection has cleared.

A *productive* cough is one which produces sputum and so helps to clear the air passages.

Sputum or phlegm

Sputum is an excretion from the lining mucous membrane of the respiratory passages. According to the nature and extent of the disease the sputum varies in amount and character. In the early stages of disease sputum may be absent, appearing later when the lesion in the respiratory tract has progressed. The sputum may be a clear white colour, when it is called *mucoid*. In such cases the sputum is usually the result of minor irritation of the respiratory passage. In more severe lesions, especially inflammatory diseases due to infection, the sputum is frankly *purulent*. Where actual destruction of tissue is present the sputum may be bloodstained owing to erosion of a blood vessel.

Some diseases of the lungs are associated with chronic widespread damage to the lung tissue, and in these cases abundant purulent sputum, often offensive and bloodstained, is present. Such diseases are bronchiectasis, lung abscess, lung cancer and advanced tuberculosis

Dyspnoea

Dyspnoea means difficulty in breathing or, as it is most usually called, breathlessness. The underlying cause in most cases is a deficiency of oxygen. Any disease which interferes with the proper uptake of oxygen stimulates the respiratory centre, so that an increase in the respirations occurs to try and overcome this oxygen deficiency. Apart from diseases primarily involving the lungs, other diseases, especially heart failure, can cause dyspnoea. In heart failure, owing to the impaired action of the heart, the circulation through the lungs becomes slower so that congestion of the lungs results and seriously interferes with the proper uptake of oxygen. In addition, any disease which makes the respiratory act painful may cause dyspnoea.

Cyanosis

When the oxygen content of the blood falls and carbon dioxide is retained in its place, the blood in the skin capillaries takes on a bluish colour known as cyanosis. In many chest diseases there is a deficient intake of oxygen which causes cyanosis. Cyanosis usually denotes a severe degree of involvement of the respiratory system.

Pain

This is usually due to the pleurisy (inflammation of the pleura) which accompanies many forms of chest disease. The inflamed layers of the pleura when rubbed together during respiration cause pain.

Haemoptysis

Coughing up blood is called *haemoptysis* and may vary from mere staining of the sputum, as mentioned above, to frank blood. The coughing up of blood is a most important sign, and in most cases denotes a serious chest disease, especially pulmonary tuberculosis and carcinoma of the lung.

DISEASES OF THE UPPER RESPIRATORY TRACT

The upper respiratory tract is usually taken to include the nose, sinuses, pharynx and trachea. Diseases affecting this part of the respiratory tract are extremely common, and many of them are described in textbooks on surgery. For instance, chronic enlargement of the tonsils and adenoids, sinusitis, etc. are not discussed here.

The common medical diseases which affect the upper respiratory tract include the following:

1. Acute coryza
2. Acute tonsillitis

3. Acute tracheitis
4. Laryngitis
5. Hay fever.

ACUTE CORYZA (The common cold)

This, as will be known, is an extremely common condition. The cause is a virus which is very infectious and spreads rapidly from person to person. One attack produces no immunity or resistance in the body, so that further attacks can and, of course, do occur.

Symptoms and signs

These will already be familiar and need little description. The essential feature is an inflammation of the nasal passages, known as *rhinitis*, which produces a running nose and sneezing. Running eyes are also common and, perhaps, a mild conjunctivitis. The inflammation often spreads to involve the pharynx and trachea and so sets up a pharyngitis and tracheitis with resulting huskiness, sore throat and cough.

Course and prognosis

Most cases clear up within a few days and the only danger is that infection may spread down to affect the lungs and thus cause bronchitis. This is likely to occur only in patients in debilitated states, especially elderly people and infants.

Treatment

A day or two at home helps to limit the spread of infection to others. Treatment is symptomatic.

ACUTE TONSILLITIS (Acute streptococcal throat)

This is a very common infection, especially in any institution where large numbers of people are closeted together. The cause is most often the haemolytic streptococcus, but other organisms can cause an acute tonsillitis.

Symptoms and signs

1. The onset is usually sudden, with a general feeling of malaise, fever and headache.

2. The patient complains of a sore throat and difficulty in swallowing. The throat is often described as feeling very dry.

3. When the throat is examined it will be found to be inflamed and red and usually white spots (*exudate*) are present on both tonsils.

4. In some cases a *peritonsillar abscess* forms which produces a large and very painful swelling in the mouth. *Quinsy* is a frequently used name for a peritonsillar abscess.

DIAGNOSIS

This is fairly obvious in most cases on account of the presenting complaint of a sore throat. Difficulties, however, often arise in the case of infants and young children. Here, even with children old enough to give an account of their symptoms, a soreness of the throat is seldom complained of. The presenting symptoms in young children are usually fever, malaise and abdominal colic; the last may give rise to a mistaken diagnosis of acute appendicitis.

Examination of the throat in sick children is therefore most important as a routine, whether or not a sore throat is complained of. The nurse should have readily available a spatula and suitable illumination (torch) for the doctor when he is examining all sick children. It is convenient here to add that, as well as the throat, the ears are always examined as a routine in all sick children. An auriscope of suitable size should therefore also be to hand.

There are two other diseases that give rise to sore throats and symptoms like those in acute streptococcal sore throat and it is important to differentiate between them:

Diphtheria. Here the symptoms are very similar except that the patient is usually more ill and toxic, and the pulse more rapid. There is also the characteristic membrane in the throat, which does not occur in most cases of acute tonsillitis. A throat swab will reveal the diphtheritic organisms.

Glandular fever. This produces a sore throat with greyish ulceration on the tonsils. Signs of fever or toxaemia are absent or mild, except in severe cases. The organisms responsible can be isolated by taking a throat swab.

Treatment

The patient is put to bed and a throat swab can be taken to find the causative organism. In cases not settling, appropriate chemotherapy may be administered.

Diet has to be light, with plenty of hot drinks, which are soothing to the throat. If the throat is very painful, especially in cases of peritonsillar abscess, kaolin poultices to the neck are very comforting.

If a peritonsillar abscess is present and does not subside rapidly on the above treatment it will need to be opened. This is done by means of sharp-pointed sinus forceps or a short-bladed knife.

ACUTE TRACHEITIS

Inflammation of the trachea may occur:
1. In association with certain of the infectious fevers, such as measles or influenza.
2. With the common cold.
3. As a primary infection in itself.

Symptoms and signs

The general signs of infection, including fever, malaise and head-ache, are present. In addition, the patient complains of a typical sore feeling behind the sternum. A dry or slightly moist cough is also common.

Treatment

Inhalations such as tincture of benzoin co. or a cough linctus may be advised.

LARYNGITIS

Acute laryngitis

CAUSES

1. Acute infectious fevers, particularly measles, diphtheria and influenza.

2. The common cold, acute tracheitis, or acute bronchitis may all cause an acute laryngitis.

Symptoms and signs

In addition to the general signs of infection, including malaise, fever and headache, there is the characteristic huskiness of voice and hoarseness. In some cases there may be almost complete loss of voice. The throat is sore and there is an accompanying dry cough.

DIAGNOSIS

The diagnosis of laryngitis is usually obvious, but it is important to distinguish those cases which are due to measles and diphtheria. The examination of the mouth will show any Koplik's spots, thus identifying the case as one of measles, as also would, of course, the presence of a morbilliform rash. In diphtheria there is in most cases the characteristic membrane present in the throat, but in a few patients this may be absent. If there is any suspicion that the laryngitis might be due to diphtheria the case is treated as such till a definite diagnosis is made. In doubtful cases a throat swab should be taken and sent to the laboratory for culture.

Treatment of acute laryngitis

The patient is nursed in bed in a well-ventilated atmosphere, but avoiding draughts. If it is thought that the laryngitis may be due to measles, diphtheria, or any other infectious fever, then proper isolation precautions are taken and, in addition, any specific treatment, e.g. antitoxin, given.

The diet should be light, with plenty of soothing hot drinks. Some patients with laryngitis find a steamy atmosphere soothing, and inhalations from an inhaler or a steam tent may be used. Friar's balsam, 4 ml to 0·5 litres of water, is the most commonly used inhalant.

Since most cases are due to a virus infection, there is no specific treatment and most cases settle in a few days. If the case is a severe one, with high temperature and signs of toxicity, penicillin or another antibiotic may be given for the possibility of a secondary bacterial infection.

Chronic laryngitis

CAUSES
1. Prolonged over-use of the voice as in singers or auctioneers.
2. Excessive cigarette smoking.
3. Tuberculous laryngitis.
4. Malignant disease of the larynx.

Symptoms and treatment

The predominating complaint is one of chronic progressive hoarseness, eventually leading to loss of voice. In all cases of chronic hoarseness an examination of the throat and vocal cords will be made by means of a laryngoscope and a biopsy taken for histological examination to exclude malignant disease. By this means the exact nature and cause of the laryngitis can usually be identified.

The treatment will naturally vary according to the cause. In those cases due to over-use of the voice, prolonged rest is usually sufficient to restore normal conditions. In tuberculous patients there is usually an advanced pulmonary tuberculous lesion as well, which requires the appropriate treatment as outlined on p. 181. Sedative lozenges are useful for the pain.

In malignant disease of the larynx, operation or radium therapy is carried out unless the disease has spread too far, in which case only palliative sedatives can be given.

HAY FEVER

Hay fever is one of the allergic diseases, like many cases of asthma and urticaria. In hay fever the patients are sensitive to the grass pollens and when they come in contact with them the typical symptoms of hay fever develop.

Symptoms and signs

1. The onset is always at a specific time of the year—in Britain in the month of May, when the new grasses grow.

2. Paroxysmal attacks of sneezing, associated with a running nose and running eyes, occur. The bouts of sneezing may last in some cases for hours on end. There is usually severe congestion of the nasal passages and eyes.

Treatment

To prevent attacks, desensitisation may be effected by means of gradually increasing doses of the offending pollens injected subcutaneously. The injections have to be started several months before the hay fever starts in May and stopped when the new grass pollens grow. The effect, unfortunately, only lasts for one or two years.

Nasal insufflators containing cromoglycate are also useful in preventing hay fever if started regularly before the pollen season.

Antihistamine tablets such as promethazine are helpful in relieving symptoms but may give rise to drowsiness. Nasal sprays containing steroids are often effective for several hours after an application.

DISEASES OF THE LOWER RESPIRATORY TRACT
BRONCHITIS

Acute bronchitis
This is a common condition often initiated by a viral infection of the upper respiratory tract with secondary bacterial infection such as *Haemophilus influenzae* or haemolytic streptococci. It is commoner in the winter months and particularly in the elderly, the frail or in those with a chronic chest disorder.

Bronchitis often occurs in children with infectious fevers, especially measles, influenza and whooping-cough.

Symptoms and signs
1. There are the symptoms of a mild fever such as malaise, headache and loss of appetite.
2. A cough is an early symptom and is associated with a moderate amount of mucoid or purulent sputum.
3. There may be soreness or pain beneath the sternum caused by an accompanying inflammation of the trachea.
4. The respirations are usually a little fast and somewhat laboured, but except in serious cases there is no severe dyspnoea or cyanosis.
5. When the chest is examined, alterations in the normal breath sounds are heard which enable the doctor to diagnose the condition.

Course
The disease usually subsides fairly rapidly in a few days with proper treatment, and is serious only in young children and elderly people where the inflammation may spread and cause a bronchopneumonia. Repeated attacks of acute bronchitis may, however, give rise to chronic bronchitis with much more serious consequences.

Treatment of acute bronchitis
The patient is put to bed and kept warm in a well-ventilated atmosphere. Light diet is given with plenty of drinks. Aspirin will probably be found useful, and on this treatment most cases will subside rapidly.

Expectorants, i.e. drugs to increase expectoration of sputum, may be ordered, especially if the sputum is thick and difficult to bring up.

More serious cases will need treatment as discussed under acute exacerbation of chronic bronchitis.

CHRONIC BRONCHITIS AND EMPHYSEMA
(Chronic obstructive airway disease)

These are two disorders which frequently exist together to a lesser or greater degree. In chronic bronchitis, there is swelling and thickening of the lining of the bronchial tree and obstruction to air entry is made worse by the presence of thick mucus. Emphysema is characterised by distension and damage of the alveolar air sacs: there is a loss of elasticity in the lungs as a whole. Chronic bronchitis and emphysema can lead to progressive disablement of the sufferer, the so-called respiratory cripple, breathless and incapacitated.

Chronic bronchitis

Chronic bronchitis is a serious cause of disability and death, more common in men than women and usually becoming manifest in middle age. Cigarette smoking is the most important single cause, though air pollution by smoke and sulphur dioxide or working in a dusty atmosphere (e.g. coal miners) could be contributory causes.

Clinical features

The onset of chronic bronchitis is usually insidious, and heralded by a morning cough (the so-called 'smokers cough'), expectoration of mucoid sputum and breathlessness on exertion. These symptoms get worse over the winter months, particularly after an upper respiratory tract infection. The cough becomes more persistent, the sputum is often purulent and the breathing more wheezy and difficult.

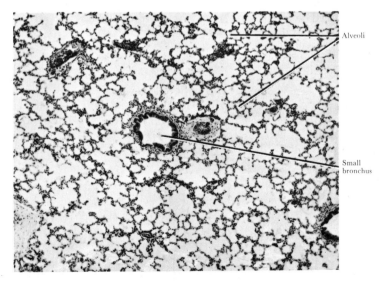

Alveoli

Small bronchus

FIG. 6.3   Section through a normal lung showing the clear empty air sacs (alveoli).

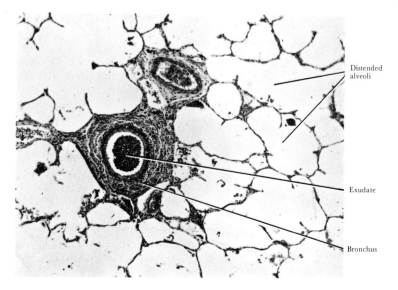

Distended
alveoli

Exudate

Bronchus

FIG. 6.4   Emphysema of the lung showing the characteristic thin-walled and distended alveoli. Bronchitis is also present, as shown by the inflammatory exudate inside the bronchus.

As the years go by, particularly if cigarette smoking is not discontinued, the disability slowly gets worse. As the airway obstruction increases, the colour becomes more cyanosed and the strain on the right ventricle of the heart may lead to congestive heart failure, the so-called *cor pulmonale*. The patient is now breathless even at rest, the phlegm more frequent and purulent, the face is cyanosed and suffused and the legs oedematous.

Acute exacerbations are brought about by episodes of infective bronchitis, leading to *respiratory failure*. The oxygen content of the blood becomes seriously depleted and there is a dangerous retention of waste carbon dioxide. This leads to deep cyanosis and mental confusion or coma. Unless vigorous measures are adopted to clear the airways and oxygenate the lungs, death will ensue.

Treatment

In the early stages:

1. Every effort must be used to persuade the patient to give up cigarette smoking entirely. He can be told, 'If you continue to smoke, your chest will get steadily worse year by year. If you give up cigarettes, there is every reason to expect a steady improvement year by year.' Smoky atmospheres should be avoided where feasible and a dusty occupation may have to be changed.

2. Chemotherapy such as co-trimoxazole tablets or tetracycline capsules should be given two or three times daily and continued for

10 days at the first sign of a chest infection or when the sputum becomes purulent.

3. Where wheeziness is present, bronchodilators may be helpful. Salbutamol is most effective, in the form of tablets or by inhaler. Wheeziness suggests an allergic response (see asthma) and in some cases steroids are helpful, usually in the form of a beclomethasone inhaler. Before prescribing steroid therapy, it is usual to perform lung function tests before and after a trial period: there is no point in giving steroids for a long term if the response to a trial does not lead to measurable improvement.

COR PULMONALE

1. Chemotherapy may need to be maintained throughout the winter months and perhaps even in the summer as well. This is because the patient's resistance to respiratory infections is very low at this stage and also because when there is so little functional respiratory reserve, even a minor chest infection can be dangerous.

2. Diuretics. Diuretics help to relieve systemic and pulmonary oedema induced by strain on the right ventricle of the heart. Bendrofluazide or frusemide are two useful diuretics in this respect. They relieve oedema of the legs and ease the breathing.

3. Oxygen. Oxygen gives symptomatic relief and increases the oxygen content of the blood. Where there is excessive carbon dioxide retention, too high an increase of blood oxygen may depress respiratory function and so lead to further CO_2 retention. Hence oxygen should be given by a Venturi mask which provides oxygen in a concentration of 28 per cent: the concentration of oxygen in air is only 21 per cent. Many patients have oxygen cylinders at home, both in the bedroom and the living room.

RESPIRATORY FAILURE

The first essential is to clear the airway.

The patient is encouraged, if he is able, to cough up phlegm and mucus. Physiotherapy can be invaluable in stimulating expectoration.

If this fails to lead an improvement, a cuffed endotracheal tube can be passed into the trachea and attached to a mechanical ventilator. By this means, the mucous secretions can be sucked out of the air passages and a mixture of air and oxygen transmitted into the lungs by the ventilator. The ventilator provides a positive pressure in an intermittent manner like that of normal breathing and this is known as *intermittent positive pressure ventilation* (IPPV). Patients in respiratory failure need continuous supervision and nursing and are often cared for in an Intensive Care Unit.

Emphysema

Whereas inspiration is an active process brought about by contraction of the chest muscles, expiration is a passive movement brought about by the elastic recoil of the lungs as the chest muscles relax. In emphysema, the alveolar air spaces are distended and enlarged and the lungs lose their elasticity. Consequently, the chest moves poorly and expiration is prolonged and difficult.

Emphysema is often associated with chronic bronchitis and is due to much the same causes. However, in some patients there is a deficiency of an enzyme (alpha-1-antitrypsin) which normally protects the structure of the alveolar walls.

Clinical features

The salient symptom of emphysema is breathlessness, gradually over the years becoming more incapacitating. Unless chronic bronchitis is present as well, cough and sputum are not troublesome. The chest moves poorly, the respiration rate is rapid and expiration is laboured and prolonged. Often the colour is good and not cyanosed.

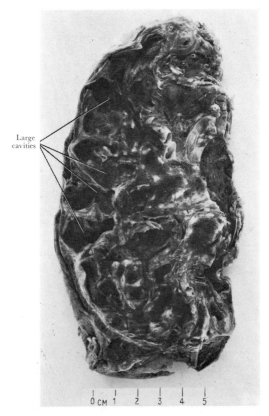

Large cavities

Fig. 6.5 Very advanced bronchiectasis showing large cavities throughout the lung.

Treatment

Treatment is mainly that of associated chronic bronchitis or the complications already discussed.

BRONCHIECTASIS

Bronchiectasis is a disorder characterised by widening and dilatation of the bronchi: these become infected and form sumps of purulent phlegm. The cause is usually unknown but may follow pneumonia or whooping cough in childhood.

Clinical features

The characteristic features of bronchiectasis are cough with the production of large quantities of purulent sputum. Often the cough occurs in paroxysms and is worse in the early mornings. There may be haemoptysis, breathlessness and loss of weight. Where the chest infection is severe, clubbing of the fingers may be noted.

DIAGNOSIS

In the early dry stage the diagnosis can be confirmed only by X-ray examination of the chest after inserting an opaque oil into the bronchi *(bronchogram)*. The bronchi can then be outlined and if they

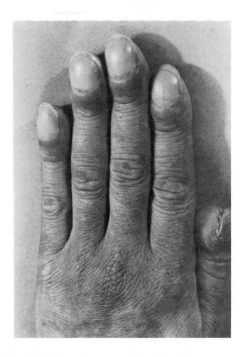

Fig. 6.6   Clubbing of the fingers in a case of bronchiectasis.

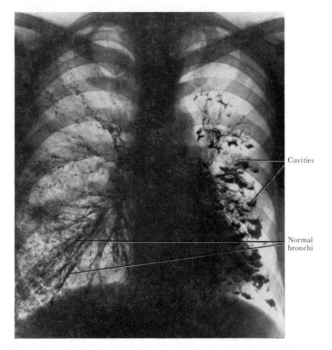

Cavities

Normal bronchi

FIG. 6.7   X-ray after the instillation of opaque iodine into the bronchi (broncho-gram). The outlined bronchi in the right lung are normal, but in the left lung bronchiectatic cavities are clearly visible.

are dilated and widened above the normal the diagnosis of bronchiectasis is confirmed. For the more advanced cases the diagnosis is usually fairly obvious, owing to the typical symptoms and signs, especially the chronic cough, copious sputum and the clubbing of the fingers.

Complications
1. Bronchopneumonia. This is the most common complication and is the usual termination of most cases.
2. Cerebral abscess. Septic purulent emboli may travel from the lungs into the arteries and to the brain to cause a cerebral abscess.

Treatment of bronchiectasis
Repeated courses of antibiotics such as ampicillin help to keep the sputum from becoming profuse and purulent.

Postural drainage is effective in preventing sputum from collecting in the dilated bronchi. If, for instance, the lower parts of the lungs are affected, then the patient is 'tipped up' so that the foul sputum is brought up more easily on coughing. The patient can be tipped up by elevating the foot of the bed with the patient lying flat on

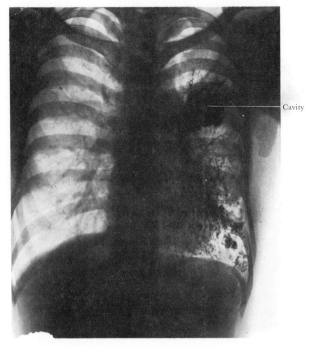

Cavity

FIG. 6.8   Bronchogram from another case of bronchiectasis showing dilatation and cavitation of the bronchi in the upper lobe of the left lung.

the bed, or else by the patient leaning forward over the edge. Special beds are available which allow easy posturing of the patient.

If the bronchogram reveals only one segment of the lung is involved and if the condition continues to be troublesome despite postural drainage, surgical resection of the affected segment of the lung can be undertaken.

LUNG ABSCESS

Abscess of the lung is a relatively uncommon condition but is seen in the following circumstances:

1. Following the inhalation of a foreign body into the lungs.
2. Due to inhalation of septic matter from the nose or throat following operations on these parts.

Symptoms and signs

There are usually signs of infection, with swinging fever, sweating and general malaise. With these symptoms there are usually a persistent cough and sputum which is characteristically foul, copious, and may be bloodstained. If the condition is allowed to become chronic, signs of bronchiectasis with clubbing of the fingers may occur.

Following the inhalation of a foreign body, or after an operation on the nose, the presence of a persistent cough and foul sputum will inevitably lead to a chest X-ray being taken. The abscess cavity will then be seen.

Treatment

Any foreign body will of course be removed by bronchoscopy. Penicillin is the drug most commonly used in lung abscess, often with very good results. Postural drainage for more chronic cases may also be very useful. If the condition does not respond to the above measures, surgical treatment to drain the lung abscess may be necessary.

PNEUMONIA

Pneumonia is an inflammatory condition of the lung caused by infection, usually bacterial or viral.

As a result of infection, the alveoli become filled with serous fluid and inflammatory cells: the area of lung involved is said to have undergone *consolidation*. As a recovery takes place, the alveolar inflammatory material is coughed up: in the early stages this sputum often contains many red cells and is rusty in appearance. Later, as the white cells invade the alveolar exudation, the sputum becomes yellow and purulent.

Lobar pneumonia

This is a pneumonic consolidation involving one or more lobes of the lung. It is bacterial in origin; usually pneumococci or Klebsiella bacilli are responsible. More common than lobar consolidation is consolidation involving patches of lung tissue, usually affecting both lungs in different areas and not confined to any one lobe. This generalised pneumonia (sometimes called *bronchopneumonia*) may be due to bacterial invasion by such organisms as streptococci or Haemophilus. It is frequently caused by virus infections or by *Mycoplasma pneumoniae*. Mycoplasma is a microorganism which lacks a cell wall and so is not bacterial: in form it can be looked on as halfway between viruses and bacteria and it is sensitive to some antibiotics.

Pulmonary tuberculosis (see p. 175) can sometimes give rise to a tuberculous pneumonia.

Pneumonia can occur in a previously healthy person due to an overwhelming infection. However, many conditions may predispose to the development of pneumonia:

1. Any chest diseases already present, such as chronic bronchitis and emphysema, lung cancer or bronchiectasis.

2. Especially in the winter months, the old and the frail are liable to respiratory infections leading to pneumonia.

3. Alcoholism and malnutrition dispose to chest infections.

4. In babies and small children, infectious fevers such as whooping cough and measles can lead to pneumonia.

5. Aspiration of infected mucus from the nose or the sinuses following a simple infection of the upper respiratory tract may lead to areas of bronchopneumonia.

Clinical features

The clinical features will depend on the type of infection causing the pneumonia (bacterial, viral or mycoplasmal) and on whether it supervenes on a chest disease already present.

Lobar pneumonia is usually caused by bacterial infections, especially pneumococci.

1. The *onset* is sudden, with a high fever (often 102° to 104° F) (39° to 40° C), and is in many cases accompanied by shivering attacks (rigors). A severe *pain* in the chest over the affected lobe of the lung is present owing to the frequently accompanying pleurisy. This pain characteristically catches the breathing so that the patient is nervous of taking a deep breath. For this reason also the *cough*, which is always present, is short and suppressed.

2. The face is flushed and *herpes febrilis* is very commonly present

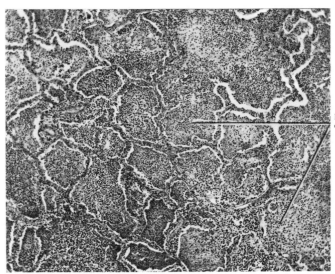

Inflammatory exudate

FIG. 6.9   Lobar pneumonia. The alveoli are completely filled with inflammatory exudate (white blood cells, fibrin and some red cells). The alveolar walls are thickened owing to congestion and oedema. The solid airless state of the lung in pneumonia is known as consolidation.

on the lips and cheek. This is a small group of vesicles clustered together which after a few days crust and resolve. Herpes febrilis is most commonly associated with lobar pneumonia or the common cold.

The respirations are rapid and the alae nasae (nostrils) may be seen to move with respiration. The pulse rate rises, but not to the same extent as the respirations.

3. After a day or so the cough becomes moist with the typical *rusty* sputum, the colour being due to altered blood. The sputum is very thick and tenacious and often adheres to the side of the sputum carton.

4. In severe cases the breathing may be very distressed and cyanosis is present. In these severe attacks delirium may also occur.

5. When the doctor examines the chest with a stethoscope, typical alterations in the breath sounds over the consolidated lobe are heard which in conjunction with the above symptoms allow a ready diagnosis to be made. X-ray examination of the chest may be carried out to confirm the diagnosis and also to watch the resolution of the pneumonia. The solid lobe shows up on X-ray as a dense shadow.

Most cases respond rapidly to treatment with appropriate antibiotics. The temperature falls after a few days, the breathing becomes comfortable and the cough becomes productive of purulent sputum.

Patients who do not get better as expected may need a change of treatment because the infection is resistant to the antibiotic being used. Other complications may be present, particularly

(a) An empyema may have formed (see p. 173). This is a purulent effusion in the pleural cavity.

(b) There may be underlying lung cancer or pulmonary tuberculosis.

The diagnosis of lobar pneumonia is reached because of the clinical features and the appearance of the chest X-ray. The sputum is sent for culture so that the organism can be grown and its sensitivity determined to various antibiotics.

Treatment

1. The patient should be propped up in bed in a comfortable position and encouraged to cough up phlegm. When pleuritic pain makes breathing difficult diamorphine may be needed despite its property of depressing the respiratory centre.

2. The antibiotic most likely to be successful in pneumococcal pneumonia is penicillin and this can be given by injection. In less severe cases, ampicillin or amoxycillin may be prescribed in capsule form by mouth.

3. In the acute phase, if breathing is difficult and the patient cyanosed, oxygen may be helpful by oxygen mask. A nervous patient will need reassurance and explanation before the mask is applied.

4. Especially in elderly patients, the help of the physiotherapist

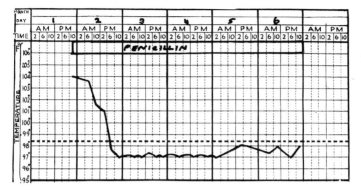

Fig. 6.10 Temperature chart from a case of lobar pneumonia showing the dramatic response to penicillin.

may be required in getting the patient to move the legs and to cough up phlegm.

Other forms of pneumonia have different characteristics according to the organism responsible for the infection.

Pneumonia due to Klebsiella bacillus tends to lead to abscess formation of the lung. It does not respond to penicillin but usually does so to gentamicin or co-trimoxazole.

Staphylococcal pneumonia sometimes follows a staphylococcal infection elsewhere in the body such as a carbuncle or osteomyelitis. It may complicate a severe attack of influenza. It may be resistant to penicillin and the choice of antibiotic may be decided by the sensitivity of the bacilli to various antibiotics after blood culture.

Pneumonia due to viruses and mycoplasma

This type of pneumonia varies considerably in severity.

The onset is usually characterised by constitutional symptoms such as general malaise, headache, sore throat, loss of appetite and temperature. These features may persist for several days before chest symptoms of cough, pleuritic pain and breathlessness become apparent. The temperature may be variable.

The diagnosis is usually made because of the typical signs and symptoms and because X-ray of the chest shows patchy shadows mostly in the lower lung fields. Confirmation can be obtained by blood tests for the presence of antibodies to particular viruses or to Mycoplasma.

Treatment

Mycoplasmal infections respond well to tetracycline or amoxycilline. Although virus infections are not sensitive to antibiotics, they are often prescribed partly because the diagnosis may be in doubt, and partly because virus pneumonias may be complicated by a bacterial infection as well.

Mycoplasma pneumonia tends to run a slow course even when treated, and both cough and X-ray shadows may persist for several weeks before complete resolution and recovery.

Secondary pneumonia

When pneumonia supervenes on a chronic chest disorder such as chronic bronchitis, emphysema or bronchiectasis, respiratory failure may ensue (see p. 163), requiring such treatment as a mechanical ventilator and oxygen.

Psittacosis (ornithosis)

This virus-type infection can be caught from parrots, canaries and budgerigars and can lead to a generalised patchy pneumonia. The onset is gradual with general malaise, a raised temperature, headache and cough. It can be diagnosed by testing the blood for antibodies and usually responds to treatment with tetracycline.

Q fever

An infection often present in animals such as sheep, cows and goats. Man becomes infected by drinking milk or inhaling dust containing the organism. It can cause pneumonia and sometimes affects the heart as well. The diagnosis is made by finding antibodies to the organism in the blood and treatment is tetracycline.

PLEURISY

The pleura is a membrane investing the lungs (the visceral pleura) and lining the inner side of the chest wall and diaphragm (the parietal pleura). Normally the visceral and parietal pleura are in smooth contact with each other, lubricated by a thin film of serous fluid. When the chest moves with respiration, this fluid prevents friction between the two layers of pleura.

Inflammation of the pleura (pleurisy) may cause friction or adhesions between the two layers. This is due to a bacterial or viral infection, and although this can occur on its own, pleurisy is commonly associated with pneumonia or with pulmonary tuberculosis.

Clinical features

1. The onset is often abrupt with raised temperature, headache and general malaise.

2. The breathing is rapid and shallow because deep inspiration leads to severe chest pain. This is due to stretching of the inflamed pleura. The patient may be in obvious distress and may grunt with each breath.

3. Coughing causes pain and so the cough is short and barking in character.

The diagnosis can be confirmed by hearing a pleural rub with the stethoscope. This is a grating sound heard over the chest and caused by friction between the inflamed layers of pleura.

Treatment

The treatment will depend on the cause. If it is bacterial, appropriate antibiotics may be prescribed. Analgesics may be necessary to relieve the discomfort. Codeine may suffice but if the pain is severe, pethidine or diamorphine may be advised though this has the danger of depressing respiration. Sometimes the application of heat in the form of a hot water bottle or poultice or electric heating pad offers comfort when placed on the chest.

Pleural effusion

Sometimes pleurisy may lead to a considerable increase of the fluid between the two layers of pleura. This pleural effusion may be large enough to compress the lung and cause embarrassment to the respiration. This can occur when pleurisy is associated with pneumonia and particularly when the pleurisy is due to pulmonary tuberculosis (see p. 175).

Carcinoma of the bronchus can invade the pleura and can cause a pleural effusion which is often bloodstained.

A pleural effusion can be part of general retention of fluid due to chronic nephritis, cirrhosis of the liver, or congestive heart failure. Oedema of the legs and ascites are also present.

Clinical features

A pleural effusion usually causes breathlessness on effort and if it is due to infection, there may be general features of a raised temperature and malaise as well.

When the chest is examined by the physician, on tapping with the finger the percussion note sounds dull instead of resonant. An X-ray of the chest will reveal the presence of fluid.

If the nature of the effusion is in doubt, aspiration of the fluid can be undertaken. A needle is inserted through the chest wall and some fluid is withdrawn for examination and culture in the laboratory.

Empyema

This term is used to describe a pleural effusion that has become infected and purulent. It is in fact a localised collection of pus in the pleural space and is most commonly associated with pneumococcal or staphylococcal pneumonia.

The empyema usually develops a week or two after the onset of pneumonia. As a rule, the patient has not been responding well to treatment. The temperature starts to rise again and the patient becomes more ill, with sweating and breathlessness. The diagnosis is suspected when the chest is examined. An X-ray confirms the presence of a pleural effusion. Aspiration must be undertaken by needling the chest and turbid purulent fluid will be withdrawn and sent for examination.

Treatment

Antibiotics must be given appropriate to the bacteria causing the infection, usually penicillin and flucloxacillin. In addition, antibiotics such as penicillin may be injected into the pleural cavity. It may be necessary to repeat the aspirations and pleural injections of penicillin on several occasions before the empyema subsides. In some cases where this treatment is not successful, surgical intervention may be necessary. Part of a rib is resected under anaesthetic, and a large tube inserted to allow drainage of the purulent material.

PNEUMOTHORAX

A small tear in the visceral pleura can allow air to escape from the alveoli into the pleural space. This is known as a pneumothorax. Sometimes, a flap is formed which allows air to enter the pleural cavity but prevents its escape. If the patient coughs a lot, more and more air is forced into the pleural space and the pressure increases. This is known as a tension pneumothorax and can cause considerable compression of the lung.

A pneumothorax can occur spontaneously in young people, probably due to the bursting of a small blister on the visceral pleura.

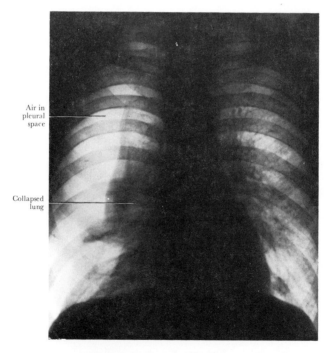

FIG. 6.11 X-ray of a case of spontaneous pneumothorax. The right lung is partially collapsed.

Pneumothorax can complicate an established chest disorder such as emphysema, asthma or pulmonary tuberculosis.

Clinical features

Sometimes the onset is marked by sudden pain in the chest and steadily increasing breathlessness. When there is a tension pneumothorax, the patient may be very breathless, cyanosed and distressed.

In many cases the only symptom is that of mild breathlessness on effort and there are no constitutional symptoms.

The diagnosis is usually suspected when the chest is examined by the physician and confirmed when a chest X-ray is taken. Air in the pleural space can be seen to compress the lung. The heart and the mediastinum may be pushed across (mediastinal shift) by the pressure of air in the pneumothorax.

Treatment

The patient is best supervised in bed in hospital, but in most cases where the symptoms are not severe, the pleural tear seals off on its own and the air is gradually absorbed through the pleura. The lung soon expands again and no further treatment is needed.

In cases of tension pneumothorax, diamorphine may be necessary to relieve pain and distress and a needle must be inserted into the pleural space to relieve the pressure by releasing the trapped air. The needle can be replaced by a catheter. This is connected to a rubber tube, the other end of which lies under water in a container to prevent air returning into the chest. When the patient coughs, air is expelled as bubbles into the water. In most cases, the pleural flap heals over after some days and the catheter can be withdrawn. The wound can be closed with a collodion dressing. Very occasionally surgical intervention is necessary to seal off the pleural tear when natural healing does not occur and the pneumothorax persists.

PULMONARY TUBERCULOSIS

Tuberculosis is the name given to the illness caused by infection with the tubercle bacillus (*Mycobacterium tuberculosis*).

There are two types of tubercle bacillus, the human and the bovine. Human tuberculosis is spread from person to person, mainly by droplet infection. Bovine tuberculosis occurs in cattle but can spread to man by drinking infected milk.

Tuberculosis can affect many parts of the body. The lungs are the organs most commonly involved, but tuberculosis can also affect the glands, the meninges, the bones, the kidneys and the joints.

Tuberculosis was a widespread disorder in the last century and was a prominent cause of death in children and young adults. There are many reasons why it is now comparatively uncommon:

1. Tuberculosis thrives when there is dirt, overcrowding, and malnourishment. Better sanitation and a better standard of living have contributed greatly to overcoming the spread of tuberculosis.

2. Tuberculosis used to affect cows and this led to milk infected

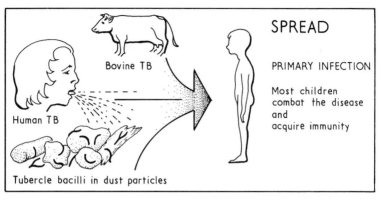

SPREAD

PRIMARY INFECTION

Most children combat the disease and acquire immunity

Bovine TB

Human TB

Tubercle bacilli in dust particles

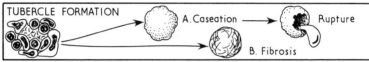

TUBERCLE FORMATION

A. Caseation → Rupture

B. Fibrosis

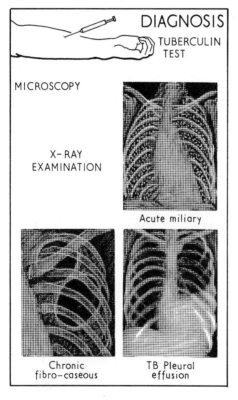

DIAGNOSIS

TUBERCULIN TEST

MICROSCOPY

X-RAY EXAMINATION

Acute miliary

Chronic fibro-caseous

TB Pleural effusion

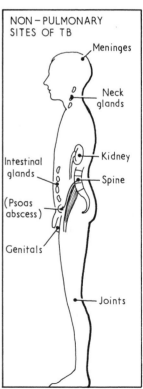

NON-PULMONARY SITES OF TB

Meninges

Neck glands

Kidney

Intestinal glands

Spine

(Psoas abscess)

Genitals

Joints

FIG. 6.12 Tuberculosis.

with bovine tuberculosis. Today, all dairy herds in Britain are free from tuberculosis and pasteurisation of milk (heating to a temperature lethal to bacteria) provides an additional safeguard.

3. Easy availability of chest X-rays uncovers cases of unsuspected pulmonary tuberculosis. Routine chest X-rays are usually taken (a) in those most likely to acquire tuberculosis, such as certain immigrant groups or those living in lodging houses, (b) in those most exposed to the disease such as nurses and hospital workers, and (c) those likely to spread the ailment such as schoolteachers or waiters.

4. Immunisation by B.C.G. vaccine protects against tuberculosis.

5. Effective chemotherapy is available for patients who have contracted pulmonary tuberculosis.

Pathology

The tubercle bacillus is known as an *acid-fast* bacillus. When specimens of sputum or other material are stained with dyes to show up bacteria under the microscope, unlike most bacilli, the tubercle bacilli do not lose colour when acid is added. This is a valuable method of identification.

The tubercle bacillus is so-called because it leads to the formation of a small rounded area or *tubercle*.

Tubercle formation

The tubercle is a collection of small *endothelial cells* and *lymphocytes* around the bacilli. 'Giant' cells typical of tuberculosis occur. These tubercles can gather together so that a wide area of tissue may be affected, and this process may then be followed by caseation and fibrosis.

CASEATION

This is a breaking down, or necrosis, of the tubercles into a soft cheesy mass which may liquefy to form tuberculous pus. What happens next depends on where the lesion is: e.g., if it is in the lungs it can rupture into a bronchus and leave behind a cavity; if in a lymph gland it can produce ulceration with discharge of tuberculous pus, forming a sinus.

FIBROSIS

Active fibrous-tissue formation can occur around the tubercles. The fibrous tissue constitutes an attempt by the body to wall off the infection and heal the lesion by scar-tissue formation.

In most cases caseation and fibrosis are present together. Marked caseation and slight fibrosis are evidence of severe infection and little effort on the part of the body to heal. Alternatively, when fibrosis is marked, then the disease is usually arrested or limited. Sometimes calcium is deposited in the caseated mass, and this calcified lesion is also usually arrested or healed.

The commonest entry of tubercle bacilli is by inhalation. When sputum is expectorated from someone with pulmonary tuberculosis,

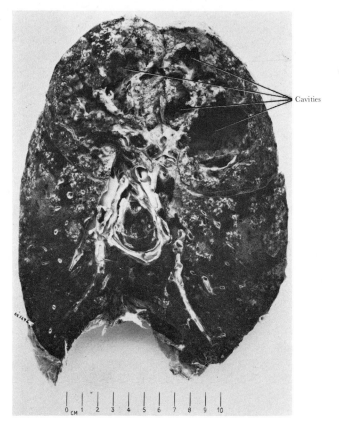

Cavities

FIG. 6.13   Advanced fibrocaseous tuberculosis of the lung showing large ragged cavities in the apex of the lung.

the tubercle bacilli can survive for many months. Infection can occur by inhaling dust which contains the bacilli or by direct droplet infection. The respiratory tract can be affected in different ways:

1. Pulmonary tuberculosis. The upper lobes of the lungs are particularly liable to be involved with infiltration and spread of the disorder to other parts of the lung. Caseation may occur with formation of cavities.

2. Infection of the pleura leads to pleurisy and pleural effusion.

3. Miliary tuberculosis. The bacteria invade the blood stream and small tubercles appear throughout the lungs and many other organs as well, especially the liver.

Primary tuberculosis

Many children or young adults are infected with tubercle bacilli without any symptoms or obvious illness. There is normally only a small area of lung or pleura involved, with enlargement of hilar glands. Healing occurs in most cases without trouble, often followed by calcification. Hence it is not uncommon in routine chest X-rays of the healthy population to find evidence of a healed primary infection in the form of a calcified focus. Further evidence that there has been a previous primary infection with tuberculosis is provided by the *tuberculin test* (Mantoux reaction).

Tuberculin is a purified protein derived from tubercle bacilli and available in different strengths. Tuberculin is injected under the skin starting with a low strength. In those who have previously been infected, a red raised area appears at the site of the injection: these subjects are designated *tuberculin positive*. Those who do not react in this way are *tuberculin negative*.

Routine tuberculin testing of schoolchildren aged about 13 shows about one in ten to be tuberculin positive. If they have X-ray evidence of lung involvement, they may need active treatment with chemotherapy.

In children who are tuberculin negative, B.C.G. vaccination is undertaken.

B.C.G. vaccination

B.C.G. (Bacillus Calmette-Guérin) is an inactivated harmless bacillus which resembles the tubercle bacillus. When B.C.G. is inoculated it gives rise to antibody formation and so protects against tuberculosis for at least 15 years.

B.C.G. is given routinely with parental consent to tuberculin-negative schoolchildren aged 13 to 15; and to those who are tuberculin negative and at special risk, for example nurses and doctors working in chest units.

Post-primary pulmonary tuberculosis

This is a progressive tuberculous involvement of the lungs, sometimes occurring many years after the primary infection. It may present in a variety of ways.

1. Clinical features of a constitutional disorder with loss of weight, loss of appetite, malaise, low grade fever, night sweats and fatigue.

2. A persistent cough, usually attributed to cigarettes, may be the first symptom of pulmonary tuberculosis.

3. Haemoptysis. There may be blood-stained sputum or the sudden coughing up of bright red blood. When an erosion of an artery in a cavity occurs, the haemoptysis may be profuse and recurrent.

4. Patients who present with pneumonia but fail to respond completely to antibiotics may have underlying chronic pulmonary tuberculosis.

5. Routine chest X-rays frequently reveal the presence of unexpected pulmonary tuberculosis. It is for this reason that a chest

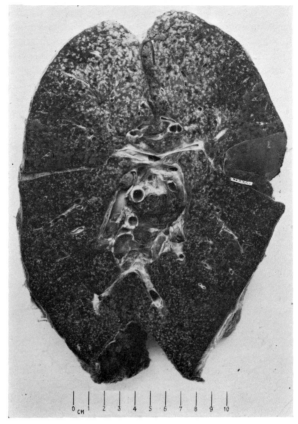

Fig. 6.14. Acute miliary tuberculosis of the lungs showing the tubercles, characteristically small and evenly disseminated throughout the lung.

X-ray is always taken in anybody who has lost weight for no known reason or has shown deterioration in general health.

Pleural effusion due to tuberculosis usually comes after the primary infection in young people. The early symptoms include:

(i) Chest pain made worse by coughing or deep breathing,
(ii) General malaise and a raised temperature,
(iii) Increasing breathlessness.

Miliary tuberculosis

This is due to widespread dissemination of small tubercles through the blood stream. The onset is usually insidious with lassitude, pyrexia, sweats and loss of weight. Headaches and drowsiness may occur if meningitis supervenes.

Diagnosis of pulmonary tuberculosis

X-ray of the chest usually provides intimation of the diagnosis but this can only be confirmed by the finding of acid-fast bacilli in the sputum. Patients must be encouraged to cough up their sputum into a disposable carton and this is then taken to the laborary for special staining (Ziehl-Neelsen technique) and examination under the microscope. The sputum will also be cultured for growth of the bacilli.

When it is not possible to obtain sputum because the patient swallows it, a gastric washing should be obtained. This is best obtained in the early morning. A Ryle's tube is passed through the nose or mouth into the stomach, 10 ml of saline is injected through the tube with a syringe and all the stomach fluid withdrawn for transmission to the laboratory.

Investigation of a pleural effusion requires aspiration of the chest and a pleural biopsy. The simplest apparatus for aspiration is a syringe with a twoway tap, one way allowing fluid to be sucked into the syringe from the chest and the other allowing the fluid to be ejected from the syringe into a bottle. The fluid is sent to the laboratory for examination of white cells (in tuberculosis they are

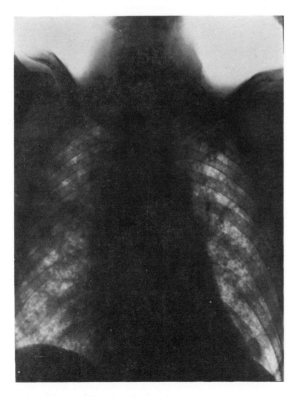

FIG. 6.15   X-ray of acute miliary tuberculosis of the lungs showing the typical fine mottling—'snowstorm' appearance.

mainly lymphocytes) and for culture to grow and identify the tubercle bacilli. A biopsy of the pleura can be obtained by the insertion of a special needle into the chest which cuts off a small piece of pleura when it is being withdrawn. The pleura examined under the microscope may show inflammatory cells characteristic of a tuberculous infection.

The tuberculin test may be used as a confirmatory test in doubtful cases since it will be strongly positive in the presence of active tuberculosis. If the test is negative, it makes the diagnosis unlikely.

Management of tuberculosis

Chemotherapy successfully cures pulmonary tuberculosis and hospital treatment is usually only advised for the first week or so to make sure the patient understands fully the details of the treatment and how and when to take the appropriate drugs. Hospital in-patient treatment is also advised—

(i) In all patients with miliary tuberculosis or pleural effusion until recovery is complete.

(ii) In ill, poorly nourished or elderly patients requiring rest and general care.

(iii) Patients with infected sputum, especially if they have children in the family at home.

(iv) Unco-operative patients with a bad social background, perhaps living in a hostel or with a history of alcoholism.

(v) Patients who have developed side effects with the drug treatment.

CHEMOTHERAPY

Since the tubercle bacillus develops resistance to most of the antituberculous drugs given on their own, at least two drugs must be given together. In the initial treatment, triple therapy (three drugs together) is prescribed. Four drugs are in common use:

1. Isoniazid. This drug is safe, effective and inexpensive. It seldom gives rise to toxic effects. Its disadvantage is that in some cases the tubercle bacille become resistant to it. It is usually given as a single dose of 300 mg each day.

2. Rifampicin. This antibiotic is bactericidal for the tubercle bacilli but can have toxic effects on the liver. If given alone, it can lose its effect after a time because the bacilli become resistant to its action. It is expensive. It should be given as a single dose of about 450 mg each morning on an empty stomach.

3. Ethambutol. This is usually given with the other two drugs as initial treatment as a single morning dose of about 800 mg each morning.

4. Streptomycin has to be given by injection and can have toxic effects on the vestibular system, causing vertigo and deafness if given to excess.

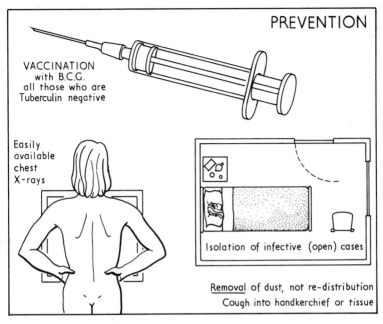

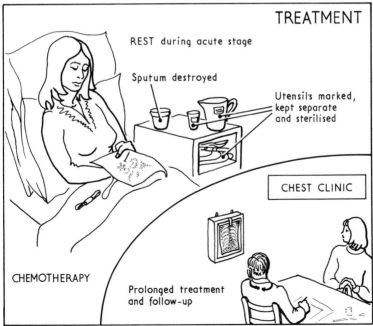

FIG. 6.16   Pulmonary tuberculosis.

THE GUIDING PRINCIPLES OF TREATMENT

1. The nature of the ailment must be explained to the patient so that his full co-operation is obtained. A successful cure depends on the patient following the treatment and attending regularly, usually at a chest clinic, for supervision and advice.

2. Treatment begins with three drugs, usually isoniazid, rifampicin and ethambutol, all given each morning as a single dose and maintained for about 2 months.

3. Treatment is then maintained with two drugs, isoniazid and rifampicin, for a further 7 months, making 9 months continuous daily treatment in all.

4. Long-term supervision, perhaps annually, is sometimes advised by the chest clinic to make sure there is no relapse.

Social aspects

Tuberculosis is a notifiable disease. Once notification has been made:

(a) Examination is made of those who have been in contact with the patient at home and at work. This may necessitate doing a tuberculin reaction and a chest X-ray.

(b) The health visitor will be informed and may visit the patient's home to see if help is needed and if the diet is adequate.

(c) Housing and sanitation facilities will be inspected.

(d) Special financial grants are available to help the patient find more suitable employment if that is necessary.

SARCOIDOSIS

Sarcoidosis is a disease which resembles tuberculosis but usually is not so serious and tends to get better without treatment. The tuberculin test is negative unless as sometimes happens tuberculosis itself supervenes. It tends to affect adults between the ages of 20 and 40.

Many organs may be affected and infiltrated by sarcoid, which under the microscope resembles tubercles but no bacilli are seen. The lungs, lymph glands and skin are frequently involved.

Lungs. The commonest symptoms are breathlessness and cough. X-ray shows a diffuse mottling of the lungs, resembling miliary tuberculosis. The condition usually improves over several months, but sometimes cortisone (or some other steroid) is necessary when progress is slow.

Skin. Pinkish nodules may appear on the face and chest. Apart from this, erythema nodosum is a common manifestation of sarcoidosis. Raised red painful areas appear on the shins and sometimes on the forearms; these may persist for several weeks before subsiding, and are sometimes associated with pyrexia and malaise (p. 492).

Glands. Enlargement of the lymph nodes in the neck and in the mediastinum may occur but, unlike tuberculosis, these glands do not suppurate.

Inflammation of the eyes (iritis) and of the salivary glands may also occur. The bones may be affected and so excess calcium appears in the urine.

Course and treatment

The disease runs a variable course, but after many months or even years the majority of patients show spontaneous recovery Steroids may be helpful in stubborn cases, and where tuberculosis occurs specific treatment, as mentioned earlier, must be used.

PULMONARY FIBROSIS AND PNEUMOCONIOSIS

Fibrosis of the lungs, like fibrosis in any tissue or organ, is a response to injury and is the predominant change occurring in chronic inflammations. Fibrosis of the lungs is seen in many chronic inflammatory chest diseases, especially in tuberculosis (fibrocaseous type) and bronchiectasis. In addition there is one other disease where fibrosis is the predominant change present in the lungs. This is called pneumoconiosis or dust disease of the lungs. Prolonged exposure to certain irritating dusts causes irritation of the lungs from constant inhaling of the fine particles of dust. The result is a dense diffuse fibrosis throughout the lungs.

The people who may develop pneumoconiosis are:

1. Anthracite coal miners (anthracosis).
2. Stone workers, gold miners and potters (silicosis).
3. Steel workers; tin, lead and iron miners (siderosis).
4. Asbestos workers (asbestosis).

In all these occupations there is a very definite liability to develop dust disease of the lungs. This causes gradually increasing dyspnoea with chronic cough and sputum. X-ray examination of the lungs reveals a typical picture of diffuse fine mottling. In many cases pulmonary tuberculosis may supervene, and this possibility presents a danger to all workers in dust occupations.

Treatment

Prophylactic measures to render the dust as harmless as possible are most important. Moistening the atmosphere with sprays, and full ventilation, with fans if necessary, are most valuable. Respirators should be worn wherever practicable.

Once the condition has arisen the patient must change his occupation or else the disease will progress, with a great risk of tuberculosis or bronchiectasis, and eventual heart failure.

ASTHMA

Asthma is a disorder characterised by attacks of wheezing and difficulty in breathing, and due to reversible narrowing of the airways. This restriction of the airway is not permanent and is due to:

(a) Bronchospasm. This is spasm due to tightening of the constricting muscles of the smaller bronchi.

(b) Congestion and thickening of the lining of the bronchial tree.

(c) Accumulation of mucus and phlegm in the smaller bronchi.

There are many factors which can cause or precipitate an attack of asthma.

HEREDITY. Especially in childhood, asthma is likely to be associated with other allergic disorders such as hay fever or urticaria. Allergic susceptibility commonly occurs in more than one member of the family, suggesting an hereditary tendency.

ALLERGY means an excessive reaction to certain environmental substances. These include pollen, plant spores, moulds, animal hairs, house dust containing mites and even certain foods. When these are inhaled by sensitive subjects, they cause spasm and swelling of the smaller bronchi.

EMOTION. Anxiety, anger, frustration and fear can all provoke an attack of asthma in those disposed to the ailment. Sometimes fear of an attack will actually precipitate one at a most unfortunate time, before an important interview or a long-awaited social event.

INFECTION. Any upper respiratory tract infection, even a heavy cold, can set off an attack in an asthmatic subject.

OTHER FACTORS may dispose to attacks in some asthmatics. These include sudden exposure to cold air: undue physical exercise: eating foods such as shellfish, chocolates or eggs: and taking certain drugs such as beta-blockers or aspirin.

UNKNOWN FACTORS. Asthma can begin later on in life and is sometimes called intrinsic asthma. In these cases, allergy does not seem to be responsible and no reason can be found for the attacks.

Clinical features

An attack of asthma usually begins fairly suddenly with wheezy respiration and a sense of tightness in the chest. When the attack is mild, the subject can usually manage to keep going, though with difficulty. When the attack is more severe, unless there is recourse to treatment, rest is essential. The duration of the attacks vary considerably, usually for a few hours.

As a rule, when asthma occurs in childhood the attacks get less frequent as the child gets older. But this is by no means always so. In some, the attacks may be frequent and some wheeziness on expiration is present all the time.

Status asthmaticus

This is the term used to describe a severe and persistent attack of asthma sometimes continuing for many hours or even days. The patient becomes exhausted and demoralised due to lack of sleep and the physical effort of breathing. There is often a cough productive of sticky mucoid phlegm. A patient admitted to hospital in status asthmaticus is cyanosed and sweating with a rapid pulse rate and sometimes a low blood pressure. This can lead to mental confusion due to lack of oxygen or even to coma with a fatal outcome.

Management of asthma

1. *Preventative measures*

ALLERGY. Careful questioning of the patient is the best way of finding out what factors bring on attacks and consequently how to avoid them. For example, if attacks occur in the spring or early summer it is likely that pollen is responsible. If they come on at night on going to bed, it might be house dust or a feather pillow. Questions should be answered from a prepared list about food, drugs, household pets and other possible provocative agents.

Skin tests seldom do more than confirm the significance of the possible factors involved. A drop each of various solutions containing the suspected provocative factor (allergen) is placed on the skin and a superficial scratch made through it. A raised wheal appears within 15 minutes if the subject is sensitive to the particular allergen.

Sometimes the asthmatic subject can avoid substances known to provoke the attacks, for example, foods, drugs, dogs or cats. Feather pillows can be changed for sorbo rubber. The bedroom should be kept clear of dust by repeated vacuum cleaning. In some cases where pollens are responsible, a course of desensitisation can be undertaken. A small amount of the allergen is injected subcutaneously and the dose increased by injections given week by week. In this way, the patient gradually builds up a resistance to the effects of the allergen, a process known as *desensitisation*.

INFECTIONS. Asthmatics should be started on an antibiotic as soon as there is evidence of an upper respiratory tract infection. If the infection is allowed to persist it may provoke an asthmatic attack.

EMOTION. Since emotional factors can precipitate asthma, the social and psychological background of the patient must be considered and discussed. The attitude of the patient to his family and his work may reveal difficulties which can be helped by discussion. Occasionally the advice of a psychiatrist may be necessary, and sometimes hypnosis has been used to give an asthmatic sufferer more confidence.

DRUGS. Cromoglycate is a drug which prevents the lining of the bronchi from reacting to allergens. To be effective it must be taken up to four times a day in the form of a powder inhalation from a special inhaler. It is not meant for treatment of an attack of asthma. It is of most use when used by patients sensitive to pollen in the months when the pollen count is likely to be rising.

2. *Treatment for attacks of asthma*

Bronchodilators are drugs which relieve bronchial spasm and are effectively given in the form of inhalers. Salbutamol (Ventolin) is supplied by a pressurised aerosol: after breathing out completely, the vapour is inhaled from the aerosol and the breath held for a moment to allow full absorption to take place. This leads to quick relief of wheeziness, but the benefits do not last long. The inhaler can be applied four times a day.

Steroid inhalations relieve the congestion of the bronchial mucosa (lining) and have a longer effect than the bronchodilators. Given in the form of aerosols containing beclamethasone (Becotide) or beta-methasone (Bextasol) they act only on the bronchi and do not have the disadvantages of cortisone given by mouth or injection (see p. 455).

A useful routine for patients with repeated mild attacks of asthma is to use the salbutamol inhaler first and when the breathing is easier, to follow this with the steroid inhalation. This allows good bronchial penetration by the steroid and keeps the breathing free for a longer time.

In mild cases, various bronchodilators, including salbutamol or orciprenaline, may be taken in the form of tablets by mouth.

Isoprenaline inhalers are effective bronchodilators but can cause tachycardia: they are no longer recommended for repeated use.

Because of the long-term effects of steroids given by mouth (see p. 458), prednisolone or other preparations of the cortisone group are only prescribed for asthma when other remedies have been proved ineffective.

3. Treatment of status asthmaticus

Status asthmaticus is an emergency and requires constant super-vision sometimes in an intensive care unit.

(a) Steroids are life-saving and should be given in adequate dosage from the moment it is clear that previous remedies have been ineffective. Steroids can be given as prednisolone by mouth, 15 mg every 6 hours initially. If the patient is too ill to take drugs by mouth, hydrocortisone 100 mg can be given intravenously.

(b) Aminophylline 250 mg may be given slowly by intravenous injections as initial treatment and gives quick relief: but the effect does not last long.

(c) Oxygen may be given by nasal catheter. In cases where cyanosis is severe and the patient confused or comatose, it may be necessary to pass a cuffed endotracheal tube and apply intermittent positive pressure ventilation (IPPV) (see p. 163). The best guide in this respect is estimation of the blood gases (P_{CO_2} and P_{O_2}).

(d) Since status asthmaticus is often precipitated by respiratory infections, antibiotics such as amoxycillin are often necessary.

(e) In no condition is good nursing care more important. Patients in status asthmaticus are frightened and exhaused and nurse can do much to give reassurance and emotional support as well as see to the physical comforts. It is important to make sure that an adequate intake of fluid is maintained and the patient is encouraged to take a light diet.

CARCINOMA OF THE BRONCHUS

Lung cancer (carcinoma of the bronchus) is now the commonest form of malignant growth in Great Britain. It is commoner in men than women and is the cause of nearly half the deaths from cancer in males. The evidence that cigarette smoking is responsible for the great increase in lung cancer is incontrovertible and indeed it has been estimated that 90 per cent of deaths from lung cancer in men result from cigarette smoking. Cigarette smokers are much more affected than pipe or cigar smokers. Those who give up cigarette smoking have lower death rates than those who continue to smoke, so that if the habit ceased the number of deaths caused by lung cancer would fall steeply in the course of time.

Pathology

Lung cancer can affect the body in three ways: by invasion of local tissues, by secondary deposits and by constitutional effects.

1. Local invasion. Bronchial carcinoma begins in the epithelial cells lining the bronchus. It invades the bronchial wall and spreads into the lung. In so doing, it may cause ulceration and bleeding from the bronchus or it may obstruct the bronchus and lead to collapse (atelactasis) of the lung (see p. 193). Infection may follow, causing pneumonia or lung abscess. Spread of the malignant cells by the lymphatic system causes the glands to enlarge.

2. Malignant cells from the growth may enter the blood stream and form metastases (secondary deposits) in other organs such as the bones, the liver or the brain. These metastases may grow themselves and invade other tissues as well.

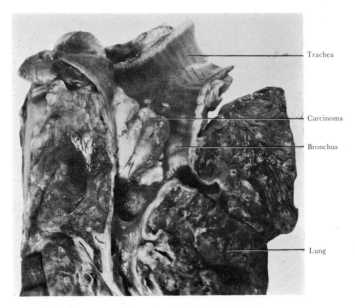

Trachea

Carcinoma

Bronchus

Lung

FIG. 6.17   Section of a lung showing a large carcinomatous growth in the bronchus of the lung just below the bifurcation of the trachea.

3. Constitutional symptoms are caused by the production of toxins and hormones by the growth. These lead to general metabolic changes and to damage of the nervous system. Production of excess hormones may lead to such disorders as Cushing's syndrome.

Clinical features

LOCAL

1. Bronchial carcinoma does not give rise to symptoms in the early stages so that the growth has normally been present for a year or more before advice is sought.

2. A cough is the commonest presenting symptom, at first ascribed to a smoker's cough. The cough becomes more persistent and is productive of purulent sputum.

3. Haemoptysis occurs sooner or later in most patients. Usually the sputum is blood-stained or contains small blobs of blood. Coughing up of free red blood is less common.

4. Shortness of breath is a prominent feature, usually associated with a productive cough. The dyspnoea can become severe when there is added infection (pneumonia) or lung collapse (atelectasis).

5. Chest pain may be caused by pleurisy or by the growth invading the ribs or the intercostal nerves. Thus the pain may be worse on breathing, or it may be persistent and gnawing, depending on the cause.

6. Wheeziness may be present due to bronchial obstruction.

7. Hoarseness of the voice may be due to pressure on the recurrent laryngeal nerve which controls the vocal cords.

METASTASES

1. Metastases in the brain may cause headaches, epileptic fits, hemiplegia or unsteadiness of gait and these may be the presenting features of a lung cancer.

2. Secondaries in the bones can lead to unexpected fractures (pathological fractures) or can be a source of unremitting pain.

3. Metastases in the liver causes enlargement of the liver and sometimes jaundice and ascites.

4. Enlargement of the glands are often painless but may lead to the diagnosis.

CONSTITUTIONAL

1. Even a small bronchial carcinoma may be associated with malaise, loss of appetite and loss of weight.

2. Clubbing of the fingers is often present and may be a clue to the diagnosis, though this occurs in other chest disorders as well, particularly bronchiectasis. The nails are curved and there is a bulbous increase in the pulp at the end of the fingers.

3. Involvement of the nervous system is common, not due to metastases but perhaps caused by a toxin from the carcinoma. It

can lead to mental confusion, peripheral neuritis and unsteadiness of movement (ataxia).

4. Endocrine disorders. Sometimes excess hormones are produced by bronchial carcinoma. Excess ACTH can cause Cushing's syndrome (see p. 450) or excess parathyroid hormone (see p. 452) can lead to hyperparathyroidism.

5. Thromboses of the veins are liable to occur with bronchial carcinoma and can cause pulmonary emboli.

Diagnosis

Loss of weight and energy, particularly if associated with cough and sputum, must always arouse suspicion of lung cancer, particularly in cigarette smokers. Examination of the chest and the presence of enlarged glands or clubbing of the fingers may reveal further evidence.

X-ray of the chest provides the diagnosis in most cases. A shadow

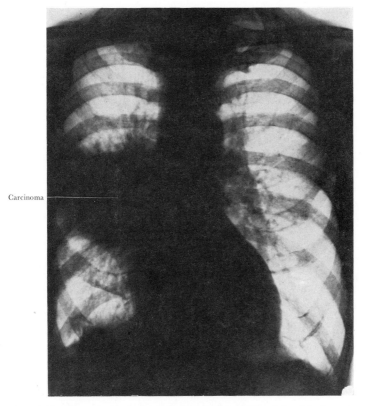

Fig. 6.18   X-ray showing a large shadow in the middle of the right lung due to a carcinoma.

in the lung associated with enlargement of the hilar glands suggest a bronchial carcinoma with lymphatic spread to the glands. Tomography (X-rays focused on one plane) may give a clearer idea of the extent of the growth.

Examination of the sputum under the microscope may reveal the presence of malignant cells, thus confirming the diagnosis. Sometimes the aid of the physiotherapist is needed to help the patient cough up a suitable specimen.

Bronchoscopy. The bronchoscope is a lighted metal tube which can be passed into the trachea and bronchi and allows inspection of the main air passages. Snippets of tissue (biopsy) can be removed from suspicious areas and examined after suitable staining under the microscope. The fibroptic bronchoscope is of smaller bore and more flexible than the fixed tube and allows inspection of the minor bronchi.

Bronchoscopy is performed in the theatre. A tablet is sucked beforehand to anaesthetise the mouth and pharynx, and the larynx is anaesthetised by spray in the theatre. As the bronchoscope is passed, the patient's neck is extended and the head is flexed and suitably supported.

When the X-ray shadow lies in the outer part of the lung it may be inaccessible to bronchoscopy. A needle biopsy may then be performed. The needle is inserted through the chest wall under X-ray guidance and a small tissue biopsy removed from the area involved. The biopsy is stained and examined under the microscope.

Treatment

1. Surgical resection of the tumour is the best treatment, usually pneumonectomy (removal of an entire lung) or lobectomy (removal of a lobe). Unfortunately this is seldom possible because at the time of diagnosis the tumour has already spread to the glands or has formed metastases. Surgical resection offers hope of survival and activity for a few years. Without operation, the average survival of bronchial carinoma at diagnosis is less than a year.

2. Radiotherapy is best used for relief of symptoms such as chest pain. A short course of irradiation may relieve the pain of rib metastases or cause to regress large glands which obstruct breathing.

3. Cytotoxic drugs. These drugs include intravenous nitrogen mustard and oral cyclophosphamide. They act by interfering with the growth processes of malignant cells without affecting healthy tissue. Unfortunately the results with lung cancer are disappointing though they sometimes cause the growth to shrink with easing of bronchial pressure.

4. In many cases, symptomatic treatment and relief of pain is all that can be achieved. A knowledge of the patient and his family background will help to decide whether he is better at home or in hospital for the terminal phase.

Prevention

Bronchial carcinoma is a distressing disorder with a bad prognosis. Since it is largely caused by cigarette smoking, nurses and doctors should do all they can to discourage this dangerous habit. All health workers should themselves set an example by not smoking and should encourage patients and their families to stop smoking. In particular, young people should be discouraged from starting the habit. Smoking advisory clinics are available to help people give up cigarettes if they lack willpower to do so on their own.

ATELECTASIS (Collapse of the lung)

Collapse of the lung is not a primary disease in itself, but is caused by any disease or condition which obstructs the bronchi or interferes with the respirations. Either blockage of a bronchus or interference with the expansion of the lungs in the respiratory movement causes the affected lung or parts of the lung to collapse into a solid airless condition. This interferes with the normal respirations and causes varying degrees of distress according to the extent of the collapsed lung area.

Causes

1. Most commonly, pulmonary collapse calling for immediate treatment is seen post-operatively. Here, sedation due to the anaesthetic depresses the cough reflex and allows thick mucus to collect, which then obstructs the bronchi, causing varying degrees of collapse. Infection of the bronchi which causes excessive mucus increases this likelihood of post-operative pulmonary atelectasis.

2. Pulmonary collapse is also always a constant danger in prolonged coma and, as in post-operative collapse, calls for energetic measures in prevention and treatment.

3. Carcinoma of the bronchus commonly causes atelectasis.

4. A foreign body lodging in a bronchus.

5. Paralysis of the respiratory muscles, as seen in poliomyelitis and diphtheritic paralysis, can cause pulmonary collapse, but this form calls for specialised treatment, usually in an artificial breathing apparatus, and is discussed under the individual diseases.

6. Again, it should be remembered that any fluid or air accumulating in the pleural cavity can cause collapse of the lung by pressure from outside.

Symptoms and signs

Most of the diseases causing pulmonary collapse are discussed under the individual headings, so only the very common form occurring post-operatively calls for special mention here.

After operation the patient is often described as being 'chesty', with a cough, pain in the chest and difficulty in breathing. If the collapse is extensive, the dyspnoea is more severe; it causes distress to the patient and is accompanied by cyanosis. In most cases a fever is present. Examination of the chest reveals the presence and extent of the atelectasis, and this is usually confirmed by an X-ray of the chest.

Treatment

PREVENTION

This is by far the most important part of the treatment. Any evidence of chest infection will naturally call for a postponement of the operation, if at all possible. Pre-operative breathing exercises in all patients subject to chest trouble are most valuable.

Routine encouragement of all post-operative patients to breathe deeply will reduce the incidence of atelectasis appreciably. In this connection also, early movement, frequent change of posture and getting the patient up as soon as possible are important. Analgesics may be prescribed to ease pain which otherwise might restrict mobility.

Tight bandaging coming up over the lower ribs is a very common cause of post-operative pulmonary collapse, and the nurse should be particularly careful to see that any bandaging does not interfere with the respiratory movements. This is of especial importance in all upper abdominal operations.

TREATMENT OF ACTUAL COLLAPSE

Deep breathing and coughing exercises every hour for a few minutes are very useful. Inhalations of oxygen are useful especially if dyspnoea or cyanosis is present. Postural drainage, by tipping the patient so that the collapsed area (usually the base of the lung) is uppermost, often dislodges a thick plug of mucus and expands the lung. This procedure is possible only in some cases, depending on the severity of the operation and the general condition of the patient. It is, however, a very useful and most effective measure whenever it can be applied. Chest percussion (or clapping) by a skilled physiotherapist is often combined with postural drainage.

Blow-bottles, or blowing up toy balloons in the case of children, also help to expand the lung and are often used in conjunction with deep breathing exercises.

If all the above measures fail to re-expand the affected area, then one of the several methods of aspiration of the bronchial tree will be necessary. Passing a firm rubber catheter through the nose and into the trachea allows suction to be applied and so dislodges the thick mucus. Even if the tube cannot be passed into the bronchi, bouts of coughing occur which may be sufficient to bring up the plugs of mucus. If the above measures fail and the collapse is severe, causing acute distress and continued cyanosis, bronchoscopy will enable the obstructing mucus to be aspirated.

PULMONARY EMBOLISM (Pulmonary infarction)

Pulmonary embolism is a most important condition, especially from a nurse's point of view, as preventive measures play a large part in minimising the frequency of the disease.

Pulmonary embolism is caused by a clot detaching itself in some part of the venous circulation, travelling in the veins, and lodging in the pulmonary artery or one of its branches. With the obstruction to the pulmonary circulation so produced, infarction of the lung or part of the lung, depending on the site of the lodgment of the embolus, occurs.

Causes

1. Venous thrombosis, especially in the large deep veins of the lower limbs and pelvis. Thrombosis in a vein occurs in several circumstances, e.g. in elderly people with slow circulation, particularly with heart failure. Prolonged rest in bed owing to a major illness or operation is also a very frequent cause.

2. Trauma to the large veins, especially in the lower abdomen during operations in this area, predispose to thrombus formation.

3. In the puerperium a venous thrombosis is often seen—'white leg of pregnancy'.

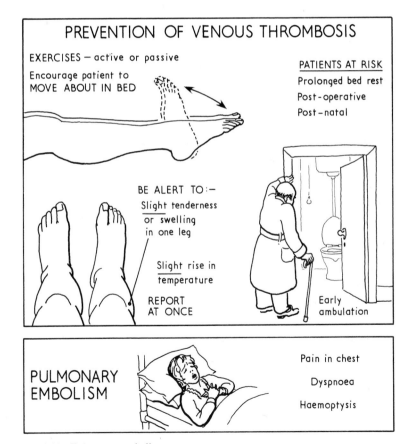

FIG. 6.19   Pulmonary embolism.

4. The contraceptive pill, probably due to its oestrogen content, disposes to venous thromboses.

5. In congestive heart failure a thrombus may form not only in one of the veins but also in the right side of the heart. This is particularly likely in heart failure associated with atrial fibrillation.

It is from thrombosis in the deep veins, particularly the calf and pelvic veins, that embolism is most likely to arise. Thrombophlebitis of the superficial veins is much less dangerous.

Symptoms and signs

The usual history and course of events is as follows: the patient may have recently undergone an operation and appear to be progressing satisfactorily, or may have had a severe illness and been confined to bed for some time. In these patients there may be evidence of a venous thrombosis in a lower limb, with swelling, tenderness and slight pain in the affected leg. On the other hand there may be no such signs, or the signs may be so slight that they have escaped notice. A low-grade fever with no obvious cause is, however, often present in deep venous thrombosis and so should be viewed with great suspicion. Suddenly the patient may collapse with cyanosis and gasping respirations and die within a few minutes. Here a large embolus, sufficient to block the main pulmonary artery and so the whole pulmonary circulation, is present.

In other cases the embolus is somewhat smaller and produces severe dyspnoea, cyanosis and great distress. Pain in the chest is common, and later a cough with frank haemoptysis develops.

In some cases, multiple small emboli reach the lung and give rise to breathlessness on effort without obvious pain or haemoptysis.

Treatment of pulmonary embolism

PROPHYLACTIC

Any measures which will avoid or minimise the risk of a venous thrombosis are very valuable. Early movement of the legs in postoperative patients and early ambulation are most important. In any long-standing or severe illness, especially in elderly people, passive and active movements of the legs must be undertaken early. The nurse should look upon this as every bit as much a part of the routine as, say, washing the patient. Of course, if there is any contraindication to movement of the limb, such as a fracture or a wound, this must be taken into consideration.

If there are signs of venous thrombosis, such as pain, tenderness, or swelling of the leg, then anticoagulant therapy with heparin and phenindione (Dindevan) is usually given. This is to prevent further spread of the thrombosis and so lessen the risk and severity of pulmonary embolism. It is important to stress that the signs of a deep venous thrombosis may be very slight, and that particular notice must therefore be taken of slight pain or tenderness in the calf, where a thrombus is especially likely to occur. This slight pain or tenderness accompanied by a low-grade fever is of particular importance, as already noted.

WHEN EMBOLISM HAS OCCURRED

A large embolus may result in sudden death. In other cases, oxygen to relieve the cyanosis and dyspnoea is of great value. Sedatives are usually needed for the pain and also to allay the acute anxiety and shock present. Pethidine or morphine are usually given. Anticoagulant drugs, such as phenindione (Dindevan), are generally given to prevent further emboli.

HAEMOPTYSIS

Haemoptysis means coughing blood, and in discussing the various diseases of the lungs it has been seen that haemoptysis is a common occurrence. Haemoptysis may be slight, so that the sputum is streaked with blood, or profuse, when several pints of pure blood are brought up.

Causes

1. *Pulmonary tuberculosis*. This used to be the commonest cause of haemoptysis, particularly in younger people. Most cases of haemoptysis are looked upon as being due to tuberculosis unless and until further investigation establishes a different cause.

2. *Congestion of the lungs* as seen in congestive heart failure, particularly in cases of mitral stenosis.

3. *Carcinoma of the bronchus*. This is the most frequent cause of haemoptysis in older people.

4. *Bronchiectasis*.

5. Certain acute chest diseases like *pneumonia* (rusty sputum) and *pulmonary embolism*.

Diagnosis

Haemoptysis has to be distinguished from haematemesis, which is the vomiting of blood. Many patients find it difficult to be sure whether they actually cough or vomit the blood. Table VI is of help in distinguishing between the two.

If the exact diagnosis, including the exact cause of the haemoptysis, is not obvious from the history or physical findings, an X-ray of the chest will usually clear up the matter. If not, bronchoscopy is performed but even then sometimes no cause can be found.

Treatment of haemoptysis

1. A slight degree of haemoptysis does not call for any treatment other than that of the causative disease.

2. Severe haemoptysis. In any case of a large haemorrhage the patient is put to bed on absolute rest, and not allowed to do anything

TABLE VI

Haemoptysis	Haematemesis
1. The blood is thick, frothy, bright red, and is coughed up.	1. The blood is dark, is usually mixed with food, and is vomited up.
2. There is a tendency to spit up small amounts of blood, often mixed with sputum, for several days after the initial haemorrhage.	2. It is usually vomited up all at once or in several large amounts.
3. Usually there are signs of chest disease or mitral stenosis.	3. There may be a history of indigestion, peptic ulcer, or other diseases of the stomach.

for himself. Fluids only will be wanted in the early stages: later a light diet is given as the general condition improves.

Most patients are best nursed in the semi-propped up position as this is the most comfortable for them.

Very few patients die as an immediate result of the haemoptysis itself, so that the patient can be reassured. As with all cases of haemorrhage this psychological treatment is most important.

To allay the anxiety and to give the patient some much-needed rest, sedatives are needed. Morphine is best avoided as it depresses the cough reflex and respiration too severely and so allows the lungs to become filled with blood. On the other hand, excessive coughing is also harmful as it can prolong haemorrhage, and so a mild sedative to reduce coughing, such as codeine sulphate (60 mg), is useful.

7 Diseases of the Alimentary System

DISEASES OF THE MOUTH

STOMATITIS

Stomatitis is an inflammation of the mucous membrane of the mouth and is a condition of particular importance to the nurse, because she can do so much to prevent it.

Causes
1. Any prolonged fever or general illness, especially in infants and elderly people.
2. Thrush (infection with a fungus, *Monilia albicans*). This commonly affects infants and elderly debilitated patients. It is also frequently associated with the prolonged use of antibiotics; these destroy the normal bacteria in the mouth and so allow the fungus to flourish in their absence.
3. A severe ulcerative stomatitis may accompany the gingivitis caused by Vincent's organisms.
4. Metallic poisoning. The continued use of mercury, bismuth or gold may give rise to a severe form of stomatitis.

Symptoms and signs
The mouth in stomatitis is red and swollen and the patient complains of soreness, especially on eating. In severe forms there may be actual ulceration, often with sloughs, and in these cases the patient is usually seriously ill and toxic. Excessive salivation and bleeding may also be present. The infection may also spread along the parotid ducts to cause inflammation of the parotid gland (*parotitis*).

In thrush white spots, very like milk clots, are seen on the mucous membrane of the mouth.

Treatment
PREVENTIVE
Most cases of stomatitis can be prevented and it is here that the nurse plays such an important role. In any fever (especially if

prolonged) or in any severe general illness, dryness of the mouth frequently results from the reduced flow of saliva. This dryness combined with reduced mastication is very liable to cause a stomatitis. For this reason every care and attention must be paid to proper mouth toilet. Apart from the essential routine cleansing of the mouth and teeth (or dentures), another most important preventive measure is to ensure that the patient drinks enough. Fruit juices are most useful in stimulating the flow of saliva.

Some cases of stomatitis are caused by unclean feeding utensils, particularly the form of stomatitis seen in infants, which is known as *thrush*, and is due to dirty feeding bottles and teats. Meticulous care in the proper sterilisation of all bottles and teats is essential, especially where a number of infants are congregated together, e.g. in hospitals or nurseries.

CURATIVE

Local treatment for an established stomatitis consists of gentle swabbing with some mild solution like soda bicarbonate, thymol or hydrogen peroxide. Local treatment must be carried out with extreme gentleness otherwise more harm than good is done. Mouth washes (potassium chlorate, thymol or weak permanganate of potash) are also useful.

In resistant cases of thrush, nystatin may be given by tablets since this antibiotic is effective against the fungus.

GINGIVITIS

Inflammation of the gums is known as gingivitis and may arise under the same conditions as cause stomatitis. The presence of decayed teeth predisposes to the development of gingivitis. A fairly common form is that caused by infection with Vincent's organisms, when the gingivitis may also be accompanied by tonsillitis (*Vincent's angina*) and stomatitis.

The treatment of gingivitis consists of proper care of the teeth and all the routine mouth toilet mentioned under stomatitis. Penicillin is most beneficial for Vincent's infections.

Bleeding from the gums is commonly present in certain blood diseases, especially leukaemia and purpura. Scurvy due to vitamin C deficiency is another cause of such bleeding.

DISEASES OF THE TONGUE

The appearance and condition of the tongue are very important in medicine. In many diseases, both local and general, the tongue is affected and proper examination of the tongue may therefore be very helpful in diagnosis and treatment. In health, the tongue is normally clean and is protruded in the midline when the patient is asked to put out the tongue. In most general illnesses, especially those associated with fever, the tongue is usually dry and coated with a thick fur. In any condition where the patient has not been taking adequate fluids the tongue tends to become dry. A very dry tongue with a hard leathery appearance is commonly seen in cases of uraemia. In pernicious anaemia the tongue loses its papillae and so becomes smooth and pale, the so-called 'bald tongue'. In acromegaly the tongue becomes very large and deeply fissured. In progressive muscular atrophy the muscles of the tongue waste away and the tongue appears shrivelled and small.

GLOSSITIS

Inflammation of the tongue (glossitis) occurs characteristically in several illnesses: (a) scarlet fever, (b) anaemias, especially pernicious anaemia, and (c) vitamin deficiency, particularly of the B complex.

The tongue in glossitis is red and looks rather glazed. The patient complains of soreness of the tongue.

The treatment of glossitis is that of the underlying cause.

Ulceration of the tongue

The commonest cause of a severe persistent ulceration of the tongue is malignant disease. Here, the ulcer is very hard and quite often the neighbouring lymph glands are enlarged and hard. Syphilis and tuberculosis are other less common causes of ulceration of the tongue.

DISEASES OF THE SALIVARY GLANDS

The salivary glands are the parotid, the submaxillary and sublingual. Their function is to aid digestion, and their secretion, saliva, also acts as a lubricant in the mastication of food. The constant secretion of saliva has a very essential cleansing effect.

The salivary glands may be affected by various diseases. The commonest are:

Epidemic parotitis (mumps)

This is an acute infectious disease caused by a virus. Both parotid glands become markedly swollen and the patient complains of difficulty in opening the mouth. There are, in addition, the general signs of a fever. Mumps is dealt with fully on page 76.

Suppurative parotitis

A suppurative inflammation of the parotid glands is usually the result of insufficient care of the mouth in the course of a severe and debilitating illness. Typhoid fever, measles and malignant cachexia are particularly prone to give rise to a septic parotitis.

Stones

Stones may form in the various salivary glands causing pain and swelling in the glands, especially after eating. The stones can usually be seen on X-ray examination. Surgical removal is necessary.

DISEASES OF THE OESOPHAGUS

DYSPHAGIA

Most diseases which affect the oesophagus give rise to the symptom, difficulty in swallowing (dysphagia).

Causes of dysphagia

Foreign body in the oesophagus. This is a common cause of dysphagia, and in these cases there is a typical history of something sticking in the throat after the patient has eaten. A fish bone is the commonest foreign body giving rise to dysphagia.

Carcinoma of the oesophagus. Carcinoma arising in the oesophagus is not uncommon, usually occurring in middle-aged or elderly people. The dysphagia is progressive, the patient complaining of increasing difficulty in swallowing foods, until finally only liquids can be taken. In the later stages the patient is wasted and anaemic from lack of nourishment.

Pressure on the oesophagus from without. The conditions which most commonly cause dysphagia through pressure on the oesophagus are:

(a) Malignant growths in the mediastinum

(b) Retrosternal goitres

(c) Aneurysms of the arch of the aorta.

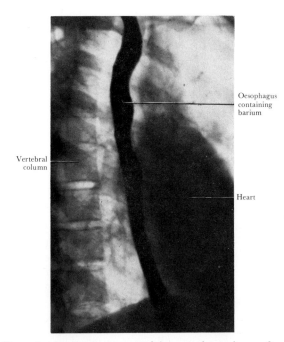

Fig. 7.1   X-ray showing the appearance of the normal oesophagus after a barium swallow. (Side view.)

Stricture of the oesophagus. This usually follows the swallowing of corrosive poisons (strong acids and caustic alkalis).

Cardiospasm (achalasia). As a result of disturbance of the nervous control of the sphincter of the oesophageal opening into the stomach, failure of the sphincter to relax and allow food to pass into the stomach is sometimes seen. Cardiospasm occurs most commonly in women; dysphagia and recurrent vomiting are the main symptoms. The symptoms are, however, not as progressive as in carcinoma.

Paralysis of the oesophageal muscles (bulbar paralysis). In polio-encephalitis and myasthenia gravis, difficulty in swallowing may arise as a result of a paralysis of the oesophageal muscles.

Hysteria. In young girls particularly, hysteria may cause a dysphagia with the characteristic sensation of a suffocating lump in the throat (globus hystericus). Another typical finding in hysterical cases is that the patient complains of equal difficulty in swallowing fluids and solids; this is never the case in non-hysterical dysphagia.

Diagnosis

When dysphagia arises after the swallowing of a fish bone or a corrosive poison, the cause is obvious. In the less acute cases an X-ray

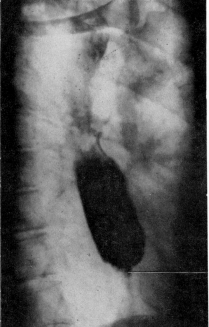

Stricture

Fig. 7.2   X-ray (barium swallow) showing barium held up by a carcinomatous stricture in the lower part of the oesophagus.

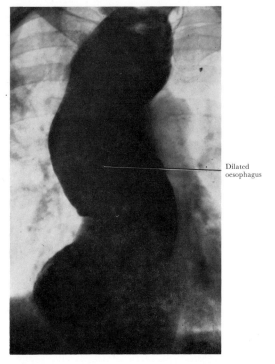

Dilated
oesophagus

FIG. 7.3   X-ray (barium swallow) showing the gross dilatation of the oesophagus in an advanced case of cardiospasm (achalasia).

is usually taken while the patient is swallowing opaque barium (*barium swallow*). By this means the site and type of the obstruction is often seen. In cases where the X-ray is not conclusive it may be necessary to pass an instrument called an oesophagoscope directly into the oesophagus, whereupon a direct view of any lesion present can be obtained.

Treatment

A foreign body is removed by operation. Cases of carcinoma were until recent years invariably fatal, but now early cases have been successfully operated on. In some cases of cardiospasm, dilatation of the sphincter by bougies is undertaken, but in others an operation to divide the muscles around the cardiac sphincter may be performed. If there is a retrosternal goitre this is removed by operation.

In many cases of dysphagia, e.g. advanced carcinoma, only symptomatic treatment can be given. In these the diet is important, as on the one hand foods cannot be swallowed, whilst on the other the patient must be given sufficient nourishment. The basis of the diet is therefore milk, which may be varied by the addition of Benger's,

Ovaltine or Horlicks. Eggs beaten up in the milk, puréed vegetables and butter are also very useful.

In the late stages of carcinoma of the oesophagus, a special tube (Mousseau-Barbin tube) can be inserted at operation and may delay complete obstruction to swallowing for a few months. Radiotherapy may be tried but is usually ineffective.

DISEASES OF THE STOMACH AND DUODENUM

DYSPEPSIA

The stomach is very readily upset both by diseases directly affecting the stomach and also by any general illness. In addition any nervous tension or anxiety frequently causes gastric upset; most people have experienced loss of appetite, vague discomfort in the stomach, a feeling of biliousness, and similar symptoms when they are under some strain, e.g. before an examination, interview or taking up a new job.

Patients use such terms as *dyspepsia* or *indigestion* to describe these symptoms and often treat themselves with alkali powders before seeking medical advice. Nevertheless, symptoms of this type often need investigation to exclude organic disease.

Pain. Varying degrees of pain occur in most diseases of the upper gastrointestinal tract and usually the pain is related to food, i.e. it tends to occur at a specific time interval after meals. Indigestible foods, such as fried fats, rich carbohydrates and spices are especially likely to give rise to pain or discomfort. The pain is most frequently felt in the epigastrium.

Nausea and vomiting. These symptoms are of common occurrence in gastric diseases. Severe pain caused by gastric lesions is particularly liable to be followed by vomiting, which often, however, relieves the pain. Recurrent vomiting, especially of blood (*haematemesis*), is a most important symptom, denoting some serious gastrointestinal disease.

Vomiting is also, however, a frequent symptom in non-gastro-intestinal diseases, and for this reason a general approach to the subject of vomiting is given on page 206.

Loss of appetite. This symptom, which occurs in both gastro-intestinal and other diseases, varies a good deal in frequency and severity. Persistent loss of appetite accompanied by progressive loss of weight may denote some severe disease such as cancer of the stomach.

Pain, vomiting and loss of appetite are the symptoms which are most often present in the more important diseases causing dyspepsia. In addition, however, the following symptoms are very frequent, particularly in the less important diseases which cause dyspepsia.

Flatulence is the distension of stomach or intestines with gas, which is then brought up or passed by rectum.

Heartburn is the well-known burning sensation which rises from the stomach to the throat. It is often accompanied by the regurgitation of a small amount of acid (sour) fluid into the mouth.

Water-brash is the term used to describe the clear fluid, like saliva, which suddenly wells up in the mouth. Water-brash is probably due to reflex salivation in response to some diseases of the stomach. The morning vomiting seen in cases of chronic gastritis, especially in chronic alcoholism, is often associated with water brash.

VOMITING

Vomiting, like pain, is a very common feature of many diseases and it is important to understand how it occurs. The actual act of vomiting consists of a contraction of stomach, abdominal and diaphragmatic muscles and a relaxation of the cardiac opening of the stomach. There is a centre, the vomiting centre, in the medulla of the brain, which controls this complicated act. This centre is closely connected with the vagus nerve, especially with the branches from the abdominal viscera.

Vomiting can be divided into three well-recognised groups:

1. Reflex vomiting

This, the commonest type, is due to stimulation of the vagus nerve. The usual causes of reflex vomiting are:

(a) *Diseases in the stomach:*

Acute gastritis
Peptic ulcer
Pyloric stenosis
Carcinoma of the stomach.

(b) *Diseases in other abdominal organs:*

Renal and biliary colic
Inflammations such as appendicitis and peritonitis
Tumours and obstruction of the intestinal tract.

(c) *Drugs (emetics).* Certain drugs irritate the stomach or stimulate the vomiting centre, thus causing vomiting, and are often used for this purpose, e.g. in cases of poisoning when it is desirable to get rid of any poison in the stomach. These drugs are called emetics and common examples are:

(i) Salt, a tablespoon in a tumbler of warm water (repeated if necessary).
(ii) Mustard, two teaspoonfuls in warm water.
(iii) Apomorphine, 7·5 mg subcutaneously.

(d) *Diseases of the ear.* The vestibular part of the ear deals with posture and equilibrium and is closely associated with the vomiting centre. Conditions affecting the vestibular apparatus often cause severe vomiting. Travel sickness and the disease known as *Ménière's syndrome* are two examples of this type of vomiting.

2. Vomiting due to direct stimulation of the vomiting centre

Various cerebral diseases can cause direct pressure on the vomiting centre. Vomiting is therefore a feature of such diseases of the nervous system as cerebral tumour, abscess and meningitis, in which increased intracranial pressure is present.

3. Vomiting due to stimulation from the higher cerebral centres

This class covers the vomiting resulting from emotional disorders, such as nervous tension, anxiety, fear and hysteria. This vomiting is often successfully controlled by chlorpromazine or allied drugs.

Finally, it should be remembered that any severe illness can by reflex toxic action give rise to vomiting.

CHARACTERISTICS OF VOMITING IN THE MORE COMMON DISEASES

Vomiting tends to be more dominant and severe in diseases of the stomach and abdominal organs. Vomiting is a feature of peptic ulcer and usually relieves the pain which is present. The vomiting is, however, not as severe as in pyloric stenosis, in which vomiting is a cardinal feature. In these cases the copious vomiting, often of food eaten the previous day, is diagnostic of stenosis. In the pyloric stenosis of infants the vomiting, apart from being copious, is typically projectile in character.

In gastric carcinoma vomiting is common, the vomit often being bloodstained and looking like coffee grounds. A more profuse haematemesis may occur, but it is not as common as in peptic ulcer; peptic ulcer is the commonest cause of haematemesis. Obstruction of the portal vein, leading to vomiting of blood, is usually the result of cirrhosis of the liver.

Acute dilatation of the stomach, which may complicate abdominal operations, is attended by most severe and copious vomiting. In acute inflammatory abdominal diseases, such as acute appendicitis, vomiting is usually associated with abdominal pain and occurs early at the onset of the illness.

In acute intestinal obstruction vomiting is persistent, and the vomit may be faecal in character. Faecal vomit is dark brown or black in colour and has a typically faecal smell.

In cerebral diseases associated with increased intracranial pressure, vomiting usually occurs with a severe headache. Vomiting is more predominant in the acute diseases causing intracranial pressure (such as meningitis) than in the more subacute diseases like cerebral tumour.

EFFECTS OF VOMITING

Vomiting is likely to have serious effects only if it is persistent and copious, as in cases of pyloric stenosis, intestinal obstruction and acute dilatation of the stomach. The main result of continued vomiting is loss of fluid and acid. The loss of fluid leads to dehydration, which causes collapse (p. 378) and in some cases acute renal failure (p. 375). The loss of hydrochloric acid in the vomit causes an alkalosis, which can lead to tetany (p. 453).

GASTRITIS

Gastritis means an inflammation of the lining mucous membrane of the stomach. It occurs in two main forms, acute and chronic.

Acute

Acute gastritis is usually caused by some severe dietary indiscretion, such as overindulgence in alcohol or eating unsuitable food. Again, bacteria ingested in food or drink may cause an acute gastritis (food poisoning).

In most cases of acute gastritis there is also an accompanying inflammation of the intestines (enteritis) and therefore, for the sake of convenience, acute gastroenteritis is disucssed under Diseases of the Intestines (p. 222).

Chronic

Prolonged dietary indiscretions, such as constantly irregular mealtimes or, particularly, eating highly spiced and indigestible foods, are a frequent cause of chronic gastritis. In many of these cases the gastritis precedes a peptic ulcer. Strong tea and coffee may also give rise to gastritis, while another frequent cause is chronic alcoholism.

In addition to the above dietary causes, certain chronic infections can also lead to a chronic gastritis, e.g. chronic sinusitis and bronchiectasis, where the continued swallowing of purulent matter may irritate the gastric mucous membrane.

The symptoms of chronic gastritis are mainly those outlined under dyspepsia. Loss of appetite with early morning vomiting are features of most cases. Flatulence and heartburn may also occur.

The treatment is, first, to clear up the cause wherever possible, i.e. to clear up any infection or correct the dietary indiscretions. Then the treatment is similar to that outlined under peptic ulcer, except that the initial period of rest in bed with a strict diet may be replaced by the more liberal post-ulcer regime.

PEPTIC ULCER

Peptic ulcer is a term used to include both gastric ulcer and duodenal ulcer.

Gastric ulcers are usually situated on the lesser curve of the stomach and as a rule only one ulcer is present. A duodenal ulcer occurs in the first part of the duodenum and is much more chronic and difficult to heal than a gastric ulcer. A duodenal ulcer is often associated with scarring of the duodenum, which can narrow the lumen and delay emptying of the stomach. The symptoms of gastric and duodenal ulcers are similar, though it is unusual for a gastric ulcer and duodenal ulcer to co-exist in the same patient.

Cause

The exact cause or causes of peptic ulcer are unknown, but certain well-recognised facotrs are present in most cases.

Age, occupation and heredity. Peptic ulcer is primarily a disease of adult life and is rare in children. Ulcers are commonest in people who have very worrying occupations or who, for whatever reason, are subject to tension and anxiety. Heredity is also a factor as peptic ulcer tends to occur in families.

Excessive acid in the stomach. It is known that ulcers never occur in the absence of hydrochloric acid: on the contrary, in the vast majority of cases of peptic ulcer there is an excessive acid secretion, i.e. hyperchlorhydria. (*Hypochlorhydria* and *achlorhydria* are terms used for diminished and absent acid secretion respectively.) The exact relation of excess of acid to the causation of ulcers is, however, not definitely known because not all people with a hyperchlorhydria develop ulcers.

Smoking does not appear to be a cause of peptic ulcer but ulcers take longer to heal and are more prone to complications in those who smoke.

Symptoms

PAIN

This is the most important symptom. It is usually felt in the epigastrium and has definite characteristics.

1. It is related to meals and especially heavy meals, coming on either after a meal or just before a meal. It tends to occur more quickly after a meal in cases of gastric ulcer than in those of duodenal ulcer.

2. It is, however, temporarily relieved by food, especially with duodenal ulcer, and the patient therefore often complains that the pain is a *hunger pain*. The pain is often described as burning in character.

3. The pain may occur at night, waking the patient from his sleep.

OTHER SYMPTOMS

Vomiting often occurs, especially if the pain is severe. Other common symptoms are heartburn and flatulence. The appetite is usually good, except in some cases of gastric ulcer where the patient may be afraid to eat for fear of bringing on the pain. There is usually no loss of weight, unlike cases of carcinoma of the stomach.

One of the most remarkable features of peptic ulcer is that the symptoms come on in attacks which may last for several weeks and then clear up completely even without any treatment, only however, to recur after an interval usually of two or three months. These recurring attacks may go on for years, becoming more severe and more frequent until eventually the patient goes to the doctor for treatment.

Physical examination of the patient usually reveals very little, except for localised tenderness to palpation in the epigastrium.

Diagnosis of peptic ulcer

The diagnosis can often be made on the basis of a typical history taken in conjunction with the finding of localised tenderness over the ulcer. The following investigations, however, are usually carried out to confirm the diagnosis.

X-RAY EXAMINATION

A specialised X-ray examination, known as a *barium meal*, will show up the stomach and duodenum and usually also any ulcer that may be present. After suitable preparation the patient is examined under an X-ray screen immediately after drinking barium sulphate (the patient must have nothing to eat or drink for six hours before the X-ray; in addition, all medicines should have been stopped). Barium is opaque to X-rays and it therefore outlines the whole stomach and duodenum. In this way an ulcer crater may be seen. Occasionally, however, even though an ulcer is present, the X-ray may not reveal it.

ENDOSCOPY (GASTROSCOPY)

The interior of the stomach can be inspected with a gastroscope. This is a flexible fibre optic instrument which when passed into the stomach and pylorus allows good vision of the stomach and sometimes the duodenum as well. The procedure is conducted in the theatre and a forceps attached to the gastroscope allows a biopsy to be taken of any regions suspicious of malignant changes.

EXAMINATION OF THE FAECES

In most cases of peptic ulcer, specimens of faeces are sent to the laboratory for examination for the presence of blood. The presence of blood in the motion is a most important sign, indicating bleeding from some source in the gastrointestinal tract. With slight bleeding from the stomach or upper part of the intestinal tract the motion may appear normal in colour to the naked eye, because any blood present is intimately mixed with the motion. For this reason the blood is spoken of as hidden or *occult*. By chemical examination, however, the blood can be detected. When faeces are sent for examination for occult blood it may be necessary to keep the patient on a meat-free diet for three days beforehand, as meat may give a misleadingly positive result.

In cases of severe bleeding from the upper gastrointestinal tract the motions become black and 'tarry' from the large amount of altered blood present. Black tarry motions from upper gastrointestinal haemorrhage are known as *melaena*.

In contrast to the effect of haemorrhage from the upper gastro-intestinal tract, blood in the motion in lower intestinal bleeding is bright red and is usually on the outside of the specimen, e.g. in carcinoma of the lower colon, haemorrhoids and colitis.

In peptic ulcer the presence either of occult blood in the faeces or particularly of a melaena means that the ulcer is active (not healed) and therefore requires strict diet and rest. In treating a case of peptic ulcer, weekly occult blood examinations are usually made as a routine measure to follow the progress of healing.

TEST MEAL

The patient fasts from the previous night and in the morning a fine narrow tube (Ryle's tube) is passed into the stomach. The resting gastric juice is removed completely by repeated aspiration with a syringe attached to the tube and sent to the laboratory for estimation. A high acid content is more consistent with a duodenal ulcer than a gastric ulcer: and a very large amount (500 ml) suggests pyloric stenosis (see later).

Treatment of peptic ulcer

The medical treatment of gastric and duodenal ulcers consists of general advice, medicaments to relieve symptoms and drugs to heal the ulceration.

GENERAL ADVICE

1. Meals should be taken at regular intervals: epigastric pain is more likely to occur when the stomach is empty. Frequent small meals are better than a heavy meal once a day. Fried foods, vinegary and highly spiced foods are best avoided though each patient soon learns which particular foods are likely to bring on symptoms. Alcoholic drinks, especially when on an empty stomach, are prone to provoke stomach pain.

2. Cigarette smoking delays the healing of peptic ulcers and should be discontinued.

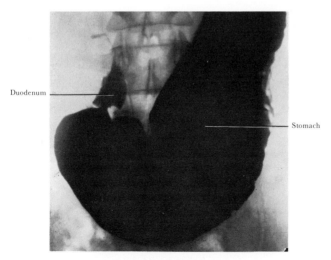

Duodenum

Stomach

FIG. 7.4   X-ray (barium meal) showing the appearance of the normal stomach.

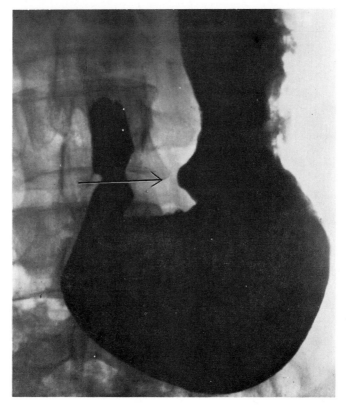

FIG. 7.5   X-ray (barium meal) showing an ulcer on the lesser curvature of the stomach.

3. Particularly aspirins, but also many other preparations pre-scribed for headaches and rheumatism, are prone to bring on ulcer pain and should be avoided.

4. Anxiety, frustration and stress are liable to provoke exacerbation of ulcer symptoms. These emotions are not easy to avoid but some-times sedation with diazepam 2 mg three times a day may help tide over a worrying episode.

5. When pain is persistent and associated with attacks of vomiting, a spell of bed rest may be effective in easing symptoms. Patients admitted to hospital with these symptoms usually settle down after a few days.

MEDICAMENTS TO RELIEVE SYMPTOMS

Alkalis usually offer quick relief of pain due to peptic ulcer. Many varieties are in common use, some prescribed by doctors, some bought at the chemist shop or supermarket. Magnesium trisilicate or aluminium hydroxide are effective alkalis and can be taken regularly between meals. They are available as tablets or as liquid medicines.

Most ulcer patients carry around with them in tablet form the particular medicament which suits them best.

Milk is often effective in relieving ulcer pain. Tablets to suck are available which combine milk and alkali (e.g. Nulacin).

DRUGS TO HEAL ULCERATION

Cimetidine is a drug which blocks the production of acid by the stomach. It should be taken in tablet form 200 mg three times a day and 400 mg at night, and in many cases leads to healing of duodenal ulcers within a month. Unfortunately the ulcer and symptoms are liable to return after a time so that further courses of the drug may be necessary.

Carbenoxolone is derived from liquorice which was observed to be helpful in patients with gastric ulcer. It is given by mouth as 50 mg tablets three times a day for three to four weeks and leads to relief of pain and healing of the ulcer even when the patient is ambulant. In some patients it causes fluid retention and headaches, usually relieved by a diuretic. It is ineffective for duodenal ulcers.

Deglycyrrhizinated liquorice (Caved-S) is a similar preparation effective for gastric ulcers.

COMPLICATIONS OF PEPTIC ULCER

1. Haemorrhage
2. Perforation
3. Pyloric stenosis
4. Malignant change.

Haemorrhage (haematemesis and melaena)

The ulcer may erode a blood vessel and thus give rise to haemorrhage. In gastric ulcers the blood is usually vomited (haematemesis), but sometimes it is passed instead through the intestines, making the motions black and tarry (melaena). Haemorrhage from duodenal ulcers usually takes the form of a melaena. As mentioned earlier (p. 220), a slight bleeding from peptic ulcer is often discovered only by chemical examination of the faeces for occult blood.

If the haemorrhage is large it is accompanied by signs of collapse and shock:

(a) The skin becomes cold and clammy.
(b) The pulse becomes very rapid.
(c) The patient is usually very restless.
(d) There is a severe drop in blood pressure.

In haematemesis the blood is dark red and may be mixed with food (compare with Haemoptysis, p. 197). When the haemorrhage is copious, blood can be clearly seen in the vomit, but if the haemorrhage is not so large the blood may be intimately mixed with food and partially digested, whereupon the descriptive term *coffee ground vomit* is often used. (In carcinoma of the stomach the haemorrhage is often in the form of 'coffee grounds'.)

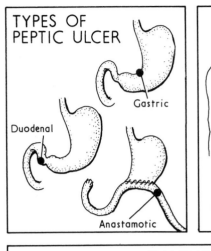

TYPES OF PEPTIC ULCER

Gastric

Duodenal

Anastamotic

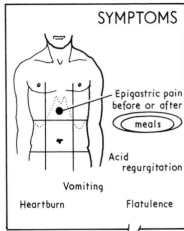

SYMPTOMS

Epigastric pain before or after meals

Acid regurgitation

Vomiting

Heartburn

Flatulence

DIAGNOSIS

HISTORY

HEREDITY
STRESS
SMOKING

Factors which dispose to excessive Hydrochloric acid and ulcer formation

Barium meal

Gastroscopy

Faecal examination for occult blood

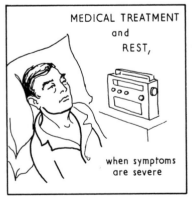

MEDICAL TREATMENT
and
REST,

when symptoms are severe

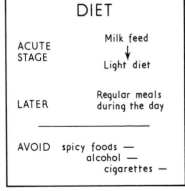

DIET

ACUTE STAGE

Milk feed
↓
Light diet

LATER

Regular meals during the day

AVOID spicy foods —
alcohol —
cigarettes —

FIG. 7.6 Peptic ulcer.

Treatment of haemorrhage

GENERAL MEASURES

If the haemorrhage is large the patient is shocked and measures to overcome this must be taken at once. The patient is kept at absolute rest; in severe haemorrhage raising the foot of the bed is very useful. Adequate warmth is necessary, but care must be taken to avoid over-heating, which only makes the condition worse. (For this reason a radiant heat cradle should be avoided.) To relieve the shock and any pain, and also to allay anxiety, a sedative such as morphine (15 mg) should be given. A half or one-hourly pulse chart is kept. This is a guide to the patient's progress, as if the haemorrhage goes on the pulse rate continues to rise. The blood pressure, too, is taken at fairly frequent intervals, a falling blood pressure, like a rising pulse, being an indication of continued haemorrhage.

If the abdomen becomes distended, as may happen with a large haemorrhage, a small enema may be ordered. To keep the stools soft and prevent straining, one or two ounces of liquid paraffin daily are useful. The patient must be warned against straining at stool as this may restart bleeding.

DIET

Whether or not the patient is given food by mouth depends on the doctor in charge. In former days the patient was usually forbidden to take anything by mouth except sips of water or milk, but in recent years a more liberal diet has been allowed. The usual practice is to allow food by mouth as for patients with an acute ulcer—that is, small frequent feeds of a bland non-irritating variety. Some patients feel like eating more than others, and in the first few days it is wise to accede to the patient's wishes within the limits of the diet mentioned.

TRANSFUSIONS

In patients with copious haemorrhage with severe shock, as revealed by a persistently rapid pulse of over 100, a systolic blood pressure below 100 mmHg and restlessness, a blood transfusion is immediately given of at least two pints or more, according to the severity of the case. Of course, before the blood is given all the usual precautions must be taken—blood grouping, determination of the Rh factor and cross-matching. A strict watch must be kept for transfusion reactions.

With patients who do not immediately require a transfusion close observation of the pulse rate and blood pressure, as already mentioned, is essential, as if the haemorrhage continues a blood transfusion may become necessary.

DRUGS

Cimetidine has a powerful effect in blocking the production of acid in the stomach. Since acid can exacerbate bleeding from the ulcer, cimetidine tablets may be useful in stemming the haemorrhage.

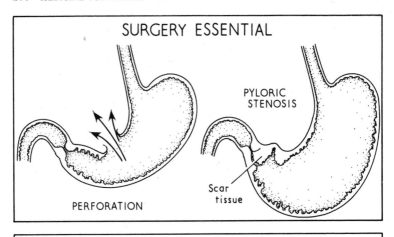

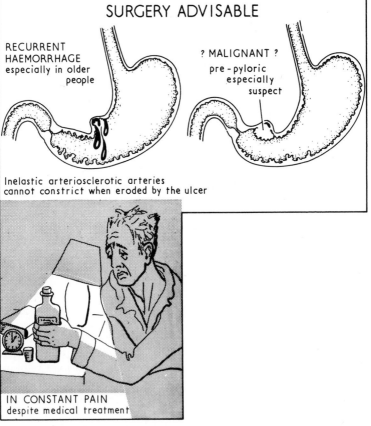

FIG. 7.7   Indications for surgical treatment of peptic ulcer.

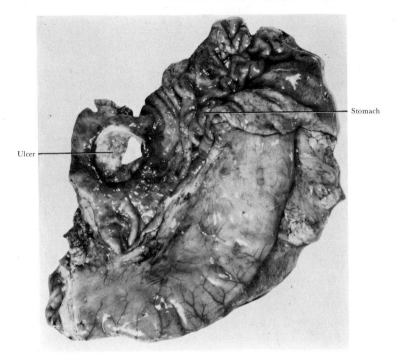

Ulcer

Stomach

Fig. 7.8 A large chronic gastric ulcer which failed to heal under medical treatment and was removed by operation (partial gastrectomy).

SURGICAL INTERVENTION

In most patients the haemorrhage subsides with the above treatment, but it does persist in a minority of cases, usually in elderly patients with large chronic ulcers. The arteries in elderly people are more likely to be arteriosclerotic and therefore do not contract down so readily in order to control the bleeding. In these elderly patients with persistent haemorrhage, surgery may be advised after the shock has been overcome with adequate transfusions of blood. Partial gastrectomy is the operation of choice.

Other causes of haematemesis and melaena

Before leaving the discussion of haemorrhage as a complication of peptic ulcer it is convenient here to mention the other causes of haematemesis and melaena. It should be remembered, however, that in 90 per cent of cases the cause is peptic ulcer.

   (a) Gastric erosion
   (b) Cancer of the stomach
   (c) Cirrhosis of the liver
   (d) Blood diseases (purpura, leukaemia, vitamin K deficiency)
   (e) Swallowed blood, e.g. from epistaxis or following operations on the nose and throat

(f) Irritating drugs such as aspirin or phenylbutazone.

When the cause of the bleeding is in doubt, fibre optic endoscopy may be undertaken in the hope that a view of the stomach and duodenum will reveal the source of the haemorrhage.

Perforation

Here the ulcer ruptures through into the peritoneal cavity, perforation being one of the common causes of an 'acute abdomen'. There is shock with severe and agonising pain. When the patient is examined the abdomen is found to be held absolutely rigid. Peritonitis can quickly supervene if an immediate operation is not performed.

Pyloric stenosis

A chronic ulcer, when it heals, produces scar tissue. If the ulcer is situated near the pylorus the scar tissue may obstruct the pyloric opening, thus causing a pyloric stenosis. In severe cases very little food may pass through into the duodenum. Usually there are the following symptoms and signs:

(a) Vomiting is frequent and copious, a history of vomiting of food eaten on a previous day being most characteristic of stenosis.

(b) The loss of weight varies with the degree of the stenosis, but it is very marked in the severe cases.

(c) Constipation is usually present.

(d) The resting juice withdrawn when a test meal is done is large in amount, perhaps as much as 500 to 700 ml.

(e) Barium meal examination will show that the stomach is very dilated and there is great delay in emptying.

The treatment for pyloric stenosis is operation, either a partial gastrectomy or gastro-jejunostomy being done.

Malignant change

Malignancy arises only with gastric ulcers, as duodenal ulcers never become malignant. When a gastric ulcer becomes malignant the symptoms become more constant and severe.

CARCINOMA OF THE STOMACH

The stomach is a common site for carcinoma, the disease arising most frequently in middle-aged or elderly people.

Symptoms and signs

Unfortunately the symptoms of carcinoma of the stomach may not appear until the growth is advanced. The symptoms may resemble those of peptic ulcer, i.e. epigastric pain, nausea and vomiting, but there are the following differences:

1. The pain is usually much more persistent, instead of recurring in the periodical attacks typical of a non-malignant ulcer.

2. Loss of appetite is an early and fairly constant symptom.

3. There is progressive loss of weight. With uncomplicated peptic ulcer, loss of weight is absent or slight.

4. Anaemia is more constant.

5. Rest and diet which rapidly clear up the symptoms of a simple ulcer have little effect on carcinoma of the stomach.

6. In most cases of peptic ulcer any slight bleeding, as detected by occult blood examination of the faeces, soon stops with rest and diet. This is not so with carcinoma; persistence of occult blood in the faeces when the patient is on rest and diet is a reason for strong suspicion of carcinoma. A haematemesis due to carcinoma usually takes the form of 'coffee ground' vomit.

7. Jaundice may be present in the very late stages owing to the spread of the growth to the liver.

DIAGNOSIS

The diagnosis is usually suspected on the above symptoms; the development, for the first time, of indigestion or gastric symptoms in middle-aged or elderly people is particularly significant. A barium meal X-ray in most cases confirms the diagnosis.

Gastroscopy is useful in distinguishing a malignant from a non-malignant gastric ulcer, particularly if a biopsy is taken for examination under the microscope. In many cases, however, the diagnosis can be confirmed only at operation, and when there is any suspicion that an ulcer is malignant, operation is performed. As mentioned earlier, duodenal ulcers never become malignant.

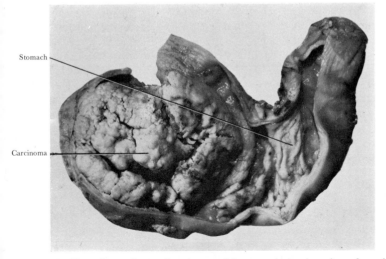

FIG. 7.9 Very advanced case of carcinoma of the stomach showing a large fungating tumour.

Treatment

The only hope of a cure is in the complete removal of the cancer by operation. Unfortunately, with the majority of patients, by the time they come to operation the cancer has spread too far to be wholly removed. The prognosis, therefore, is usually bad except for the few patients who come to operation early.

PYLORIC STENOSIS

It has already been seen that one of the possible complications of peptic ulcer is pyloric stenosis. Another well recognised form of stenosis is:

Congenital hypertrophic pyloric stenosis

This form of stenosis occurs in the first few weeks of life, and nearly always, for some unknown reason, in boys. The pylorus becomes thickened and hypertrophied from muscle spasm, until eventually a severe degree of stenosis is present.

Symptoms and signs

1. The infant is usually perfectly normal for the first week or so of life, after which persistent vomiting after nearly every feed begins. The vomiting is typically described as being **projectile** in nature, the feed being forcibly expelled for some distance.

2. The baby is hungry and greedy for his feeds.

3. Constipation is always present and the stools are usually small and dark green in colour ('hunger' stools).

4. From the lack of nourishment the baby loses weight and becomes dehydrated, the skin becomes pinched and the eyes and fontanelle become sunken.

5. If the baby is examined under a good light and during a feed, *peristaltic waves* will be seen in the upper abdomen. These waves are due to the contractions of the stomach forcing the food against the stenosed pylorus.

In most cases a firm, hard contracting tumour is felt in the pyloric region. This tumour is the hypertrophied pylorus.

DIAGNOSIS

The diagnosis is usually easily made on the characteristic symptoms and the finding of visible peristalsis and a pyloric tumour. It is essential to stress that the baby must be examined during or after a feed. The only other condition likely to be confused with this is one where, instead of a definite stenosis being present, there is spasm of the pylorus, causing similar symptoms. In these cases the infant is usually a girl and the symptoms are not so severe, rapidly responding to medical treatment.

Treatment of congenital pyloric stenosis

MEDICAL

In early cases medical treatment may suffice. This consists of:

(a) Daily gastric lavage to empty the distended stomach.

(b) Antispasmodic drugs, given either as drops (Eumydrin) or as lamellae placed on the tongue (Pylostropin). The drops and lamellae, which are both atropine preparations, are given 15 to 20 minutes before each feed. The dose of Eumydrin is 1 to 3 drops of the alcoholic solution.

(c) If dehydration is present, extra fluid should be given sub-cutaneously.

SURGICAL

In those cases where medical treatment has been tried and failed, and at once in all severe cases, an operation to relieve the stenosis is performed. *Ramstedt's* operation, which is usually done under a local anaesthetic, is a simple procedure. An incision down to the mucous membrane is made into the hypertrophied pylorus, thus relieving the stenosis.

Post-operative feeding is very important. Glucose saline is given several hours after the operation starting with 5 ml doses hourly, and after four such doses, increasing to 10 ml. Milk feeds, preferably with breast milk, are given eight to ten hours after the operation, commencing with 15 ml every one and a half hours. Twenty-four hours after the operation the milk feeds are increased to 60 ml three-hourly, and to 90 ml three-hourly after 48 hours. After this the appropriate diet for the infant's age is given.

One of the greatest post-operative dangers is gastroenteritis and therefore every care must be taken in regard to cleanliness in feeding. An enteritis can also arise from too rapid an increase in the post-operative feeds.

DIAPHRAGMATIC HERNIA (Hiatus hernia)

This is a common disorder particularly in overweight middle-aged women. Part of the stomach protrudes through the oesophageal opening (hiatus) of the diaphragm into the thorax. The hernia is not necessarily permanent but can slide into the thorax especially when the patient bends forward after a heavy meal. Reflux of gastric acid into the oesophagus occurs giving rise to a burning discomfort in the upper abdomen and behind the sternum in the chest. Congestion in the hernia can give rise to bleeding and anaemia.

The diagnosis of hiatus hernia can be confirmed by a barium meal X-ray with the patient tilted downwards on the X-ray table to demonstrate the hernia above the diaphragm.

To avoid symptoms the patient should:

1. Reduce weight and abstain from heavy meals.

2. Avoid tight clothes around the abdomen.

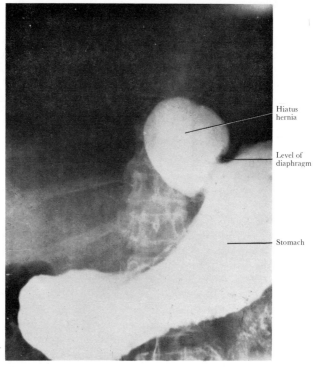

Hiatus
hernia

Level of
diaphragm

Stomach

FIG. 7.10   Hiatus hernia. The herniated portion of the stomach can be clearly seen
lying in the thoracic cavity above the diaphragm.

3. Avoid lying or sitting in a hunched up position especially after
meals.

Antacids are helpful in relieving discomfort and particularly antacid
preparations combined with a viscous alginate (Gaviscon) which coats
the lower end of the oesophagus.

An operation to repair the opening in the diaphragm is necessary in
patients with severe symptoms who do not respond to medical measures.

DISEASES OF THE INTESTINES

Disorders of the intestines may give rise to colicky pain, to constipation or to diarrhoea.

Abdominal colic

Pain is a constant feature of most intestinal diseases and is usually
'colicky' in nature. By this is meant pain which gradually increases
in intensity and then completely eases off. The pain comes and goes
in frequent spasms. Pain in intestinal disease may, however, also
be of a more persistent nature.

Constipation

Constipation means delay in the evacuation of the bowels. It is important to remember, however, that the bowel habit varies considerably from person to person. Constipation may not be present even if the bowels are opened only once in two days or even longer. When definite constipation is present the motions passed are not only infrequent but also usually hard and dry.

Causes

These are extremely numerous. The most usual are as follows.

1. *Habit.* Normally the desire to empty the bowel is experienced after a meal owing to the reflex bowel action called the gastrocolic reflex. In most people the gastrocolic reflex is most active after breakfast. If the desire to defaecate is ignored the reflex impulse soon loses its force, and as a result the faeces are retained. The retained faeces then become dry and hard from loss of water and so more difficult to pass. Thus a vicious circle develops.

Habit constipation is seen most often in people who rush off to work or to school without allowing sufficient time for a proper evacuation of the bowel. 'Habit constipation' is by far the commonest type met with.

2. *Inadequate fibre.* If the diet contains too little fibre (see page 386), the faeces become too small to excite normal peristaltic action and so constipation results. Foods containing a high fibre content resist complete digestion and form sufficient bulk to stimulate the intestinal peristalsis. They include green vegetables, fruit, salads, wholemeal bread, rough cereals and bran.

3. *Any acute general illness*, especially if accompanied by fever.

4. *Local causes in the intestines.*

(a) Any inflammation of the rectum, e.g. haemorrhoids or anal fissures, may result in constipation owing to the pain caused by evacuation.

(b) Megacolon (see p. 236).

(c) Tumours of the bowel may cause obstruction and thus lead to constipation. The constipation caused by tumours of the intestines often alternates with diarrhoea.

(d) Adhesions or bands, especially after operations, may cause obstruction.

Treatment

Any organic cause, such as anal fissures, tumours, adhesions, etc., must be treated by the appropriate surgical measures. The treatment of constipation resulting from an acute general illness is dealt with on page 11. In the commonest types of constipation, due to faulty habits and bad diet, correction of these usually leads to rapid improvement.

In the initial stages of treatment, drugs to help evacuation of the bowel (purgatives, aperients) may be used but should be discontinued as soon as possible.

In more severe cases of constipation, especially in children or in the elderly, the lower bowel is filled with inspissated faeces and a suppository or an enema may be used to induce evacuation. A glycerin or bisacodyl (Dulcolax) suppository can be inserted into the rectum but should be allowed time to dissolve before defaecation is attempted. Where this fails, an enema of warm water or warm normal saline can be used.

Very hard faeces may be softened by an olive oil enema, 100 to 250 ml of warm oil being left in the rectum for several hours if possible. A soap and water enema afterwards is useful.

Diarrhoea

When unformed stools are passed, diarrhoea is said to be present, Diarrhoea is a common and important symptom of intestinal disease, its severity and nature varying according to the disease. It is impossible here to give all the causes of diarrhoea, but a classification of the main causes is useful.

Causes of acute diarrhoea
  (a) Acute gastroenteritis
        (i) Alcoholic
       (ii) Dietetic
      (iii) Food poisoning
       (iv) Chemical poisoning
        (v) Infective gastroenteritis of infants
  (b) Enteric fevers
  (c) Dysenteries
  (d) Functional (simple nervous diarrhoea).

Causes of chronic diarrhoea
  (a) Inflammatory diseases
        (i) Ulcerative colitis
       (ii) Regional ileitis (Crohn's disease)
      (iii) Diverticulitis
       (iv) Tuberculosis
  (b) Carcinoma of the bowel
  (c) Coeliac disease and sprue
  (d) Vitamin B deficiency (pellagra)
  (e) Thyrotoxicosis.
  (f) Irritable bowel syndrome.

For the purpose of diagnosing the cause of diarrhoea, and also of watching the effects of treatment, the character of the stools is of great importance and a summary of the main characteristics of the stools in the different diseases is given at the end of the chapter. First, however, in the following pages, some of the individual diseases causing changes in the stools are dealt with.

ACUTE GASTROENTERITIS

Acute inflammation of the stomach (Gastritis, p. 208) is often accompanied by inflammation of the small intestine (enteritis), so giving rise to the condition called gastroenteritis. It is convenient to discuss the disease under two heads: (1) in adults and (2) in infants.

1. Gastroenteritis in adults

The predominant symptoms in all cases are acute vomiting and diarrhoea, often accompanied by abdominal colic and perhaps fever. Acute alcoholism is a frequent cause of acute gastroenteritis, as also is overindulgence in highly spiced or other unsuitable foods. Food infected with the Salmonella (food poisoning) organism is also responsible for many outbreaks of acute gastroenteritis; reheated pies and sausages and duck's eggs are common sources of infection. Food poisoning is discussed on page 83. Rarer causes of acute gastroenteritis are arsenical or mercurial poisoning. Severe enteritis may also occur during the administration of broad-spectrum antibiotics, such as the tetracycline antibiotics (p. 56).

In most cases of gastroenteritis the symptoms soon subside. All that is necessary is to keep the patient on a fluid diet till the vomiting and diarrhoea stop and then to give a bland non-irritating diet for a few days. In any case that does not settle within a day or so or whenever several cases occur together, the stools must be sent to the laboratory to find out whether any organisms of Salmonella food poisoning, dysentery or enteric fever are present. In all such cases strict isolation procedures must be carried out, especially with regard to disposal of stools.

2. Gastroenteritis in infants

Gastroenteritis presents a special problem when it arises (as it frequently does) in infants, because it may have a serious effect on the baby and also in many cases is extremely infectious.

The digestive system of an infant is very easily disturbed, not only by diseases of the gastrointestinal tract itself but also by disease of any other part of the body. Gastroenteritis of infants is therefore often divided into two groups: (a) cases due to disease outside the gastrointestinal tract—parenteral gastroenteritis; and (b) those due to diseases of the gastrointestinal tract itself—enteral gastroenteritis.

(a) *Parenteral gastroenteritis.* Any general infection of an infant may be accompanied by vomiting and diarrhoea, e.g. measles, whooping-cough, bronchitis, pneumonia, etc. In all these conditions the primary disease is obvious. There are, however, certain infections in which vomiting and diarrhoea are the predominating signs and, therefore, unless specifically looked for, the existence of the primary disease may in these cases not be realised. Thus infections of the ear (otitis media), the urine (pyelitis) and the throat (tonsillitis) may all appear to be cases of gastroenteritis.

Parenteral gastroenteritis usually responds to treatment of the primary disease, but where the vomiting and diarrhoea are severe it may be necessary to give weaker milk feeds. In the less common cases where the gastroenteritis is very severe, with dehydration also present, the treatment is the same as for acute infectious gastroenteritis.

(b) *Enteral gastroenteritis.* Gastroenteritis in infants which is due to disease in the gastrointestinal tract is often caused by improper feeding. Simple overfeeding may upset the infant's digestive system and so give rise to colic, vomiting and diarrhoea, whilst too strong a milk mixture or excessive use of sugar in the feeds is also a common cause of gastroenteritis. These dietetic forms of gastroenteritis usually rapidly respond to correct feeding.

Much more serious are the acute forms of gastroenteritis caused by intestinal infections, the commonest of which are acute bacillary dysentery (usually due in infants to the Sonne organism) and acute infective gastroenteritis (summer or epidemic diarrhoea). Severe enteritis may develop during the administration of the tetracycline antibiotics (p. 56). Acute bacillary dysentery is discussed on page 82.

ACUTE INFECTIVE GASTROENTERITIS OF INFANTS
(Summer diarrhoea)

CAUSE AND INCIDENCE. The cause is unknown but is probably some as yet undiscovered organism (although in some cases coliform bacilli have been identified as the cause). Acute infective gastroenteritis is most highly infectious to other infants, and if a case occurs in a ward or nursery it can spread with lightning rapidity to the other children. It is most prevalent in the summer months when the weather is hot, and for this reason is often known as summer diarrhoea. In an epidemic there may be many serious cases with fatal results. Again, it can complicate other diseases in infants, especially whooping-cough and measles. Infection is probably spread through lack of cleanliness in preparing a feed, bad hygienic conditions, overcrowding and flies.

Symptoms and signs

1. The disease is usually seen in children under 2 and is particularly serious in infants under 1 year. It is a much less common and serious disease in breast fed as opposed to artificially fed infants.

2. The onset may be very abrupt, the infant being well one moment and in a matter of hours seriously ill. The severity of the attack varies from a mild rapidly cured condition to a fulminating fatal disease.

3. The infant vomits his feeds and this vomiting is persistent. Diarrhoea sets in quickly and the stools are characteristically frequent, watery and green in colour. In severe cases the stools may be a bright orange colour and extremely frequent.

4. The infant is very lethargic and signs of dehydration rapidly appear in any severe case, i.e. the eyes become sunken, the fontanelle depressed and the skin when pinched remains in a fold. The whole aspect of the child is one of severe toxicity and lethargy. Fever may also be present.

5. Bronchopneumonia is a common complication.

Treatment

Acute infective gastroenteritis must be treated as a *medical emergency* for two reasons:
1. To prevent spread to other children.
2. To prevent the disease becoming worse with the consequential great risk of a fatal outcome.

1. TO PREVENT THE SPREAD OF THE DISEASE

The strictest isolation precautions must be taken at once. The first signs of green watery stools in a child in any institution calls for immediate isolation. This point cannot be stressed too much and its importance must be fully understood. Full isolation technique as described on page 61 must be undertaken. Gowns, masks and gloves must be worn, and the nurse must pay particular attention to washing her hands after attending to the infant. A receptacle containing a disinfectant, in which to put all soiled napkins and linen, must be placed beside the cot. The nurse who attends to the child's toilet should not also handle bottles, teats or the feeding utensils either of the affected infant or other children.

2. CURATIVE MEASURES

(a) *Warmth.* The infant must be nursed in a warm well-ventilated room. Adequate warmth is essential.

(b) *Initial period of starvation.* This is necessary in all cases, and during this time only boiled water, glucose water or some such solution as Hartmann's is given by mouth. The total amount of fluid required in the 24 hours should be calculated on the basis of 165 ml of fluid per kg body-weight plus an additional amount of 150 to 450 ml to overcome any existing dehydration. Thus an infant of 4·5 kg needs 4·5 × 165 = 750 ml approximately of fluid plus the amount necessary to overcome the dehydration.

These feeds must be given in small frequent amounts to prevent recurrence of the vomiting and also to avoid tiring the infant. To carry out these measures will call for all the skill and attention that the nurse can give. Usually the feeds are given at three or four hourly intervals.

(c) *Treatment of dehydration.* To infants with severe dehydration, i.e. with marked lethargy, sunken eyes, depressed fontanelle and pinched skin, fluid must be given by the intravenous route as soon as possible. Delay in giving intravenous fluid in these cases can be fatal. Intravenous therapy is also necessary in those cases where even boiled water is not tolerated by mouth. Half-strength saline, glucose-saline and Hartmann's solution are the usual types of fluid given intravenously.

(d) *Feeding.* After the preliminary period of starvation, which usually varies from 12 to 36 hours according to the persistence of vomiting and the frequency of stools, milk feeds are started. At first one part of milk diluted in three or four parts of water is given, as the infant will not tolerate stronger feeds. If the infant keeps down the feeds, then the concentration of milk in each feed is gradually increased until finally the infant is taking full strength milk mixtures appropriate to his age. It usually takes approximately two to three days to re-establish normal feeds.

Breast milk is the ideal milk for an infant, but when an infant who is artificially fed is recovering from an attack of gastro-enteritis, it is best to keep him on a half-cream milk for a short period as too much fat is not well tolerated.

(e) *Drugs.* Different antibiotics have been used with success in some cases of infective gastroenteritis. Oral neomycin has proved of value in cases due to coliform organisms. Oral streptomycin, chloramphenicol and the tetracycline antibiotics may be useful in others.

ULCERATIVE COLITIS

In ulcerative colitis there is severe inflammation with ulceration of the mucous membrane affecting the rectum and the whole colon. The cause is not known.

Symptoms and signs

1. The disease is most common in young and middle-aged people. It is a chronic condition which may temporarily clear up spontaneously or under treatment, only to recur.

2. Chronic diarrhoea, with watery stools containing blood and mucus, is the main complaint. In severe cases the stools may be as frequent as ten to twenty a day and may consist entirely of blood and pus with no faecal matter.

3. Abdominal colic sometimes accompanies the diarrhoea and the abdomen may be very tender to the touch.

4. In a severe case, the patient is toxic, wasted and anaemic.

DIAGNOSIS

The diagnosis is usually easily made on the characteristic symptoms and confirmed by *sigmoidoscopy.* A sigmoidoscope is a flexible tube with a light attached, by means of which the lower colon can be seen. In cases of ulcerative colitis the mucous

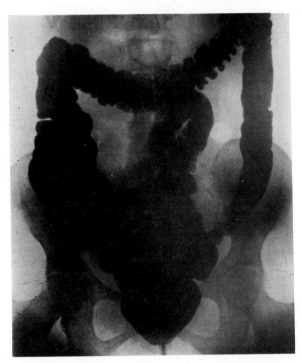

FIG. 7.11   X-ray (barium enema) showing the appearance of the normal colon.

membrane will appear grossly inflamed and ulcerated. A sigmoido-scopy is also an important means of excluding other causes of chronic diarrhoea with the passage of blood in the stools, especially carcinoma of the lower colon. A rectal biopsy can be taken and the small fragment removed can be examined under the microscope: the mucosa (lining of the bowel) can be seen to be abnormal and inflamed.

A barium enema X-ray will show the extent and degree to which the colon is affected. The colon looks narrowed and does not contract normally.

The stool must be examined in the laboratory to exclude disorders such as amoebic dysentery. The blood picture must also be taken to reveal the extent to which the patient is anaemic.

Complications

1. *Haemorrhage.* Moderate bleeding from the bowel is common in ulcerative colitis but occasionally a massive and life-threatening haemorrhage can occur.

2. *Perforation.* In acute cases, the bowel becomes distended and erosion of the mucosa may lead to perforation and peritonitis.

3. *Carcinoma.* After many years, chronic ulcerative colitis may give rise to carcinoma of the colon.

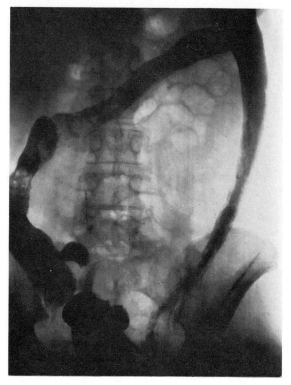

Fig. 7.12 X-ray (barium enema) from a severe case of chronic ulcerative colitis showing the narrowed tubular appearance of the colon and the absence of the normal haustral markings.

Treatment of ulcerative colitis

Ulcerative colitis can be a chronic disorder and even when apparently cured for many years is liable to relapse. However, many patients never have further trouble after the initial attack so there is every reason to adopt an optimistic attitude. Some patients with ulcerative colitis have underlying anxiety as to the nature of their illness and as to their future. The nurse should report fears expressed by the patient. Records must be kept of the nature and number of stools passed and whether the stools contain blood or mucus. In acute cases the fluid intake and output should also be monitored.

REST

In an acute phase, particularly when the temperature is raised and the diarrhoea is severe, the patient should be nursed in bed, usually in hospital. The period of bed rest will be determined by progress and in a severe case several weeks may be necessary.

DIET

In the acute phase, the diet is likely to be determined by what the patient can manage so that heavy meals should be avoided. In the long term, a diet containing sufficient protein and high in roughage is more likely to be beneficial than the low residue diet previously recommended. Adequate fibre in the diet (see page 386) adds bulk to the intestinal contents and is less likely to lead to loss of fluid and undue intestinal contractions. The patient soon learns that some types of food give rise to diarrhoea in her case and so will avoid them.

DRUGS

1. Cortisone and other steroid preparations are the most effective remedy in the acute phase. Prednisolone given by mouth in adequate doses reduces the inflammation of the colonic mucous membrane with relief of constitutional symptoms and control of the diarrhoea. Unfortunately, when prednisolone is taken for long periods, side effects prove troublesome (see page 458) so that steroids are not advised for long-term treatment.

When the rectum is particularly involved, prednisolone can be administered in the form of a suppository or as an enema. The enemata are supplied in plastic containers with nozzle attached. The patient can be taught to insert the lubricated nozzle into the rectum, best done while lying on the left side, and the solution then squeezed in. The nozzle and bag are then discarded and the patient lies on her front for about half an hour before going to sleep.

2. Sulphasalazine (Salazopyrin) is a combination of a salicylate and a sulphonamide and is effective as long-term treatment for suppressing

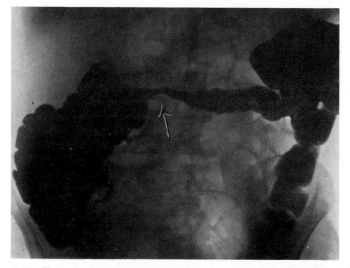

FIG. 7.13   X-ray (barium enema) showing an obstruction with narrowing of the gut in the region of the hepatic flexure of the colon, due to a carcinomatous stricture.

diarrhoea and abdominal colic in ulcerative colitis. It is given by mouth, usually 1 g three times a day initially and the dose can be reduced gradually if symptoms do not recur. The drug sometimes gives rise to nausea.

3. Diazepam 2 mg three times a day, is very useful for allaying the anxiety and nervous tension seen in these patients.

4. Codeine and belladonna are useful to relieve the abdominal colic. Hot stupes and hot-water bottles also help to relieve abdominal pain.

5. Iron is given for the anaemia.

6. Vitamins. The diet should contain all the necessary vitamins, but if necessary extra supplies of vitamins should be given. Vitamins B and K are particularly likely to be deficient.

BLOOD TRANSFUSIONS

Blood transfusions may in some cases bring about a useful remission of symptoms. Anaemia delays healing of the ulcerated bowel. Transfusions may, therefore, be tried in severe cases who have become anaemic and are not responding to the other measures mentioned above.

GENERAL MEASURES

Owing to the chronic and relapsing nature of the illness and the anxiety factor which is usually present, patients with ulcerative colitis demand all the understanding and continual reassurance which the doctor and the nurse can give. A sympathetic and kindly nurse can do much to help these patients through a tiresome and trying illness.

SURGICAL MEASURES

Surgery is indicated:
(a) Where medical treatment, after adequate trial, has failed and the patient suffers chronic ill-health.
(b) In long-standing cases where carcinoma is suspected.
(c) In cases of intestinal obstruction due to strictures formed in healing of the ulcers.

The surgical treatment usually carried out is removal of the affected portion of the colon (*colectomy*), leaving the patient with a permanent *ileostomy*. The patient wears a permanent appliance over the opening and the bag is emptied two or three times a day. The patient can lead a normal and active life and can take a full diet.

CROHN'S DISEASE (Regional ileitis)

Crohn's disease is difficult to distinguish from ulcerative colitis in many cases because the symptoms are often similar. It affects mainly the terminal ileum but also the colon, and leads to areas of thickening and rigidity of the bowel. Strictures and adhesions are common so that loops of bowel become matted together to form palpable masses which obstruct bowel movement.

Signs and symptoms

As with ulcerative colitis, chronic diarrhoea and abdominal colic are common symptoms. In addition, however, intestinal obstruction may occur with severe pain and vomiting. These symptoms may be associated with fever and considerable loss of weight. Bleeding from the rectum is not uncommon, sometimes associated with abscess formation in the rectum or anal region.

DIAGNOSIS. A barium enema X-ray may show areas of the colon or ileum to be narrowed and thickened.

Treatment

DIET

In some patients the diarrhoea may respond to milk restriction but in general the diet is as in ulcerative colitis.

DRUGS

Codeine (60 mg three times daily) may help the diarrhoea.

Steroids such as prednisone can be used to tide the patient over a severe attack.

SURGERY

Surgery may become obligatory when intestinal obstruction or abscess formation occurs and indeed the majority of patients with Crohn's disease require surgery at some stage of the ailment. The obstructed area of bowel has to be resected but unfortunately in some patients the condition recurs after a time in some other part of the bowel.

IRRITABLE BOWEL SYNDROME

This term is applied to many patients, commonly young women, who complain of frequent attacks of diarrhoea, abdominal discomfort, flatulence and a sense of distension in the abdomen. Investigations including examination of the stools, sigmoidoscopy and barium enema do not reveal any organic disease and the disorder is regarded as emotional in origin.

Reassurance and explanation are often helpful and a discussion as to possible social or domestic stresses may give a lead as to the nature of the disorder.

CARCINOMA OF THE COLON

Carcinoma of the colon is usually dealt with in full in textbooks on surgery, but as the condition may be seen in medical wards during the preliminary stages of investigation, a brief word on the disease is advisable here.

Carcinoma of the colon is most frequently seen in middle-aged or elderly people, but it can arise in young people.

Symptoms and signs

The main symptom is an increasing degree of constipation which characteristically alternates with bouts of diarrhoea. Abdominal colic is usually present. If the growth is in the rectum or sigmoid colon, bright red blood may be passed with the motion. If the carcinoma is higher up, the blood in the faeces is not usually visible to the naked eye, but may be detected by a chemical examination for occult blood.

In some patients the first sign of an intestinal growth may be an attack of acute intestinal obstruction with vomiting, absolute constipation, abdominal distension and pain. In advanced cases of carcinoma of the colon, wasting and anaemia are present.

Diagnosis

This is usually made on the symptoms of alternating constipation and diarrhoea, abdominal colic and, in many cases, the presence of visible or occult blood in the faeces. If the carcinoma is in the rectum a digital examination will reveal a palpable hard mass. A sigmoidoscopy will detect a growth situated in the pelvic or sigmoid colon.

An X-ray examination (*barium enema*) is most useful in confirming the diagnosis, and the barium is usually held up at the site of the growth.

The treatment of carcinoma of the colon is surgical, consisting of removal whenever possible.

MALABSORPTION SYNDROME

This condition is due to failure of the small intestine to absorb the products of digestion. Fat appears prominently in the stools, so that the condition is often called *steatorrhoea*; but this is only one aspect of malabsorption, since glucose, vitamins, minerals and other foodstuffs are also poorly absorbed. Three clinical states are included under this heading:

1. *Coeliac disease*, occurring mainly in children but also in adults. This has been shown to be due to an intolerance of gluten, a protein in wheat and certain other cereals. As a result of this idiosyncrasy the small intestine fails to function properly when gluten is present in the diet.

2. *Idiopathic steatorrhoea* in adults. Here the cause of the malabsorption is usually unknown, though damage to the small intestine by such diseases as tuberculosis or malignant infiltration may sometimes give rise to this condition.

3. *Tropical sprue*, occurring especially in India and China, is also of unknown origin.

Symptoms and signs

1. The patients are undernourished, wasted and easily fatigued. Loss of appetite is a marked feature. Children with coeliac disease show abdominal distension and fail to grow and thrive.

2. The characteristic feature is a chronic diarrhoea with very large, bulky, pale, offensive stools. The appearance of the stools is due to the large excess of fat which they contain.

3. Many complications may arise which are best described according to their cause:

(a) Deficient absorption of the following *vitamins*:

    (i) Folic acid and vitamin B_{12}, resulting in a pernicious (macrocytic) type of anaemia.

    (ii) Vitamin D—causing rickets in children and osteomalacia in adults. The vitamin D deficiency is also responsible, in conjunction with a deficient absorption of calcium, for the tetany seen in sprue.

    (iii) Vitamin B complex—causing a sore tongue (glossitis) and peripheral neuritis.

    (iv) Vitamin K resulting in prothrombin deficiency and haemorrhagic manifestations.

(b) Deficient absorption of *minerals*:

    (i) Iron, causing a hypochromic anaemia.

    (ii) Calcium, causing tetany and softening of the bones (osteomalacia).

(c) The combination of the deficient absorption of fats, carbohydrates, minerals and vitamins causes the lack of growth and infantilism seen in children with coeliac disease.

Treatment

During the active stages of the disease, bed rest is essential to rapid recovery. Diet is of the utmost importance. In coeliac disease the main essential is to exclude the wheat protein, gluten, and this is achieved by cutting out from the diet all articles made with wheat flour and by using instead corn flour or soya bean flour. When gluten is excluded from the diet, children with coeliac disease are able to tolerate fat in the diet to a much greater degree. In sprue, it has not yet been proved that a gluten-free diet is as beneficial as in coeliac disease.

The diet in idiopathic steatorrhoea and coeliac disease should contain a high protein, low starch and low fat content as well as excluding gluten. All the missing vitamins must be given, especially A, D, B complex and K. Calcium should also be added to the diet. Food is best given in small amounts at frequent intervals, the amount being gradually increased as the condition improves.

Folic acid (and in some cases vitamin B_{12}) is most useful, especially when a macrocytic anaemia is present. If a hypochromic anaemia is present this denotes a deficiency of iron, and ferrous succinate or ferrous gluconate will be given.

ACUTE INTUSSUSCEPTION

Acute intussusception (which almost invariably arises in infants) is described in surgical textbooks, but mention is made of the condition here because it can be mistaken for acute bacillary dysentery in infants. In intussusception, part of the intestine becomes invaginated into the intestine immediately below it. The invaginated part of the intestine can then travel onwards for a considerable distance in the gut. The result of intussusception is to produce an acute intestinal obstruction. An intussusception usually starts in the region of the lower end of the ileum near the ileocaecal valve.

Symptoms and signs

1. Breast-fed infants under 1 year are usually affected.

2. The onset is sudden with abdominal colic, the infant having attacks of screaming and drawing up its legs.

3. Vomiting starts early and is severe and repeated.

4. After the first motion the infant passes only pure blood and mucus from the bowel—the 'red-currant jelly' stool.

5. A typical sausage-shaped tumour is usually palpable in the abdomen. This tumour is the invaginated portion of the intestine. On rectal examination the lower end of the invaginated bowel may in some cases be felt. The finger when withdrawn will be covered in blood.

Diagnosis and treatment

Intussusception must be distinguished from the other acute illnesses in infants in which blood and mucus are passed in the stools. Acute bacillary dysentery (usually due to the Sonne bacillus) is the condition which is most likely to be confused with acute intussusception. In the dysentery cases, however, the vomiting and the screaming attacks of colic are slight or absent and an abdominal tumour is not felt.

The treatment of intussusception is immediate operation to relieve the obstruction. The invaginated portion of intestine is 'milked back', great care being needed to prevent the bowel tearing. If, as happens in some cases, the bowel is gangrenous, then resection of the gangrenous part is necessary.

TUBERCULOSIS OF THE INTESTINES

Tuberculosis of the intestines falls more conveniently into the same section as tuberculous peritonitis (p. 241).

MEGACOLON

Megacolon, which is also known as *Hirschsprung's disease*, is a relatively rare condition. It occurs both in children (when, for some unknown reason, it is nearly always boys who are affected) and adults. In megacolon, due to disturbance in the nerve supply, part of the colon in the rectosigmoid region becomes narrowed and thickened with the result that the bowel above the contracted segment becomes enormously dilated.

The cardinal signs of megacolon are extreme constipation and abdominal distension. In children the symptoms date from soon after birth, and in severe cases the abdomen becomes enormously distended with coils of bowel visible through the abdominal wall. Evacuation of the bowel may take place only at intervals of weeks, and in these severe cases death can ensue from toxaemia and intestinal obstruction. X-ray examination (barium enema) reveals the grossly distended large bowel.

Treatment of megacolon consists of resection of the narrowed segment of the colon (rectosigmoidectomy).

INTESTINAL WORMS (Helminths)

Worms often inhabit the intestinal tract. Those most commonly found in Western countries are:

1. Threadworms
2. Roundworms
3. Tapeworms.

In tropical countries there are many other types of worms as well which cause serious ill-health, with severe anaemia as a particular feature.

Threadworms

Threadworm infection is extremely common, especially in children, the tiny white worms being seen in the faeces or around the anus. Marked perianal itching is present. The child becomes infected by swallowing the eggs (ova). Continuous reinfection takes place through the child scratching the anus and thereby infecting the hands.

Treatment

As most of the children and even adults in the family are usually infected with threadworms at the same time, it is most important for all members of the family to be examined and for those infected to be treated together: failing this, reinfection will take place.

1. ERADICATION OF THE WORMS. A suitable anthelmintic⸴ (drug which kills worms) is given after the bowels have been well opened by a mild purgative. Piperazine is at present the drug of choice. Piperazine citrate (Antepar) is given in doses of 50 to 75 mg for each kilogram of body-weight daily for seven days. The maximum dose for an adult is 1 g twice daily. With piperazine adipate (Entacyl) the usual dose is 200 mg for each year of age up to a maximum of 1·2 g daily for patients over the age of six. Alternatively piperazine may be given in one single large dose of 3 g for a child aged two to five years. A useful preparation for this purpose is piperazine combined with Senokot (Pripsen).

2. PREVENTION OF REINFECTION. This is most important. The anal region must be properly cleansed after each motion and mercury ointment applied. The hands must be washed after visiting the toilet. The child's nails must be cut short, while painting with iodine will prevent the fingers being sucked and so causing reinfection. Wearing gloves at night also helps to prevent scratching. The underclothes, night attire and linen should be boiled after all infected members of the family have been treated.

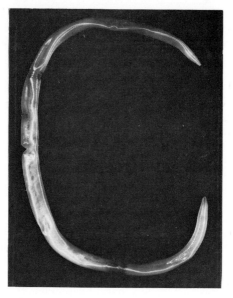

FIG. 7.14   Roundworm.

Roundworms *(Ascaris lumbricoides)*

Roundworm infection results from eating or drinking contaminated food (particularly raw vegetables and salads) or water. The worms mainly inhabit the intestines, but occasionally invade the bile ducts, liver or trachea. In adults the main symptoms are abdominal pain, diarrhoea or constipation, while in infants, enuresis (bed-wetting) and convulsions are common. With many patients the first sign is the presence of the worms in the motions. Piperazine is usually given in a single large dose up to a maximum of 3 g for an adult.

Tapeworms

Tapeworm infection occurs in both adults and children. There are two common types: *Taenia saginata* derived from infected cattle and *Taenia solium* from infected pigs. Man becomes infected through eating infected meat or pork which has been insufficiently cooked. Adequate cooking of meat and pork destroys the worms.

Tapeworms grow to a length of many feet. The worm, which has a flat white appearance, is made up of a head and individual small segments which usually drop off in turn and are passed in the faeces. The symptoms of tapeworm infection are slight, usually consisting of excessive appetite, mild abdominal colic and perhaps some loss of weight.

Treatment

There are several effective anthelmintics available for the treatment of tapeworm.

1. Niclosamide (Yomesan). Two tablets (each 0·5 g) are chewed and swallowed with a few sips of water before breakfast, and a further two tablets are taken similarly an hour later. The worm tends to disintegrate so that the head (scolax) cannot as a rule be identified in the stools.

2. Mepacrine. For the day before treatment the patient is kept on a light diet and a saline purgative is given in the evening. Only fluids are taken next morning and two doses of 0·5 g of mepacrine are given at an hourly interval. Two hours after the second dose, a saline purgative (e.g. 15 ml magnesium sulphate) is given. The head of the worm can be identified in the stools on the day of treatment.

3. Dichlorophen (Anthiphen). Four tablets (each 0·5 g) are given three times a day on two consecutive days.

4. Filix mas (male fern) is an old-fashioned remedy most suitable for *Taenia solium*. The patient has to be prepared for 48 hours by fluid diet and saline purges, and felix mas then administered in three separate doses of 2·5 ml at intervals of a quarter of an hour. A further purge is then given, and the scolax can be found in the subsequent motions.

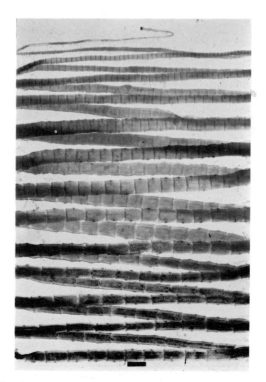

Fig. 7.15   Tapeworm.

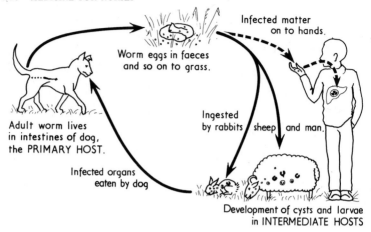

Fig. 7.16   Hydatid cysts.

Hydatid cysts

Hydatid disease is rare in this country but is seen in visitors from abroad, particularly Australia and the Middle East. The worm, taenia echinococcus, is small (about 0·5 cm long) and lives in the intestine of the dog. The eggs which it passes in the faeces contaminate material ingested by man, sheep and rabbits, who are the intermediate hosts. The ova are transferred into a larval state in the intestine. The larvae penetrate the intestinal wall and enter various organs, especially the liver, where cysts are formed. Dogs eat the infected viscera of sheep and rabbits, the worms develop in the dog (primary host) and so the cycle continues.

Clinical features

Cysts in the liver may grow to a great size leading to abdominal swelling and discomfort: sometimes pressure on the bile ducts causes jaundice.

The diagnosis should be suspected in a patient from abroad with a large liver. Surgical treatment is sometimes needed to remove the cyst.

DISEASES OF THE PERITONEUM

PERITONITIS

Inflammation of the peritoneum (peritonitis) is often seen as the result of a spread of infection from the intestinal tract or pelvic organs. Most cases of acute peritonitis are caused by such surgical conditions as acute appendicitis, perforated peptic ulcer or acute salpingitis (inflammation of the Fallopian tubes). Rarer types of acute peritonitis are those due to perforation of a typhoid ulcer in the intestines and the primary pneumococcal peritonitis usually resulting from a generalised blood-stream infection.

Apart from the above forms of acute peritonitis, which are mainly surgical problems, there remains tuberculous peritonitis, which is essentially a medical condition and is, therefore, dealt with in more detail.

Tuberculous peritonitis

Tuberculous peritonitis is often seen in children as a result of the drinking of infected milk. The bovine tubercle bacilli penetrate the intestinal wall to reach the mesenteric lymph glands, whereupon the tuberculous glands frequently set up a tuberculous peritonitis by direct spread of the infection.

In adult women, tuberculous peritonitis is not uncommonly caused by the spread of infection from tuberculosis of the Fallopian tubes (tuberculous salpingitis).

Symptoms and signs

Tuberculous peritonitis varies in its onset from a slow gradual process to a much more acute attack.

1. Abdominal pain and signs of general ill-health are the main features in the early stages. Loss of weight and appetite with a persisting low-grade fever are usually present.

2. Constipation often alternating with diarrhoea occurs.

3. The abdomen may be distended owing to the presence of a large amount of fluid in the peritoneal cavity (*ascites*). This form of tuberculous peritonitis is spoken of as the ascitic type. In other cases the abdomen is not distended with fluid but is characteristically described as doughy to the touch.

Course and treatment

Treatment, as in all forms of tuberculosis, consists of rest and a prolonged course of chemotherapy. The general treatment is as outlined on page 182 and the outlook is good.

The ascites seldom becomes so great that a paracentesis abdominis has to be performed to relieve the distension.

ASCITES

Ascites is the presence of fluid in the peritoneal cavity, and may be caused by many different types of disease bearing little relation to each other. It is convenient, therefore, to summarise the main types of ascites according to the causative diseases.

Causes of ascites

Congestive heart failure

This is the commonest cause of an ascites and the fluid present is part of a general oedema. Oedema of the legs and a 'sacral pad' are

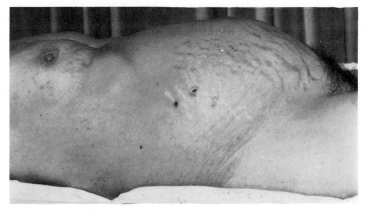

FIG. 7.17 Ascites. The abdomen is grossly distended. The two puncture marks from the paracentesis can be clearly seen.

also present. The ascites in heart failure may require tapping (paracentesis abdominis), when the fluid removed will be clear yellow in colour.

Diseases of the peritoneum

1. Tuberculous peritonitis. The ascites is accompanied by a general wasting, fever and diarrhoea. The fluid seldom needs tapping.

2. Secondary carcinoma of the peritoneum caused by spread (metastases) from other organs, particularly the ovaries, stomach and intestines. Malignant peritonitis causes a rapid and large ascites that needs frequent tapping. The general condition of the patient is poor, severe wasting and anaemia being present. Treatment is directed towards the patient's comfort but in some cases cytotoxic drugs (such as nitrogen mustard) or radioactive gold can be injected into the peritoneum in the hope of counteracting the malignant cells.

Diseases of the liver

1. Carcinoma of the liver, usually the result of spread from other organs such as the lungs, stomach or intestines.

2. Cirrhosis of the liver. Ascites is present in the late stages of most cases of cirrhosis. It is caused by pressure on the portal vein from the fibrous tissue in the liver. Enlarged veins are often present in the abdominal wall (caput medusae).

Nephritis

Ascites, as part of a general oedema, is sometimes present in cases of nephritis, particularly in the oedematous forms of chronic nephritis.

CHARACTER OF THE STOOLS IN DISEASE

Number

The number of stools passed in the day varies from person to person. On an average the bowels are opened once a day, but constipation is not necessarily present if the bowels are not opened daily. Frequent motions which are also semiformed or watery are seen in diarrhoea.

Colour

Normal stools are dark brown owing to the presence of stercobilin (altered bilirubin).

1. *Pale stools* are seen:
    (a) When no bile reaches the intestine, e.g. the clay-coloured stools of obstructive jaundice.
    (b) If excessive fat is present, e.g. in the malabsorption syndrome.
    (c) In patients on a purely milk diet.
2. *Black stools* are due to:
    (a) Administration of iron, bismuth or charcoal.
    (b) Altered blood from bleeding in the upper intestinal tract, i.e. the black tarry stools of melaena.
3. *Green stools.* The stools may be green in colour when there is severe acute diarrhoea due to inflammation of the small intestine. Green stools are particularly characteristic of the acute infective gastroenteritis of infants.

Consistency and formation

1. In constipation the stools are hard, dry and often in the shape of round balls known as scybala.
2. In all types of diarrhoea the stools are unformed, whilst in extreme cases the stools are watery and contain little faecal matter. For instance, in the tropical disease, cholera, where diarrhoea is intense, the stools are watery, colourless and contain mucus—the 'rice-water' stools of cholera.
3. Stools containing a great deal of mucus are 'slimy' in appearance.
4. Ribbon-shaped stools are seen in intestinal obstruction, e.g. in carcinoma of the bowel.
5. In typhoid fever the stools are characteristically described as 'pea-soup' stools.

Abnormal substances in the stools

Undigested food and curds. In diarrhoea undigested particles of food may appear in the stools. During infancy, curds may be seen when the protein or fat is not properly digested. Protein curds are yellow or white in colour and large and hard—sinking in water. Fat curds are also yellow or white, but are smaller and softer—floating in water. In patients on a milk diet, curds due to undigested protein may appear in the stool; if so, citrate should be added to the milk or the amount reduced.

Blood. The appearance of the stool with blood in it varies according to the site of the bleeding in the gastrointestinal tract and also, of course, according to the amount of blood present.

(a) A large haemorrhage from the upper part of the gastro-intestinal tract (usually due to peptic ulcer) produces black tarry stools—*melaena*. A small haemorrhage from the upper gastrointestinal tract causes little change that is visible to the naked eye and chemical tests are necessary to detect the presence of blood (*occult blood*).

(b) Blood from the large intestine is usually bright red in colour. If the bleeding is in the upper part of the large intestine the blood may be partially mixed with faecal matter. Bleeding from the rectum (usually due to haemorrhoids, carcinoma or anal fissure) produces a streaking of the outside of the motion.

(c) Blood accompanied by mucus or pus is seen in severe inflammation of the intestines, e.g. in dysentery and ulcerative colitis. In very severe cases no faecal matter may be present, the stools consisting of blood and mucopus only.

(d) Pure blood and mucus with no faecal matter are passed in acute intussusception in infants, producing the 'red-currant jelly' stool characteristic of intussusception.

Mucus. The presence of mucus in the faeces indicates disease, usually an inflammation in the large bowel. Mucus, which gives the stool a 'slimy' appearance, may be on the outside of the motion or mixed with it. Mucus may be present alone in less severe degrees of inflammation of the large bowel, but it is usually accompanied by blood in such diseases as ulcerative colitis and dysentery. As already stated the 'red-currant jelly' motion of acute intussusception consists of pure blood and mucus.

Pus. Pus, either as pure pus or muco-pus, is present in the stools in severe inflammation and ulceration of the large bowel, i.e. in severe cases of dysentery and ulcerative colitis.

Parasites. The commonest parasites found in the faeces in Western countries as opposed to tropical countries are the intestinal worms, especially threadworms, roundworms and tapeworms.

SUMMARY OF SOME ROUTINE PROCEDURES UNDERTAKEN IN DISEASES OF THE ALIMENTARY SYSTEM

1. Faeces examination

(a) For occult blood.

    (i) In peptic ulcer, to exclude haemorrhage and to follow progress of healing in cases of haemorrhage.

    (ii) In all suspected cases of bleeding from the gastro-intestinal tract, especially carcinoma of stomach and bowel.

(b) Bacteriological examination. In cases of acute diarrhoea, particularly when the presence of enteric, food-poisoning and dysentery organisms is suspected..

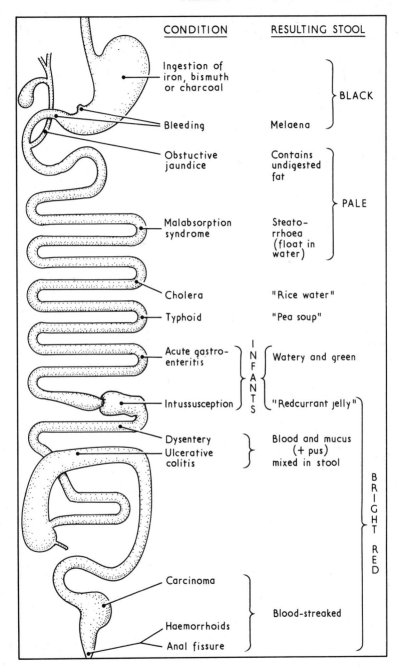

Fig. 7.18   Characteristics of the stools in various ailments.

(c) For parasites. In cases of intestinal worms.

(d) Fat estimation. In the malabsorption syndrome. (In normal people the daily excretion of fat in the stools seldom exceeds 5 g.)

2. X-ray examination

(a) Barium swallow, to exclude any disease of the oesophagus, particularly when dysphagia is a symptom.

(b) Barium meal, in cases of dyspepsia, to confirm or exclude peptic ulcer, carcinoma of stomach and pyloric stenosis.

(c) Barium enema, to diagnose particularly carcinoma of the intestines; also in cases of colitis, diverticulitis, persistent chronic diarrhoea and constipation.

3. Test meal

(a) In peptic ulcer, where excess of acid is usually present.

(b) In carcinoma of the stomach, where an achlorhydria is common and blood may be present in the gastric specimens.

(c) In the diagnosis of certain anaemias, especially pernicious and simple achlorhydric anaemias, wherein achlorhydria is always present.

(d) To estimate the amount of resting juice and delay in emptying in cases of suspected pyloric stenosis.

4. Sigmoidoscopy

In the diagnosis of chronic diarrhoea, particularly in cases of ulcerative colitis and carcinoma of the lower colon.

5. Oesophagoscopy

(a) In the diagnosis of dysphagia, especially to exclude carcinoma of the oesophagus.

(b) To remove a foreign body lodged in the oesophagus.

6. Gastroscopy

The fibre-optic gastroscope is flexible and easy to pass. It enables the operator to perform a biopsy of any suspicious area under direct vision.

(a) In the diagnosis of gastric ulcer and gastric carcinoma.

(b) In the diagnosis of anastomotic ulcer.

7. Colonoscopy

In the diagnosis of polyps, carcinoma or inflammatory disease especially in the sigmoid and ascending colon.

8 Diseases of the Liver, Biliary Tract and Pancreas

ANATOMY AND PHYSIOLOGY

Both anatomically and physiologically the liver and biliary systems are intimately connected. The liver, which is situated beneath the right leaf of the diaphragm, is composed of two main types of cells:

1. The hepatic cells, which are the main excretory cells of the liver.
2. The Kupffer cells, which are entirely different from the hepatic cells and belong to the specialised system known as the reticulo-endothelial system.

Running between the liver cells are the small bile capillaries which merge together to form larger ducts which ultimately form one large duct—the common hepatic duct. The common hepatic duct joins with the cystic duct from the gall-bladder to form the common bile duct which opens into the duodenum. The gall-bladder acts as a reservoir where the bile can be stored and where it is also concentrated.

MAIN FUNCTIONS OF THE LIVER

1. Bile metabolism

(a) BILE PIGMENTS. The red blood cells have a normal life of about 120 days, after which they become worn out and are destroyed by the reticulo-endothelial system. In the course of their destruction bile pigments are formed of which the pigment *bilirubin* is the most important. This bilirubin is excreted by the hepatic cells of the liver into the biliary tract and eventually emptied into the duodenum. In the intestine the bilirubin is, in a changed form, known as stercobilin, and gives the faeces their normal dark brown colour. In the absence of stercobilin the faeces are pale. In addition to being excreted in the faeces a small amount of the biliary pigment stercobilin is reabsorbed back into the blood stream from the intestines, to be partially excreted in the urine. This small amount of pigment which is excreted in the urine is given the name urobilin, although it is in fact identical with stercobilin. In normal health the amount of

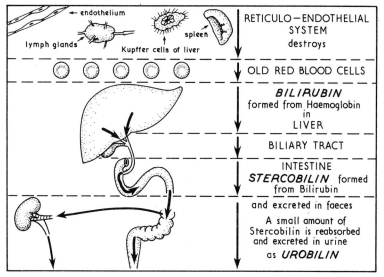

FIG. 8.1   Normal bile pigment formation and circulation.

urobilin present in the urine is too small to be found on ordinary routine examination.

(*b*) BILE SALTS. These are formed by the hepatic cells and together with the bile pigments pass into the common hepatic duct, are stored in the gall-bladder and are eventually emptied into the duodenum. The bile salts are most important in aiding the proper absorption and digestion of fats and also in the absorption of vitamin K.

2. Metabolism of carbohydrates

The liver plays a very important role in the metabolism of carbohydrate foodstuffs, as it stores glucose in the form of glycogen to be used as necessary by the body. The liver is thus a great storehouse of energy, as glucose is one of the most important foodstuffs for providing energy.

3. Metabolism of protein

The liver plays an important role in the metabolism of proteins, during which process urea is formed. Urea is excreted as a waste product by the kidneys.

4. Storage of vitamin B_{12}

The liver is the main storage place for vitamin B_{12}, which is essential for the proper formation of the red blood cells.

5. Formation and storage of prothrombin

Vitamin K which is present in certain foods and also manufactured by bacteria in the bowel is absorbed from the intestines to form prothrombin in the liver. Prothrombin is essential for the proper clotting of blood.

JAUNDICE

Before discussing individual diseases affecting the liver and biliary tract it is advisable to explain the main causes and types of jaundice. This is because jaundice is a very common and frequently the predominating sign in most diseases of the liver and biliary tract. Jaundice is the term given to the yellow discoloration of the skin and conjunctiva caused by an excess of bile pigment in the blood stream. This yellowish colour is the clinical sign of jaundice.

TYPES OF JAUNDICE

Jaundice can be divided into two main types, according to the manner in which the excess of bile pigment develops in the blood, known as obstructive and haemolytic.

Obstructive jaundice

In this type excess of bilirubin occurs in the blood stream owing to a blockage or disease in some part of the liver or biliary passages. As the bile cannot pass down its normal channel it is reabsorbed back into the blood stream, thereby giving rise to jaundice.

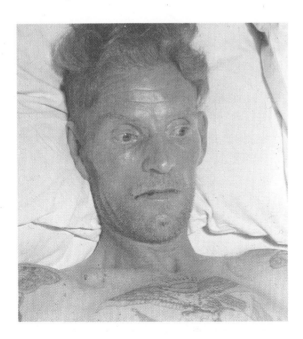

Fig. 8.2   Jaundice.

Causes

1. Obstruction in the ducts
   Gall-stones
   Stricture.
2. Obstruction and pressure on the ducts from outside
   Carcinoma of the head of the pancreas
   Secondary carcinoma in the lymph glands.
3. Obstruction or disease in the liver
   Inflammatory diseases, i.e. hepatitis
   Certain drugs, especially chlorpromazine
   Cirrhosis of the liver
   Carcinoma of the liver.

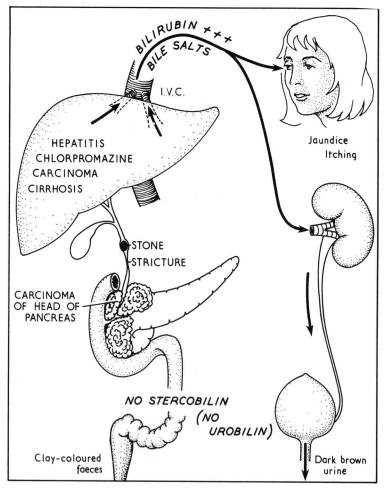

FIG. 8.3   The main causes and features of obstructive jaundice.

Symptoms and signs

1. The jaundice is usually very deep and easily recognisable. It is generally first noticed in the conjunctiva.

2. The faeces are pale. This is because the bilirubin is not reaching the intestine owing to the obstruction. As a result the normal dark brown colour of the faeces, which is due to the bile pigment, is replaced by a clay colour.

3. The urine is dark brown in colour owing to the presence of bilirubin.

4. Pruritus or itching of the skin. The well-marked itching of the skin seen in obstructive jaundice is caused by the accumulation of the bile salts in the blood.

5. In long-standing cases of obstructive jaundice the absence of bile salts, which prevents the absorption of vitamin K from the bowel, leads to prothrombin deficiency. This deficiency causes a prolonged blood clotting time. Prothrombin deficiency is the cause of the excessive bleeding sometimes seen in operations on cases of obstructive jaundice.

Haemolytic jaundice

In haemolytic jaundice the excess of bile pigments in the blood, which gives rise to the jaundice, is not due (as in obstructive jaundice), either to disease in the liver or to obstruction in the biliary passages but to excessive destruction (haemolysis) of the red cells.

Jaundice does not necessarily develop with haemolysis of the red cells because the liver can cope with a certain excess of bile pigments. When the haemolysis goes beyond a certain level, however, the overworked liver cannot deal with the resultant large excess of bile pigment and therefore the bile accumulates in the blood and jaundice develops.

The causes of haemolysis of the red blood cells which may give rise to haemolytic jaundice are fully discussed under Haemolytic Anaemias (Chapter 10).

Symptoms and signs

The factor common to both obstructive and haemolytic jaundice is the presence of excess bile pigment in the blood giving rise to staining of the skin and conjunctiva. There are, however, several differences between the two types of jaundice apart from the different causes. In haemolytic jaundice:

1. As there is no obstruction either in the liver or biliary tracts the bile pigment, stercobilin, is present in the faeces, which are not therefore clay-coloured as in obstructive jaundice. Indeed, as there is an excess of bile formed, the stools are often darker than usual.

2. Bile salts do not accumulate in the blood as in obstructive jaundice and therefore itching of the skin does not arise. (As the bile salts are formed in the liver and there is no obstruction they are excreted in the normal way.)

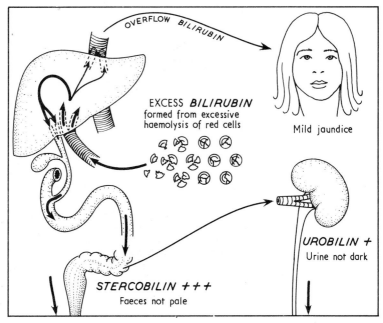

FIG. 8.4   The mechanism of haemolytic jaundice.

3. As there is an excess of the bile pigment, stercobilin (urobilin), in the intestine, there is also a great increase in the amount of stercobilin (urobilin) absorbed from the intestine and excreted in the urine. In haemolytic jaundice, therefore, excess of urobilin is found in the urine but bile itself does not appear.

It is convenient to note here that the commonest causes of jaundice seen in clinical practice are:

(a) Gall-stones, usually in middle age.
(b) Acute infective hepatitis, commonest in younger people.
(c) Carcinoma, especially carcinoma of the head of pancreas, especially in elderly patients.
(d) Drugs such as chlorpromazine which affect the liver.

INDIVIDUAL DISEASES OF THE LIVER

INFECTIOUS HEPATITIS

Infectious hepatitis is an acute inflammation of the liver caused by a virus infection. Two strains of virus have been identified.

Virus A

When present this virus is excreted in the patient's stool. Contaminated water, shellfish or vegetables can provide the source of infection. The incubation period of virus A hepatitis is from 3 to 6 weeks, usually a month.

Virus B

This strain gives rise to serum hepatitis, so-called because it can be spread by inadequately sterilised syringes or needles that have been used for taking blood specimens from an infected patient. Cases have been reported following immunisation, tattooing or acupuncture. Even simple contamination of the fingers with infected blood can lead to hepatitis and outbreaks among nurses and doctors have occurred in units (such as haemodialysis units) which deal with frequent blood transfusions. Since the virus can persist in the serum for many years, all prospective blood donors are tested for this virus before blood is taken. Infection with virus B can be detected by the presence of an antibody first found in an Australian aborigine and called Australian (Au) antigen. Blood with a positive Au antigen cannot be used for transfusion since it would transmit the virus to the recipient.

The use of disposable syringes and needles has done much to reduce the risks of serum hepatitis and special containers should be available on the ward and in outpatients for the disposal of materials likely to be infected.

The incubation period of virus B hepatitis is about 3 to 6 months.

Symptoms and signs

The onset is usually gradual over a matter of days, with marked loss of appetite and nausea as the predominating symptoms, the sight of food, especially fats, being enough to cause nausea or even vomiting. There is a general feeling of being off-colour, with headache and slight pyrexia.

After a few days of these symptoms the urine becomes dark owing to the presence of bile, and the faeces clay-coloured. The conjunctiva and skin become yellow.

The severity of the attack varies: usually it is mild, but in a small percentage of cases the attacks are severe and fulminating, with delirium, high fever and intense jaundice. These cases are exactly the same as those of acute yellow atrophy, where severe liver necrosis is present.

Diagnosis and course

The diagnosis is usually simple. The absence of any severe pain or history of previous attacks of pain usually distinguishes it from the common type of jaundice caused by gall-stones.

Various liver function tests are available which can show whether the jaundice is caused by damage and obstruction in the liver, as in cases of hepatitis, or by obstruction outside the liver, e.g. gall-stones or carcinoma of the head of the pancreas, in which case there is no actual damage to the liver itself. The drawback with these tests is that the liver has to be fairly severely damaged before the tests are positive.

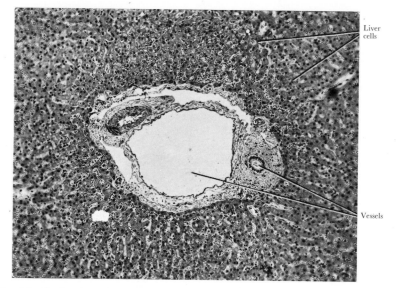

Liver
cells

Vessels

FIG. 8.5   Section through a normal liver.

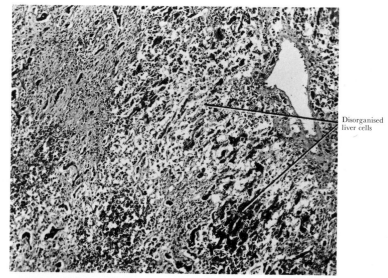

Disorganised
liver cells

FIG. 8.6   Hepatitis. The liver cells have been destroyed and their normal orderly pattern disarranged.

Sometimes a liver biopsy is necessary to determine the diagnosis. A needle is inserted into the liver and a fragment withdrawn. This specimen is examined under the microscope and will show whether the liver cells are inflamed, or whether the damage is due to obstruction. The differentiation is most important for operation may be necessary if obstruction is the cause.

Usually the jaundice subsides in a matter of weeks. Complete recovery occurs in most cases, but in a small minority the jaundice may persist for months or years. The condition known as *chronic active hepatitis* may follow infective hepatitis, though other unknown causes may be responsible. It is a disorder commonest in young women. The liver remains enlarged and the jaundice fails to subside, most patients not surviving more than five years.

Treatment

1. Even in the mildest cases the patient should be put to bed, because rest in bed lessens the damage to the liver and hastens convalescence.

2. As the patient has very little appetite in the early stages, the diet must be very light. Fats are usually not tolerated and so should be omitted. Glucose provides adequate calories and places no strain on the liver, and so is particularly useful, particularly when nausea and vomiting are present. It can be given in flavoured drinks or in milk. The diet can gradually be increased as the jaundice lessens and the appetite improves.

3. When the jaundice is deep and slow to improve, a course of cortisone or prednisone will hasten recovery.

WEIL'S DISEASE (Leptospirosis)

Weil's disease is uncommon except in people whose work brings them in contact with rats (e.g. workers in sewers, miners and fish curers), as the responsible organism, a spirochaete, is excreted in the urine of infected rats. Infection in many may occur by contamination of food or through abrasions in the skin.

Symptoms and signs

1. The disease varies in severity from moderately severe attacks to acute fulminating cases which gravely damage the liver, i.e. acute yellow atrophy.

2. Signs of severe fever with prostration and, in some cases, delirium are present. Severe conjunctivitis is often a feature.

3. An obstructive form of jaundice, with pale stools and dark urine, develops about the fourth day. In addition to the bile in the urine heavy albuminuria is also usually present.

4. In severe cases haemorrhages from the nose, bowel, kidneys or into the skin (purpura) develop. These haemorrhages are often so predominant that Weil's disease is also known as *infective haemorrhagic jaundice*.

Treatment

Treatment is on the lines of that for acute infective hepatitis, with copious fluids and abundant glucose. In addition, the tetracycline antibiotics and penicillin have been found effective in some cases.

CIRRHOSIS OF THE LIVER

In cirrhosis of the liver there is a degeneration of the liver cells and also a dense infiltration of the liver by fibrous tissue, so that the liver cells become strangled and die. The process is usually slowly progressive until in the end the liver ceases to function and death ensues. Cirrhosis is frequently the result of prolonged alcoholism (portral cirrhosis) but it can occur in abstemious people for unknown reasons. Long-standing obstruction of the bile ducts can also lead to liver damage and this is then known as biliary cirrhosis.

Portal cirrhosis

Heavy drinking over the years leads to degeneration and fibrosis of the liver cells, but probably lack of protein and vitamins in the diet is as important a factor as the toxic effects of alcohol. Alcoholics seldom take an adequate diet. In non-alcoholics the cause of cirrhosis is usually obscure, though some cases may be due to imperfect healing of a previous hepatitis.

Symptoms and signs

Most of the symptoms and signs are the result of the obstruction of the various parts of the liver and biliary tract by the contracting fibrous tissue. This may obstruct:

1. The portal vein—causing
   (*a*) Ascites
   (*b*) Congestion of the veins in the intestinal tract (especially

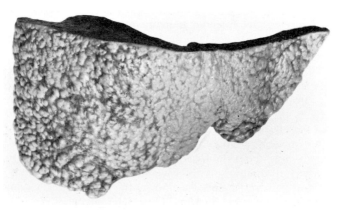

FIG. 8.7 Cirrhosis of the liver showing the typical granular appearance resulting from the excessive fibrous tissue.

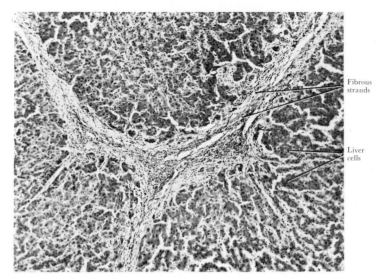

Fibrous
strands

Liver
cells

FIG. 8.8   Cirrhosis of the liver. Section of the liver to show the dense strands of fibrous tissue present. The liver cells are beginning to degenerate.

those in the stomach and rectum), leading to a haematemesis or to the development of haemorrhoids.

2. The bile ducts, causing an obstructive jaundice. The intensity of the jaundice is, however, usually slight.

The patients often complain of severe dyspepsia. Haemorrhage, most often in the form of haemorrhoids or a haematemesis, is common. The general health is affected and in the late stages the patients become confused in mind and wasted in body. Ascites is a characteristic feature of the disease.

Once the condition has advanced beyond the early stages the patients become progressively worse, eventually bed-ridden and die in coma from liver failure.

Treatment

Where cirrhosis is due to alcohol every effort must be made to persuade the patient to give up drink completely. As his co-operation is essential if success is to be achieved, the situation must be explained clearly to him. He may well need special treatment in this respect, and sometimes psychiatric advice is necessary. He must have a full and nutritious diet and may require injections of concentrated vitamins.

In the more advanced stage, ascites can be reduced by diuretics such as chlorothiazide or frusemide, sometimes with the addition of aldactone. These diuretics are usually successful in disposing of the retained ascitic fluid but occasionally paracentesis becomes necessary.

When the patient becomes confused or comatose, protein in the diet must be avoided entirely since the damaged liver cannot metabolise protein adequately. Glucose and fluid may have to be administered intravenously. To prevent absorption of toxic material from the bowel which the liver can no longer detoxicate, the bowel is sterilised by giving neomycin or other antibiotics.

Haematemesis frequently occurs in cirrhosis. The flow of blood in the portal vein is obstructed and so the oesophageal veins (which empty into the portal vein) become distended and bleed easily. When the haematemesis is severe, blood transfusions must be given. The bleeding may be controlled by injections of pitressin which cause the veins to constrict.

Biliary cirrhosis

This type of cirrhosis usually occurs in middle-aged women and is not associated either with alcohol or hepatitis. The cause is unknown.

Symptoms and signs

The onset is gradual, usually presenting with itching of the skin (pruritus) and jaundice. The liver and spleen are enlarged. The jaundice slowly deepens and the course of the illness is progressively downhill over a few years.

Treatment

Treatment is similar to that described for portal cirrhosis.

CARCINOMA OF THE LIVER

Carcinoma of the liver is very common because malignant growths in various organs of the body very often spread to the liver, so causing a secondary carcinomatosis of the liver. A *primary* carcinoma of the liver (i.e. where the growth starts in the liver) is known as a *hepatoma* and is liable to arise in patients with cirrhosis.

Symptoms and signs

With most patients there is a history or evidence of the primary growth. For instance in cases due to spread from carcinoma of the stomach a history of epigastric pain, vomiting and loss of appetite is usual; in cases of carcinoma of the bronchus of the lung there is usually a cough and perhaps haemoptysis. By the time the primary growth has spread to involve the liver the progress of the illness is rapid and death is not far off.

The specific signs of liver involvement are:
1. An enlarged, stony-hard liver, palpable in the abdomen.
2. Ascites, which may need frequent tapping; the fluid withdrawn is serous or bloodstained.
3. Obstructive jaundice.

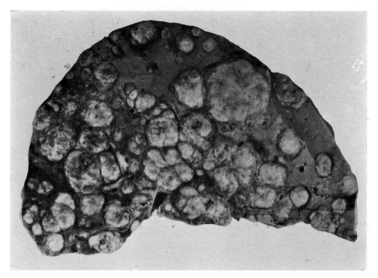

Fig. 8.9   Secondary carcinomatous deposits in the liver from a primary growth in the stomach.

Treatment

Palliative treatment is directed towards the patient's comfort. Tapping the ascites may relieve uncomfortable abdominal distension and analgesics may be necessary for pain.

DISEASES OF THE BILIARY TRACT

CHOLECYSTITIS AND GALL-STONES

Cholecystitis occurs in both acute and chronic forms and with most patients gall-stones are present. *Acute cholecystitis* causes severe pain in the right side of the upper abdomen in the region of the gall-bladder, and it characteristically radiates around the lower costal margin. Fever, nausea and vomiting accompany the pain. Acute cholecystitis is one of the causes of an 'acute abdomen' and is commonest in middle-aged overweight women.

Chronic cholecystitis is one of the causes of chronic dyspepsia, with recurrent flatulence, heartburn, nausea and pain in the epigastrium as the main symptoms. Gall-stones are commonly present and may give rise to attacks of *biliary colic*. Bouts of agonising pain occur in the epigastrium, radiating around to the back and often referred to the tip of the right shoulder. Sweating and vomiting accompany the pain.

In addition to biliary colic, gall-stones may cause obstructive jaundice by blocking the common bile duct.

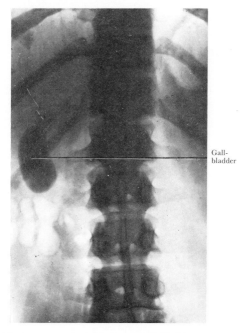

Gall-
bladder

FIG. 8.10   X-ray (cholecystogram) of the normal gall-bladder.

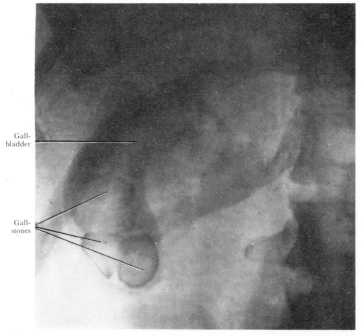

Gall-
bladder

Gall-
stones

FIG. 8.11   Gall-stones. In this case the stones were radio-opaque and were visualised on a straight X-ray.

DIAGNOSIS. In the diagnosis of chronic cholecystitis and gall-stones an X-ray examination is usually performed. As most gall-stones are radio-opaque a plain film of the gall-bladder may reveal the presence of the stones. In some cases it is, however, necessary first to give a dye which is excreted in the bile and thus outlines the gall-bladder (*cholecystogram*). By this means it is possible to see whether the gall-bladder is functioning properly and also to determine whether or not stones are present.

Treatment

Acute cholecystitis is often due to an infection of the gall bladder and responds to antibiotics such as tetracycline. In cases in which gall-stones are causing symptoms an operation to remove the stones is usually necessary. Occasionally gall-stones are not radio-opaque because they are formed of cholesterol. Cholesterol stones can be dissolved medically by giving chenodeoxycholic acid (Chendol capsules) by mouth three times a day, but the treatment must be continued for at least a year.

Cases of chronic cholecystitis in which gall-stones are not present may respond to medical treatment. The patients are put on a diet similar to that used in the after-treatment of peptic ulcer, especial care being taken to omit all fried, fatty and rich foods.

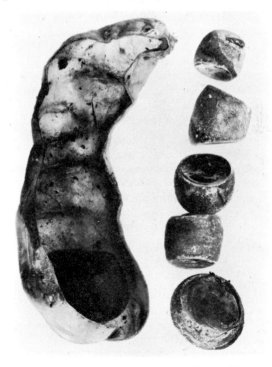

FIG. 8.12   A large distended chronically inflamed gall-bladder filled with gall-stones (same patient as Fig. 8.11).

Tumours

Tumours of the gall-bladder and bile ducts are rare and cause a progressive obstructive jaundice, cachexia and death. A progressive obstructive jaundice is, however, frequently caused by a carcinoma of the head of the pancreas, which obstructs the common bile duct as it passes through the head of the pancreas.

The progressive nature of the obstructive jaundice in carcinoma of the head of the pancreas may be contrasted with the cases due to gall-stones, in which the obstructive jaundice is intermittent and accompanied by biliary colic.

Often the cause of obstructive jaundice remains in doubt despite X-rays and cholecystogram. Other techniques may then be used to establish the diagnosis.

Ultrasound. This is a procedure employing high-frequency sound waves which penetrate body tissues but are deflected by abnormal structures and provide a photographic picture of the deflection. The investigation does not incommode the patient and is capable of revealing enlarged bile ducts or a growth in the pancreas or the liver.

ERCP (Endoscopic retrograde cholangio pancreatography). In this specialised technique a cannula is introduced into the duodenum via the mouth and thence into the biliary and pancreatic ducts. Radio-opaque dye is then injected into the cannula to outline these ducts on X-ray so that any obstruction or dilatation of the ducts can be visualised.

CAT scan (computerised transverse axial tomography). The scanner is a very expensive apparatus available only in special centres. By computerising numerous X-rays taken simultaneously at different planes, it is capable of detecting small structural abnormalities.

DISEASES OF THE PANCREAS

The pancreas is a flat elongated gland lying on the posterior wall of the upper abdomen. It serves two main functions. It produces pancreatic juices which it discharges via the pancreatic duct into the duodenum to help digest food in the intestine: and it provides insulin directly into the blood from the islets of Langerhans (see p. 411).

ACUTE PANCREATITIS

Inflammation of the pancreas often occurs in association with gall-stones or with an excessive intake of alcohol.

Clinical features

The onset is often sudden with very severe unremitting pain in the upper abdomen, passing through to the back. Vomiting may be persistent and in severe cases the patient is in shock with pallor, sweating and restlessness: the pulse is rapid and the blood pressure low. The abdomen is tender even with light pressure. The diagnosis, suspected on clinical grounds, is confirmed by the finding of a high level of amylase in the blood. Amylase is one of the digestive enzymes produced by the pancreas and is released into the blood when the pancreas is inflamed.

Treatment

Acute pancreatitis presents as an emergency. Diamorphine or pethidine may be necessary to relieve pain. Fluid should be given by intravenous drip when the patient is vomiting or in shock. Records will be taken of the fluid intake and output, the pulse, the blood pressure and the temperature which may be subnormal in the early stages. Antibiotics may be prescribed to prevent infection of the damaged pancreas though there is no evidence that a bacterial infection is responsible for acute pancreatitis.

In most cases, the condition subsides over a few days or a week.

CHRONIC PANCREATITIS

The story is characterised by intermittent bouts of abdominal pain, usually causing vomiting, loss of weight and appetite and loose stools containing a high fat content (steatorrhoea). Damage of the islet cells may lead to diabetes (see p. 412). The serum amylase is often raised during an attack.

Treatment

The fat content of the diet should be restricted and alcohol avoided. Diabetes may require insulin. Strong pancreatin tablets contain extracts of hog pancreas and help better digestion of the food. They should be taken with each main meal.

9 Diseases of the Central Nervous System

ANATOMY AND PHYSIOLOGY

Nowhere else in medicine is knowledge of the relevant anatomy and physiology so important in understanding diseases of the part as in the central nervous system. The nurse should, therefore, before reading this chapter on Diseases of the Nervous System refresh her knowledge of the anatomy and physiology. It is intended here merely to outline briefly the main parts of the nervous system which are especially important in understanding neurological diseases.

The central nervous system can be divided into the following parts:

    I. Motor system
    II. Reflexes
    III. Sensory system
    IV. Special senses.

MOTOR SYSTEM

The motor system can be conveniently divided into two main parts—the upper and lower motor neurone. A neurone is a nerve cell and the fibre which arises from it.

UPPER MOTOR NEURONE

The starting point of the motor pathway is the nerve cell (Betz cell) in the motor cortex of the frontal lobe of the cerebrum. It is called the motor cortex because all the motor cells which supply motor power to all the muscles of the body are situated here. The nerve fibres originating in the Betz cells travel downwards in a compact bundle or tract called the *pyramidal tract*, which is therefore the great main motor tract of the nervous system.

The pyramidal tract passes downwards through the internal capsule, midbrain, pons and into the medulla. Here the pyramidal tract from the right side crosses over to the left side to travel downwards in the lateral part of the spinal cord, ending opposite the second lumbar vertebra. The pyramidal tract from the left cerebral motor cortex similarly crosses over in the medulla to the right side. Because the motor fibres cross over in this way a disease in the right motor cortex or right pyramidal tract above the point of crossing of the tracts produces its effects on the left side of the body.

Individual fibres continually leave the pyramidal tract in its passage through the spinal cord, and these fibres end around the

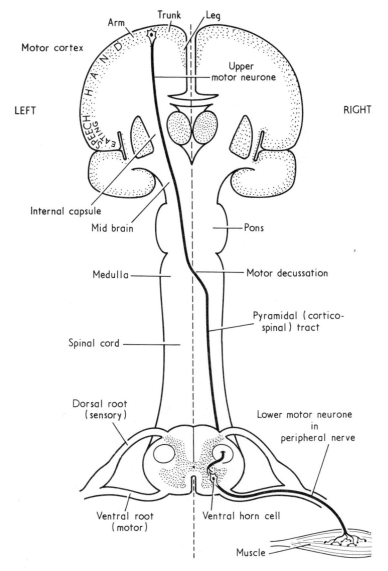

FIG. 9.1   The motor system.

anterior horn cells situated in the central grey matter of the cord. The upper motor neurone consists therefore of the nerve cell in the motor cortex and its fibre, which passes down in the pyramidal tract to its termination around the anterior horn cell. The pyramidal tract is thus made up of individual upper motor neurone fibres.

LOWER MOTOR NEURONE

The lower motor neurone fibres (known as the anterior motor roots) start in the anterior horn cells and leave the spinal cord to join up with the posterior roots. The latter are sensory fibres which end around the posterior horn cells. The combined motor and sensory fibres form what are known as the peripheral nerves, which leave the vertebral canal through the intervertebral foramina to end in whatever part they supply.

We shall see later that this division of the motor system is extremely important, in that a disease affecting the upper motor neurone produces a different set of signs from those produced by a disease affecting the lower motor neurone. This difference in the signs helps in clinical practice to locate the exact site of the disease in the nervous system. Before, however, we can understand the difference between an upper and lower motor neurone lesion it is necessary to consider the reflexes.

THE REFLEXES

The reflexes are peculiar motor actions which usually occur without any conscious effort. There are many different types of reflex, but expecially important are the deep tendon reflexes and the superficial reflexes.

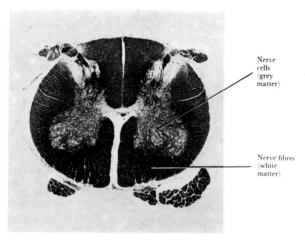

Nerve
cells
(grey
matter)

Nerve fibres
(white
matter)

FIG. 9.2   Section of a normal spinal cord. The central mass of grey matter (nerve cells) can be clearly distinguished from the surrounding white matter.

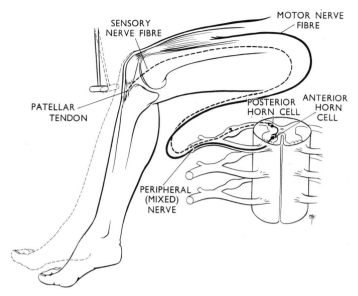

FIG. 9.3   The reflex pathway of the knee jerk.

DEEP TENDON REFLEXES
   Knee jerk
   Ankle jerk
   Arm jerks.

   To explain the deep tendon reflex action we shall consider the knee jerk. When the tendon over the knee is tapped an impulse travels up the sensory fibre in the peripheral nerve supplying the knee tendon, enters the spinal cord through the posterior sensory root and so into the posterior horn cell. From here the impulse (unlike all non-reflex sensory impulses which go up towards the brain) travels directly across the spinal cord to the anterior horn cell, thence out in the anterior motor root and down the motor fibre of the peripheral nerve to the quadriceps muscle. This motor impulse causes the quadriceps muscle to contract and the typical jerk of the knee results.

   The important point in this reflex pathway is that the impulse goes only through the *lower* motor neurone and does not use the *upper* motor neurone pathway. As a result, as we might expect, loss of the deep tendon reflexes occurs only in diseases affecting the lower motor neurone pathway.

SUPERFICIAL REFLEXES
   These reflexes are as important in the study of neurological disease as the deep reflexes, but they are very complex actions, and it is proposed only to mention the main types and the changes that affect them as a result of disease in the central nervous system.

The *abdominal reflexes* are elicited by stroking or scratching the skin of the abdominal wall, when a flickering of the underlying abdominal muscle occurs. These reflexes, unlike the deep tendon reflexes, use the *upper* motor neurone in their reflex arc. For this reason loss of the abdominal reflexes is seen only with lesions affecting the upper motor pathway.

The *plantar reflex* is a most important reflex which like the abdominal reflexes uses the *upper* motor pathway for its reflex arc. It is elicited by stroking the sole of the foot, when normally the big toe will turn downwards (flex). In diseases of the upper motor pathway this reflex is altered and the big toe turns upwards (extends). The abnormal response therefore is called an extensor response. It is also commonly called Babinski's sign, after the discoverer of this change in the plantar reflex.

Common symptoms and signs in diseases of the motor pathway

We have so far discussed the path taken by the motor impulses which activate the various muscles and organs of the body so that the body can perform the various actions required in everyday life. We have also described the important reflexes which use this motor pathway. We are therefore in a position to understand the common symptoms and signs which occur in diseases affecting the motor system.

First, it must be repeated that the motor path is divided into two main divisions and that according to which part is affected so a different set of signs is produced. These differences in the effects produced by diseases affecting the upper motor neurone and those affecting the lower motor neurone are of great importance to the doctor, as they enable him to approximately locate the site of the disease in the nervous system. It is also of value to the nurse to understand the principal signs of neurological diseases, as she will every

TABLE VII

Changes in the affected limbs	In upper motor neurone disease	In lower motor neurone disease
1. Paralysis (loss of power)	Present, often not complete. Tends to affect *whole limbs*	Present, usually complete. Affects *groups of muscles* in a limb or limbs
2. Tone of muscles	Stiff and rigid (spastic)	Limp (flaccid)
3. Wasting of muscles	Usually slight	Usually marked
4. Tendon reflexes	Present (usually exaggerated)	Absent
5. Abdominal reflexes	Absent	Present
6. Plantar reflex	Extensor response (Babinski's sign present)	Normal flexor response
7. Sensation	Usually only slightly disturbed	Sensory disturbances more evident

day in the course of her ward duties see the doctor examining the nervous system by testing reflexes, noting the power in the muscles and also observing the tone, i.e. whether they are stiff (spastic) or limp (flaccid).

The main differences between an upper motor neurone disease and a lower motor neurone disease are in the reflexes and in the tone and degree of wasting of the muscles. As pointed out above, because the deep tendon reflexes use only the lower motor pathway, upper motor neurone lesions do not abolish these reflexes as do the lower motor neurone lesions. On the other hand, the two important superficial reflexes, the abdominal and the plantar, use the upper motor neurone and so are affected in the upper motor neurone lesions only.

The more severe wasting and loss of tone in the lower motor lesions are due to the more complete interference with the motor and the muscle tone fibres which occurs in lower, as opposed to upper, motor neurone lesions.

Common types of paralysis

We have just seen that the main effect of a lesion in the motor pathway is a paralysis (loss of power), which varies in form according to the site of the disease. In addition, however, to the differences between the types of paralysis produced respectively by upper and lower motor neurone lesions, the extent of the paralysis will also vary according to the actual site and severity of the disease in either the upper or lower motor pathway.

The following are the common types of paralysis with their main causes.

Upper motor neurone types

Hemiplegia. This is a paralysis of one side of the body, and when complete includes the lower half of the face, arm and leg. A complete hemiplegia is caused by disease affecting all the motor fibres in one pyramidal tract which supply the opposite side of the body. When a patient has a stroke, the brain is damaged by a haemorrhage, thrombosis or embolism usually in the region known as the *internal capsule*, where the pyramidal tract lies. The most frequent result of a stroke therefore is a hemiplegia. Other diseases which commonly affect the pyramidal tract to cause a hemiplegia include multiple sclerosis and cerebral tumour.

In a hemiplegia the paralysis is spastic in form with increased deep tendon reflexes because the upper motor pathway is affected.

Paraplegia. Paralysis of both the lower limbs is called a paraplegia. In most cases of paraplegia the paralysis is spastic and is caused by a disease which affects both pyramidal tracts. The diseases multiple sclerosis and general paralysis of the insane (one form of syphilis affecting the brain) are frequently associated with a spastic paraplegia.

Again, pressure on the spinal cord by tumours or by tuberculous disease of the spine also often cause a spastic paraplegia.

Injuries to the spine, especially fracture dislocations, may give rise to a paraplegia. In these cases the damage to the spinal cord is usually very severe and involves most of the tracts in the spinal cord, including both the upper and lower motor and sensory pathways. The resulting paraplegia is usually a complete flaccid paralysis, with extensive sensory loss accompanied by disturbances in bladder function (retention or incontinence of urine).

Monoplegia. Paralysis of the whole of one limb is called a monoplegia. In apoplexy the lesion may not be sufficiently extensive to cause a complete hemiplegia, and in these cases a monoplegia is often the form of paralysis present.

Lower motor neurone types

Individual peripheral nerve paralysis. Lesions of the individual nerves are usually seen as a result of wounds or other injuries. The resultant paralysis is a typical example of a lower motor neurone lesion, with complete loss of power in the part affected, loss of deep reflexes, loss of sensation and severe wasting. Common examples of this form of peripheral nerve lesion are paralysis of the radial nerve (causing dropped wrist), paralysis of the ulnar nerve and brachial plexus birth injuries in infants.

Peripheral neuritis means a general involvement of the peripheral nerves causing weakness and altered sensation in the limbs. It is common in diabetes and in alcoholism. It sometimes is associated with carcinoma of the bronchus. Less commonly it can be caused by deficiency of vitamin B or by certain poisons such as lead or arsenic.

In addition to the above types of lower motor neurone paralysis there is another common form caused by the disease, acute anterior poliomyelitis, where the lesion is in the actual anterior motor horn cell. This causes a paralysis of various muscles or groups of muscles in one or more limbs.

SENSORY SYSTEM

There are various forms of sensation such as touch, pain and the feeling of heat and cold. The sense of position of a limb or joint is also important. The different sensory impulses arise in the skin, muscles and joints, and are carried backwards (upwards) in the sensory fibres which run together with the motor fibres in the peripheral nerves. The sensory fibres enter the spinal cord through the posterior spinal root (sensory root) and end around the posterior horn cell, which is situated in the grey matter of the spinal cord. From here start a new set of sensory fibres which run upwards in the spinal cord in many different tracts (sensory tracts) to end in cells in different parts of the brain. The main sensory cells are grouped together in the sensory cortex in the parietal lobe of the cerebrum, just behind the motor cortex. The sensory fibres cross over as do the motor fibres.

Disturbances in sensation are much more prominent in lesions of the peripheral nerves than in lesions of the brain. Such disturbances of sensation include:

Anaesthesia	Loss of sensation of touch
Analgesia	Loss of sensation of pain
Hyperaesthesia	Increased sensation of touch, causing tenderness
Paraesthesia	Sensation of pins and needles

SPECIAL SENSES

The special senses include sight, speech, hearing, smell and taste. Special areas exist in the brain which deal with the specialised reception and interpretation of these sensations. For instance, the sight areas are in the occipital lobes and hearing in the temporal lobes. Speech is different from the other senses in that it has centres on the left side of the brain only. Therefore only diseases affecting the left side of the brain produce speech disturbances. The term *aphasia* is used to describe disturbances in speech resulting from a brain lesion.

CONTROL OF THE BLADDER

Control of micturition in adults is a complex act which is often disturbed in diseases of the central nervous system. Sensory fibres convey pain and a sense of distension upwards to the brain, where there sensations are interpreted and controlled by the person's will. If it is desired to empty the bladder impulses travel downwards to relax the sphincter muscles and contract the detrusor (expelling) muscles. Disturbance of this voluntary control of bladder action is often present in central nervous diseases.

Incontinence of urine, often with incontinence of faeces, is present in most cases of coma, whatever the cause. When the patient becomes conscious, bladder control is usually quickly regained. In elderly people incontinence of urine may also arise in any severe illness and may persist for some time.

Instead of incontinence of urine, retention of urine may be seen in cases of coma. Spinal cord injuries, especially where caused by fracture-dislocation of the spine, are commonly accompanied by retention of urine, which may persist for weeks or months.

It should be noted that in some cases of retention an *overflow* dribbling of urine may occur which may be mistaken for a simple incontinence without retention. The importance of distinguishing between the two must be stressed because an unrelieved retention of urine can cause severe and lasting damage to the kidneys. In cases of overflow dribbling of urine caused by retention of urine the distended bladder can be felt and often seen as a firm round swelling in the midline of the abdomen just above the pubes.

It must be realised that local disease in the bladder and prostate also frequently causes incontinence or retention of urine. Indeed an enlarged prostate is the commonest cause of retention.

The importance of the care of the bladder will be dealt with under the different diseases affecting this organ.

SUMMARY OF THE COMMON SYMPTOMS AND SIGNS IN NEUROLOGICAL DISEASES

The exact site of the disease in the central nervous system determines the part to be affected. Also, according to whether it is mainly a motor, sensory or special sense area involved, so the signs will be mainly motor, sensory or 'special sense' in type. Certain of the more common symptoms and signs seen in central nervous system diseases will be briefly summarised.

1. Diseases affecting the motor pathway produce loss of power (paralysis) as the predominating sign. The paralysis varies in extent, depending on the site and severity of the disease. Common forms of paralysis include hemiplegia, paralysis of one side of the body; paraplegia, paralysis of both lower limbs; and monoplegia, paralysis of one limb.

2. Changes in the muscles, such as wasting and in tone, either spastic or flaccid, are important signs of motor lesions. The exact degree and type of change depends, as described earlier, on whether the upper or lower motor neurone is affected.

3. Changes in the reflexes, especially the deep (tendon) reflexes and the abdominal and plantar reflexes, occur in lesions of the motor pathway. Again, the type of change in the reflex depends on whether an upper or lower motor neurone lesion is present.

4. Disturbances in sensation are common, particularly in diseases of the peripheral nerves. Changes in the sensation of touch (anaesthesia and hyperaesthesia) and in the sensation of pain (analgesia) are common disturbances. Paraesthesia in the form of 'pins and needles' is also frequently met with.

5. Disturbances in sight, hearing, speech and other special senses depend on lesions directly affecting the specialised areas and nerves in the brain which deal with these senses.

6. Control of the bladder is often affected in certain neurological diseases, leading to incontinence of urine or to retention.

7. Other signs common to many neurological diseases include:

(a) TREMORS. These are disordered rapid movements of muscles leading to a shakiness of the parts affected. There are many different types of tremor, such as *intention tremor* where the tremor occurs only when the affected limb performs or intends to perform any action. Fine tremors also occur in toxic diseases as well as in neurological diseases, as in thyrotoxicosis and alcoholism. In diseases of the nervous system the tremors are usually coarse and very obvious. Such diseases as paralysis agitans, disseminated sclerosis and general paralysis of the insane are usually associated with obvious tremors.

Nystagmus is a tremor of the eyeballs which causes a to-and-fro movement of the eyes, which is especially marked when the patient looks to one or other side. It occurs in such conditions as disseminated sclerosis and diseases affecting the cerebellum.

(b) TROPHIC LESIONS. When the sensation of pain is lost, ulceration of the skin and damage to the joints commonly follow. Perforating ulcers on the feet occur in diabetic neuritis and also in tabes dorsalis. In the disease known as syringomyelia, where loss of pain is a marked feature, severe ulceration of the fingers is a prominent sign.

Charcot's joints, where gross arthritis and derangement of the joints are present, are most frequently seen in tabes dorsalis and syringomyelia. This is because injury to a joint which has lost the sense of pain passes unheeded and therefore eventually with continued use or with repeated injuries, however trivial, gross destruction of the joint develops.

Pressure sores, which are a form of trophic lesion, are liable to occur in cases of paralysis but, as will be stressed in the nursing of a paralysed patient, can be prevented in most patients by careful nursing.

(c) ATAXIA. This term means inco-ordination of movement and particularly applies to the gait or walking. Various types of gait characteristically occur in different neurological diseases. A patient with the disease known as paralysis agitans can be at once picked out by means of the typical shuffling, short-step gait. The patient with tabes dorsalis walks with a wide, stamping, staggering gait, usually aided with sticks. The gait in the common form of paralysis, hemiplegia (wherein one half of the body is affected), is also typical. Here the patient drags one leg, and the arm on the paralysed side does not swing but is held close to the side.

(d) REACTION OF DEGENERATION. When muscles are paralysed certain changes develop in their reaction to stimulation with an electrical current. These changes, the reaction of degeneration, are often used for diagnosis and also to estimate the possibility of recovery in paralysed muscles.

DISEASES OF THE MENINGES
MENINGITIS

Meningitis (inflammation of the meninges) is the most common and important disease affecting the meninges.

Types of meningitis

1. Pyogenic meningitis. This includes several types of meningitis,

of which the commonest are meningococcal, pneumococcal, influenzal, streptococcal and staphylococcal meningitis, caused by various pus-forming organisms.

2. Tuberculous meningitis.

3. Virus meningitis.

Symptoms and signs

Most of the symptoms and signs are the same in all forms of meningitis, and are due to the inflammation of the meninges causing increased intracranial pressure. These common symptoms and signs will be given first, and afterwards the special features of the different types will be mentioned.

1. ONSET. This is in most cases sudden, with the one exception of the tuberculous type. The patient is severely ill and toxic, with a high fever. The pulse is relatively slow in relation to the height of the temperature.

2. HEADACHE. This is very constant and persistent. It comes on early and is associated with vomiting.

3. VOMITING. The combination of severe headache and vomiting is always suggestive of an intracranial lesion.

4. The patient is drowsy and irritable, and often delirious. He lies in a characteristic attitude, curled up in bed and turned away from the light, as photophobia (dislike of light) is present. He resents being touched or disturbed and, if a child, cries with a high-pitched cry.

5. CONVULSIONS OR FITS. These are common, especially in infants.

6. NECK RIGIDITY. There is a marked stiffness of the neck, and any attempt to flex the head is strongly resisted. This rigidity of the neck muscles is due to the inflamed meninges. As bending the neck stretches the meninges and so causes pain the patient holds the neck rigid to prevent this pain.

7. KERNIG'S SIGN. This is the resistance met with on attempting to straighten the flexed knee, as here again straightening the flexed knee by stretching the inflamed meninges in the spinal cord causes pain.

Special features of the individual types of meningitis

Meningococcal meningitis. This is the most common form of pyogenic meningitis and is also known as cerebrospinal fever. It is acute in onset and often very severe. Meningococcal meningitis often occurs in epidemics.

Pneumococcal and influenzal meningitis. Both these types are very acute and severe in their onset and course.

Streptococcal and staphylococcal meningitis. In many cases of these types of meningitis there is often evidence of infection in the ear (otitis media), mastoid (mastoiditis) or sinuses (sinusitis), the meningitis developing as a result of spread of the infection to the meninges.

Tuberculous meningitis. Tuberculous meningitis differs from all the other types in that the onset is gradual, often one or two weeks elapsing before the characteristic picture of meningitis appears. After the meningococcal form it is the most common type met with.

Virus meningitis. This type of meningitis is usually less severe than the pyogenic forms.

Course

If untreated the patient lapses into coma, becomes delirious and incontinent and death usually supervenes, except in virus meningitis. In pyogenic meningitis chemotherapy has, however, dramatically improved the outlook. In tuberculous cases recovery, when it occurs, is much slower, taking many weeks.

Diagnosis

The symptoms and signs of meningitis are in most cases so definite that the condition will be at once suspected. To confirm the diagnosis a *lumbar puncture* will be done. Here a special needle with stilette is inserted, *under the strictest aseptic technique,* between the fourth and fifth or third and fourth lumbar vertebrae, piercing the dura mater and passing into the subarachnoid space. On the withdrawal of the stilette the cerebrospinal fluid (CSF) flows through the needle. A normal cerebrospinal fluid comes out drop by drop at a certain pressure (which can be measured by a special mano-meter, such as Greenfield's) and, most important, normal fluid is always crystal clear.

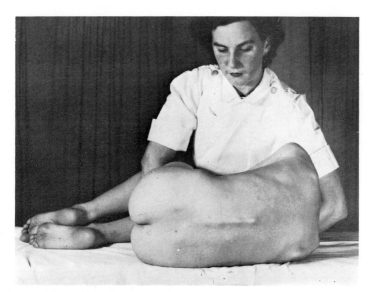

Fig. 9.4   The position of the patient for lumbar puncture. The spine must be fully flexed.

In all types of meningitis the fluid, being under pressure, spurts out and is definitely cloudy. In all pyogenic types of meningitis the fluid is not only cloudy but usually frankly purulent, and at once the diagnosis of meningitis can be made. By examining the fluid in the laboratory and culturing the organism the exact type of meningitis—meningococcal, pneumococcal, influenzal, etc.—can be ascertained. With a purulent cerebrospinal fluid, treatment is immediately started as for a pyogenic meningitis without waiting for the result of the culture.

In the early stages of tuberculous meningitis the fluid is only slightly cloudy, and therefore the diagnosis of meningitis may not be obvious from the naked-eye appearance of the cerebrospinal fluid. Confirmation may therefore have to await the results of the laboratory examination.

Treatment of meningitis

NURSING

Patients with meningitis are severely ill and toxic, thus requiring the most skilled nursing. They resent all interference, so that great patience on the part of the nurse is needed in order to make sure that the patient gets sufficient fluids. In the early stages the patient will be able to take only fluids with glucose, but as soon as specific treatment has had effect light diet will be possible. The patient is best nursed in a subdued light on account of the photophobia. Quietness is essential as noise is badly tolerated.

SPECIFIC TREATMENT

Pyogenic meningitis. The introduction of the sulphonamide drugs and antibiotics has completely changed the outlook in pyogenic meningitis. Before these drugs were used the majority of cases of meningitis died. Now the vast majority recover. Depending on the severity and type of infection, it is usual to give penicillin intravenously, 2 million units every 2 to 4 hours. Chloramphenicol may be given in addition. Penicillin (10,000 to 20,000 units) is sometimes given by the intrathecal route, but great care is necessary if penicillin is used in this way owing to the irritating effect of concentrated doses of penicillin on the meninges.

Tuberculous meningitis. Before the introduction of streptomycin and isoniazid all patients with tuberculous meningitis died. Chemotherapy has, however, resulted in the complete recovery of most patients, especially when treatment is started early. Streptomycin, para-aminosalicylic acid and isoniazid are given in a prolonged course lasting for at least six months. Isoniazid appears to be a very valuable drug in tuberculous meningitis as it easily

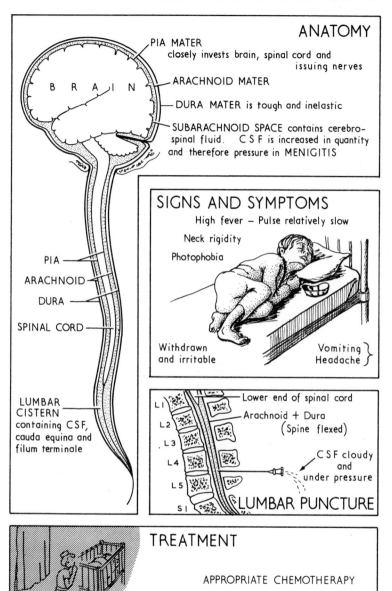

ANATOMY

PIA MATER closely invests brain, spinal cord and issuing nerves

ARACHNOID MATER

DURA MATER is tough and inelastic

SUBARACHNOID SPACE contains cerebro-spinal fluid. C S F is increased in quantity and therefore pressure in MENIGITIS

B R A I N

PIA
ARACHNOID
DURA
SPINAL CORD

LUMBAR CISTERN containing C S F, cauda equina and filum terminale

SIGNS AND SYMPTOMS

High fever – Pulse relatively slow

Neck rigidity

Photophobia

Withdrawn and irritable

Vomiting
Headache

L1
L2
L3
L4
L5
S1

Lower end of spinal cord

Arachnoid + Dura
(Spine flexed)

C S F cloudy and under pressure

LUMBAR PUNCTURE

TREATMENT

APPROPRIATE CHEMOTHERAPY

Fluids + +
Quietness
Dim light
Patience

FIG. 9.5 Meningitis.

penetrates the cerebrospinal fluid. In serious cases, streptomycin may be given intrathecally, i.e. into the cerebrospinal fluid by a lumbar puncture needle.

VASCULAR DISEASES OF THE BRAIN
STROKES

Causes

A stroke is an extremely common catastrophe and may be caused by three different lesions in the cerebral arteries, all of which produce a similar clinical picture, so that they can be conveniently grouped together.

1. *Cerebral thrombosis.* In elderly people the cerebral arteries are affected by arteriosclerosis in which the lining of the arteries become thickened and roughened. The flow of blood is obstructed and clotting occurs. This clot (thrombus) blocks the artery and deprives part of the brain of its blood supply.

2. *Cerebral haemorrhage.* Hypertension frequently causes rupture of

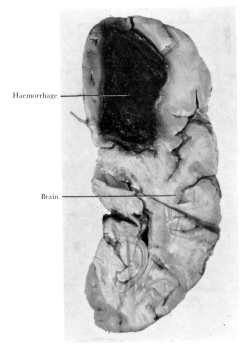

Haemorrhage

Brain

Fig. 9.6   Section of the brain showing a large cerebral haemorrhage. The patient had severe hypertension.

a cerebral artery, producing haemorrhage into the brain and the clinical picture of a stroke. Cerebral haemorrhage from hypertension and cerebral thrombosis from arteriosclerosis are the two commonest causes of stroke.

3. *Cerebral embolism*. An embolus, or detached clot, may lodge in one of the cerebral arteries and produce a stroke. This variety of stroke is seen in diseases where a clot forms on the left side of the heart and is carried up in the blood stream to lodge in one of the cerebral vessels. The diseases which most frequently cause a clot in the left side of the heart are:

(a) Mitral stenosis with atrial fibrillation
(b) Subacute bacterial endocarditis
(c) Coronary thrombosis.

Symptoms and signs

1. The symptoms and signs of cerebral thrombosis, haemorrhage and embolism are all exactly the same except for the onset. In thrombosis this is a matter of hours or even days, while in embolism the onset is very sudden. In haemorrhage the onset is also fairly sudden, over a few hours only. There is usually a history of preceding hypertension in cases of cerebral haemorrhage, while in cases of embolism the patient may be under treatment for mitral stenosis, coronary thrombosis or bacterial endocarditis.

2. In mild cases, which are usually due to cerebral thrombosis, the first sign of a stroke may be the onset of the paralysis without unconsciousness, but in many cases the patient becomes drowsy and lapses into *coma* or alternatively goes into coma with extreme suddenness. While the patient is unconscious the breathing is usually very deep and stertorous and the pupils dilated; incontinence of urine and faeces is also present.

3. The patient in severe cases may die without regaining consciousness. In other cases, when the patient regains consciousness paralysis is usually present, generally taking the form of a complete *hemiplegia* (i.e. paralysis of one side of the body, including the face, arm and leg). The degree of paralysis may, however, vary from a complete hemiplegia to a monoplegia, where only one limb is affected.

4. The pyramidal (motor) pathways crowd together in a small area of the brain known as the internal capsule (Fig. 9.1). This area receives its blood supply from a branch of the middle meningeal artery, and this is the small artery which is prone to rupture or blockage by a thrombosis or embolus. When this happens the pyramidal tract is interrupted with consequent paralysis of one side of the body.

If the site of the lesion is on the right side of the brain the paralysis occurs on the left side of the body because, as already mentioned, the pyramidal motor tracts cross over in the medulla to

CAUSES

Middle meningeal artery (usually)

Cerebral......
......thrombosis

...haemorrhage

...embolism

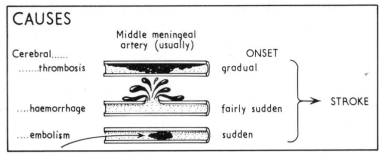

ONSET
gradual

fairly sudden → STROKE

sudden

ONSET
In severe cases
may be COMA

Pupils dilated

Breathing deep and stertorous

Incontinent

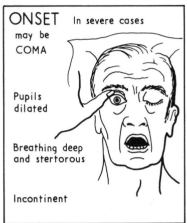

LATER
If damage to left side of brain,

Aphasia

Right-sided hemiplegia

N.B.
Patient mobilised as early as possible

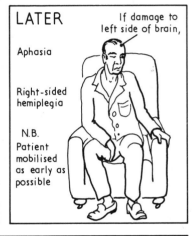

NURSING — COMA   Limbs in optimal position

Clear airway   Passive movements

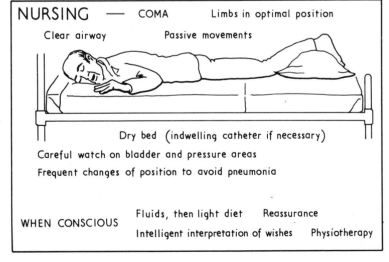

Dry bed (indwelling catheter if necessary)
Careful watch on bladder and pressure areas
Frequent changes of position to avoid pneumonia

WHEN CONSCIOUS   Fluids, then light diet   Reassurance

Intelligent interpretation of wishes   Physiotherapy

Fig. 9.7 Strokes.

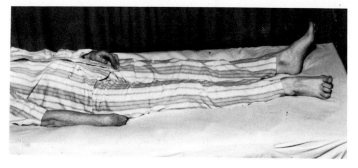

Fig. 9.8   Right hemiplegia. The leg is externally rotated and the foot is dropped. The paralysed arm is adducted and the hand curled under the body.

supply the opposite side of the body. If the lesion is on the left side of the brain, the speech centre may also be involved with resulting disorder of speech (aphasia) as well as a right hemiplegia.

Course

If the patient remains in a coma for over two days recovery is unlikely. In other cases the patient often regains some power of movement in the paralysed limbs. The degree of recovery, which varies considerably, may be almost complete with one patient and extremely limited with another. In the latter case the patient becomes bedridden for the remainder of his life, with the ever constant danger of pneumonia, pressure sores, or urinary infections which threaten all paralysed patients.

Treatment of strokes

NURSING

During the stage of coma the nursing of the patient is of the utmost importance. As in any case of coma with paralysis certain dangers are very prone to arise which, if possible, must at all costs be prevented.

1. A clear airway must be maintained so that the patient does not become asphyxiated through the paralysed tongue falling back in the mouth. The patient's head is best put on the side, and if necessary an airway should be inserted. If there is any difficulty over drainage of the mouth secretions, the patient is best nursed in the prone or semiprone position. The nurse will recognise asphyxia by the presence of cyanosis.

2. Pressure sores are very liable to develop in any prolonged coma, especially in elderly people, and particularly if paralysis is also present. In apoplexy the vast majority of the patients are elderly, and as paralysis is nearly always present, pressure sores are extremely liable to occur. For this reason preventive measures, such as attention to the skin over the pressure areas and frequent

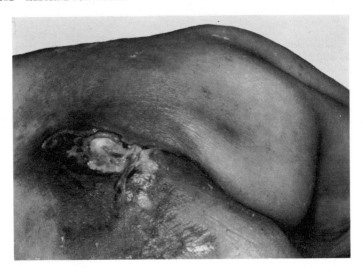

Fig. 9.9   Pressure sore.

changing of the patient's position, are particularly important. A rubber mattress is also most useful and every effort should be made to maintain a 'dry bed'.

3. Frequent changing of the patient's position, which must be done with great care and gentleness, will also help to avert another prevalent danger—pneumonia. If pneumonia should develop, penicillin or one of the other antibiotics will be given.

4. Careful watch on the bladder is necessary. As has already been stated, either incontinence of urine (which is more usual) or in some cases retention of urine with a distended bladder may occur. In cases of retention when the bladder becomes grossly distended an overflow dribbling of urine can occur. A large distended bladder is felt as a tense rounded tumour in the midline of the abdomen above the pelvis. In either case, an indwelling catheter with closed drainage bag attached is the safest way to prevent infection of the urinary tract and to keep the patient dry.

5. The question of providing warmth to the patient will naturally arise and, as with all unconscious patients, the greatest care must be taken with hot-bottles to ensure that they do not burn the patient. All patients are apt to be restless when recovering from the coma, and the covers of hot-water bottles can be easily kicked off, with resulting burns. It is best, therefore, not to use hot-water bottles with any comatose patient and to supply any necessary warmth with sufficient bedclothes.

6. When the patient has recovered consciousness fluids can be given by mouth; later, when the patient's condition has improved, light diet is given.

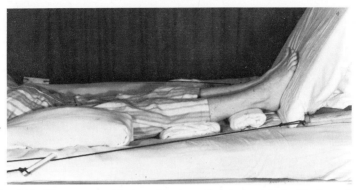

FIG. 9.10 The correct positioning of the lower limb in hemiplegia. The large firm pillow against the thigh prevents external rotation of the whole leg. The pillow just below the knee slightly flexes the knee and relaxes the muscles. The small pillow under the ankles prevents pressure on the heels and the foot-board overcomes the foot-drop.

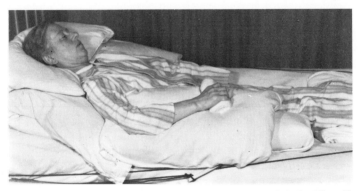

FIG. 9.11 The correct positioning of the upper limb in hemiplegia. The pillow prevents adduction of the arm and the hand-roll keeps the fingers and thumb opposed to each other.

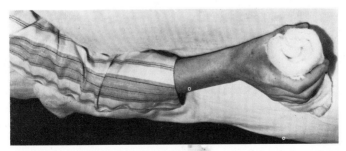

FIG. 9.12 Close-up view of the hand with the hand-roll in place to show the proper positioning of the fingers, thumb and wrist.

TREATMENT OF THE PARALYSED LIMBS

All weight must be taken off the paralysed limbs by bed-cradles.

The paralysed limbs must be put in the best position for the prevention or minimisation of deformities. The affected leg should be prevented from rotating outwards by the proper use of sandbags or firm pillows. The leg should be in a position of extension with the knee slightly flexed to relax the muscles. A small pad or pillow, placed under or just below the knee, helps to maintain this position. To prevent pressure on the heels a small flat pillow should be placed under the ankles. On no account must heel rings be used to prevent pressure sores as they themselves cause pressure. A foot-board or pillow at the end of the bed will help to prevent foot-drop.

A small pillow should be placed in the axilla on the affected side to prevent adduction of the arm and to relax the muscles. To prevent flexion of the fingers a soft rubber sponge or firm roll of cotton-wool should be placed in the hand so that the fingers and the thumb are opposed to each other. The sponge or hand-roll acts as a useful resistance against which the patient can later undertake active movements.

It is essential to put the paralysed limbs through a full range of passive movements several times a day from the very start of the illness. Passive movements help to prevent arthritis and fixation of the joints.

AFTER CARE

The whole stress of treatment of hemiplegia is to mobilise the patient as early as possible. The patient must not be kept in bed if he is able to sit in a chair and active movements and exercise must be organised, usually by the physiotherapist. Walking is no longer a reflex activity. It needs a conscious effort of will by the patient to control the paralysed limb and the experience is often a distressing one, needing constant reassurance and encouragement. With the aid of a Zimmer walking frame or a four-legged stick (see Fig. 9.13), the patient can be educated to balance himself and to gain confidence.

If the hemiplegia is on the right side, speech disturbance (*aphasia*) is likely to be present. A patient so affected is greatly upset to find he cannot express himself and nurse will take care to offer reassurance and try to anticipate his needs. A speech therapist will be able to help the patient to articulate his words and to speak slowly.

Occupational therapy has the major role to play in rehabilitation. The occupational therapist can prepare the patient for the various day-to-day tasks needed on return to home. Climbing the stairs, using the bath and the lavatory, eating and preparing of meals, all these functions, previously accepted without thought, now become matters of effort and re-learning. A visit to the home by the therapist

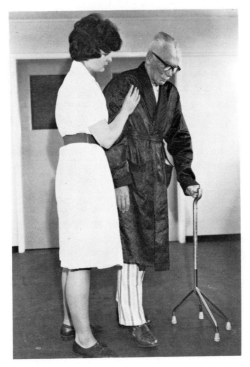

Fig. 9.13   Right hemiplegia. Mobilising the patient.

will reveal any unexpected difficulties that need to be provided for. Discussion with the family by the nurse, the doctor and the social worker may help to restore confidence. In doubtful cases, a trial visit home for a day or a weekend before discharge from hospital should be arranged. In many areas, Rehabilitation Centres provide special facilities for the further education of the hemiplegic patient.

MEDICAL TREATMENT

1. Hypertension is the most important predisposing cause of a stroke and if high blood pressure is found, treatment is indicated by such drugs as propranolol and a diuretic (see p. 104). Too great a reduction in blood pressure is not advised since this might diminish the cerebral circulation.

2. If the stroke has been caused by an embolus from atrial fibrillation, anticoagulant therapy (p. 114) can be used to prevent further clot formation and digoxin can be used to slow the heart rate.

SUBARACHNOID HAEMORRHAGE

Haemorrhage into the subarachnoid space of the brain is usually caused by extensive cerebral haemorrhage. Injury to the brain, especially a fracture of the skull, may also cause subarachnoid haemorrhage. In addition, in young people especially, a subarachnoid haemorrhage may occur without injury or haemorrhage into the brain substance, and in these cases rupture of an unsuspected cerebral aneurysm is usually the cause. Small aneurysms of the cerebral arteries (*berry aneurysms*) are not uncommon and are a result of congenital weakening of the arterial wall. These aneurysms may never give rise to symptoms unless they rupture.

Symptoms and signs

1. The patient is either a young adult or in the middle span of life. In older people subarachnoid haemorrhage is more likely to be due to hypertension and arteriosclerosis than to a congenital aneurysm.

2. The onset is usually sudden with intense headache and vomiting. If the haemorrhage is large the patient may be comatose and convulsions may be present.

3. The pulse is slow. Neck rigidity is a characteristic feature.

4. The urine often contains albumin and sometimes sugar as well.

5. In some cases paralysis, often of the cranial nerves, may develop.

Diagnosis

The picture of intense headache, vomiting, neck rigidity and slow pulse resembles that of a meningitis except for the absence of fever. A lumbar puncture, however, will establish the diagnosis, as in subarachnoid haemorrhage the cerebrospinal fluid is heavily bloodstained and not purulent as in meningitis.

Angiography is also very helpful in the diagnosis and localisation of a cerebral aneurysm and is always done before any operative procedure. A radio-opaque dye is injected into the carotid artery and an X-ray of the skull then taken. The dye outlines the blood vessels and may show up the aneurysm. Angiography is also used in the diagnosis and localisation of cerebral tumours (p. 296).

Treatment

At the present time it is believed by many that the best hope of a cure lies in immediate surgery after angiography has been carried out to localise the aneurysm. Either the carotid artery is ligatured or the aneurysm is removed if it is accessible.

Patients treated medically must be nursed at complete rest, everything being done for them to eliminate the least possible strain. The patient remains in bed for about six weeks. Recurrence of rupture of the aneurysm is not uncommon and often takes place two to three weeks after the initial attack.

MIGRAINE

Migraine is a form of paroxysmal headache often occurring in more than one member of a family. Thus mother and daughter may both

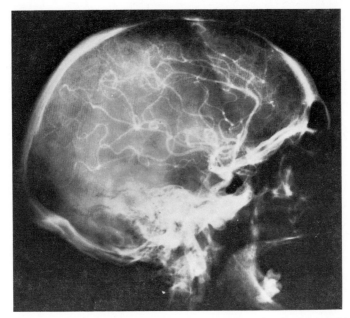

FIG. 9.14 Cerebral angiogram in a normal person. The opaque dye is injected into the carotid artery so that the carotid artery and cerebral blood vessels are clearly outlined.

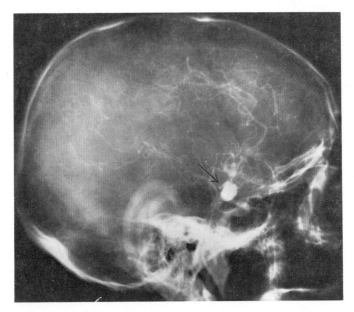

FIG. 9.15 Cerebral angiogram showing a large aneurysm.

suffer from migraine. Migraine has various characteristics, but not every migraine sufferer has all these symptoms.

1. The headache is often preceded by an *aura*. This usually consists of a visual disturbance with flashes of light, zigzags of varying colours, or even partial loss of vision; or a sense of numbness and tingling on one side of the face or body. This aura may last for up to half an hour and is followed by the headache.

2. The headache is often throbbing in character, worse on one side of the head, and frequently associated with anorexia, nausea or vomiting. The headache may last many hours or rarely for several days, the so-called *status migrainous*.

3. Migraine sufferers are often over-conscientious and perfectionist. Attacks of migraine are most likely to occur at times of relaxation after spells of intense activity or stress, particularly at the weekends.

4. Attacks of migraine can be precipitated in different subjects by different trigger factors. Certain foods (e.g. chocolate, cheese, alcohol), certain drugs (e.g. contraceptive pill), strong light, excessive exercise, emotional upsets or pre-menstruation may dispose to a migraine attack.

Pathology

Migraine is thought to be due to changes in the cerebral blood vessels. In the aura stage, the vessels become constricted and narrowed while the throbbing headaches are associated with a subsequent fullness and dilatation of the vessels.

Treatment

1. Migraine subjects should learn what trigger factors are liable to precipitate an attack and how to avoid them.

2. Sometimes when migraine becomes very frequent and due to stress, a course of sedation, perhaps diazepam 2 mg three times a day, may help to reduce the frequency of the attacks.

3. Clonidine (0·025 mg four times a day) prevents spasm of the cerebral vessels and is sometimes successful in preventing attacks if taken regularly.

4. If given at the first intimation of an attack, an injection of ergotamine 0·25 mg administered subcutaneously by the patient himself can be most effective in preventing the attack from developing. Ergotamine given in this way prevents the dilatation of the blood vessels associated with the headache but is usually less effective when given by mouth in tablet form.

Other causes of headache

1. Headache is often a feature of any general illness and many common infections are ushered in by a headache.

2. Tension headaches occur in nervous subjects when under stress. The headache is often described as 'like a tight band round the head':

It is sometimes at the back of the head. There is no aura and it is not associated with vomiting. It usually responds to simple analgesics.

3. Despite a popular misconception, hypertension does not usually cause headaches. However, if the blood pressure is very high, headaches and vomiting may occur.

4. Cerebral tumours may present with headaches and the physician always has this possibility in mind when confronted with a patient who has begun to get episodes of headache. Investigation may be necessary to make sure of the diagnosis.

5. Temporal arteritis (see page 472). This inflammation of the temporal arteries is commonest in elderly women and the headache is associated with malaise, pyrexia and sometimes mental confusion.

DISEASES OF THE PERIPHERAL NERVES

Lesions of the peripheral nerves are frequently seen. Wounds or other injuries often produce a paralysis of the radial, ulnar or peroneal nerves.

Birth injuries are dealt with on page 318. The remaining common disease affecting the peripheral nerves is known as peripheral neuritis.

PERIPHERAL NEURITIS (Polyneuritis)

Causes
1. Poisons (arsenic, lead, mercury, gold, benzol, etc.)
2. Chronic alcoholism
3. Diabetes mellitus
4. Vitamin B deficiency
5. Acute infective polyneuritis
6. Carcinoma, especially carcinoma of the bronchus
7. Diphtheria.

Symptoms and signs
1. Usually the larger nerve trunks of the arms and legs are affected, resulting in diminution of power or even a complete paralysis. The typical result of this loss of motor power is a dropped wrist or foot. The muscles affected show some wasting.

2. Sensory disturbances are present usually in the form of pins and needles in the hands and feet. In some cases, however, severe pains in the arms and legs may occur with marked tenderness of the muscles. Alternatively, there is usually some degree, varying from mild to severe, of loss of sensation to pain and touch.

3. The tendon reflexes both in the legs (knee and ankle jerks) and the arms are absent. This is because the reflex arc has been interrupted. In fact all the signs present are typical of a lower motor neurone lesion, with severe loss of power, marked sensory

disturbances, wasting of muscles and loss of the deep tendon reflexes.

4. In some cases the cranial nerves, such as the facial are affected.

Features of the different types

1. *Alcoholic neuritis.* This mainly affects the legs, causing weakness of the feet and ataxia (inco-ordination) of gait. Sensory disturbances are common and the muscles of the legs are very tender to the touch.

2. *Diabetic neuritis (neuropathy).* This usually leads to loss of sensation in the feet and legs with absent reflexes. Occasionally pain in the legs can be very severe, especially at night.

3. *Acute infective polyneuritis (Guillain-Barré syndrome).* The cause of this form of peripheral neuritis is probably a virus infection, with all the usual symptoms of fever, headache and malaise, which is followed by paralysis of the arms and legs. In some cases the paralysis may spread to affect the respiratory muscles with the danger of asphyxia developing. The cranial nerves may also be involved, particularly the seventh, causing a facial paralysis.

4. *Diphtheritic neuritis.* Serious infections of diphtheria may lead to paralysis of the limbs and the muscles of respiration.

5. *Carcinoma of the bronchus.* This can give rise to peripheral neuritis with weakness of the limbs and ataxia, even before signs in the chest develop. This is not due to secondary deposits but is probably a toxic effect of the carcinoma.

Treatment of peripheral neuritis

1. In an acute case the patient is put to bed. Care must be taken to avoid injury to the affected limbs, and in this respect bed-cradles are very valuable. Particular attention to the skin and pressure areas is most important to prevent pressure sores.

2. The foot-drop usually present must be corrected by the use of a foot-board or pillow against the feet, or, alternatively, well-padded light splints may be used. Passive movements to prevent fixation of the joints must be started from the onset.

3. If the case is acute, with a good deal of tenderness and pains in the muscles, active movements will be postponed until the symptoms subside. Analgesics for the relief of pain are usually needed.

4. All the appropriate specific measures will be taken, such as the giving of vitamin B in the vitamin-deficiency cases, control of the diabetes and the withdrawal of any poisons.

5. The use of a respirator will be necessary in those cases of respiratory paralysis due to acute infective polyneuritis.

SCIATICA

The term sciatica is given to the common pain which occurs along the distribution of the sciatic nerve. It is most commonly due to pressure on the nerve by a prolapsed intervertebral disc (p. 470), but it can be due to malignant tumours of the vertebrae or of the pelvic organs. Hence sciatica is a symptom which merits careful investigation.

Symptoms and signs

The characteristic symptom in sciatica is pain along the distribution of the sciatic nerve. The pain is felt in the back and down the back of the thigh to the ankle. Anything that causes stretching of the sciatic nerve produces the pain so that the patient walks with a limp to avoid lifting the leg. The ankle jerk is usually absent, and in some cases there is a loss of sensation in the area supplied by the sciatic nerve.

Treatment

Treatment will depend on the cause of the sciatica.

COMMON DISEASES OF THE CRANIAL NERVES

The cranial nerves, which arise from the brain and run their course almost entirely within the skull, are frequently affected by diseases affecting the brain, especially any lesion which causes pressure in the skull. Only the more common and important diseases affecting the cranial nerves will be discussed.

THE OPTIC NERVE

The optic nerve conveys the visual impulses from the retina of the eye back to the sight centre in the occipital lobe of the brain. The optic nerve is of extreme importance in the diagnosis of certain diseases of the central nervous system because it is the one nerve which can actually be seen. By means of an instrument called an ophthalmoscope a clear picture of the whole of the retina of the eye, including the actual optic nerve (optic disc), can be obtained.

Normally, the optic disc is seen as a white circular area with a distinct margin. In cases of increased intracranial pressure, however, oedema or swelling of the optic nerve (*papilloedema*) develops and the optic disc becomes swollen and the margins blurred. Papilloedema is a most valuable sign of increased intracranial pressure.

Optic neuritis

A neuritis of the optic nerve may be caused by excessive alcohol and tobacco. Syphilis and multiple sclerosis also cause an optic neuritis. The symptoms are those of dimness of vision or in severe cases, partial blindness.

Optic atrophy

Atrophy, or wasting, of the optic nerve fibres, may follow a severe papilloedema or optic neuritis. Syphilis is especially prone to cause this effect. Total blindness results from complete optic atrophy.

Examination of the eye with an ophthalmoscope is of importance not only in disease of the central nervous system but in certain other diseases too which may show characteristic changes in the retina. Hypertension frequently causes haemorrhages and white spots (exudates) in the retina, and also oedema of the optic disc. Diabetes and chronic nephritis also produce similar changes.

THE OCULAR NERVES

The third, fourth and sixth cranial nerves supply the muscles of the eyes responsible for the movement of the eyeball. The iris muscle of the eye, which causes contraction and dilatation of the pupils, is also supplied by these nerves.

In addition, these nerves supply the muscle which raises the upper eyelid.

Diseases which affect the ocular nerves can produce any of the following signs:

1. Drooping of the upper eyelids known as *ptosis*.
2. Squint (*strabismus*), often associated with seeing double (*diplopia*).
3. Unequal pupils.

The diseases which most commonly affect these nerves to produce the above signs include syphilis, brain tumours and aneurysms, encephalitis (inflammation of the brain) and myasthenia gravis.

THE FIFTH NERVE (Trigeminal)

A lesion of the fifth nerve which is sometimes met with is *trigeminal neuralgia,* where paroxysms of extremely severe pain occur in the distribution of the fifth nerve, i.e. over the jaw, cheek and forehead. The slightest touch in these areas may bring on an attack.

Treatment of trigeminal neuralgia is often difficult. Bad teeth or sinus infection must be attended to if present. Carbamazepine (Tegretol) is often effective in relieving the pain during an attack. In severe cases section of the nerve root or an injection of alcohol into the nerve has to be carried out.

THE SEVENTH NERVE (Facial)

A paralysis of the facial nerve is frequently seen as part of a hemiplegia, of which the most common cause is a cerebral thrombosis. In a hemiplegia, only the lower half of one side of the face is paralysed. In contrast to this, paralysis of the whole of one side of

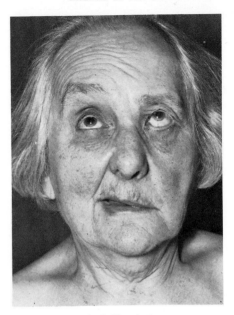

Fig. 9.16   Left-sided facial paralysis (Bell's palsy).

the face including the forehead is often seen in the condition known as *Bell's palsy*.

The exact cause of Bell's palsy is not known, but it usually follows exposure to cold and is supposed to be due to inflammation or neuritis of the facial nerve. The condition usually clears up in a few weeks without any special treatment but occasionally leaves permanent weakness of the affected side of the face. ACTH injections are sometimes used in the acute phase.

A facial paralysis is sometimes seen after operations on the mastoid owing to injury to the nerve during the operation. Finally, a transitory facial paralysis may arise in infants owing to a birth injury, especially in cases of forceps delivery.

THE EIGHTH NERVE (Auditory)

The eighth nerve has two main functions, one dealing with hearing and the other with the maintenance of equilibrium and proper posture of the body. Diseases of the auditory, or hearing, part of the nerve commonly cause deafness and buzzing in the ears (*tinnitus*). Diseases of the division of the nerve dealing with equilibrium cause severe attacks of giddiness, during which all objects may appear to spin around. In severe attacks the patient may fall and vomiting may also occur. These attacks are known as *vertigo*. Motion sickness (sea-sickness, car-sickness) with its nausea, vomiting and vertigo is probably caused by the undue motion affecting the eighth nerve.

Ménière's disease is commonest in elderly people and is associated with tinnitus (noises in the ears) and progressive deafness. It gives rise to bouts of sudden, terrifying, and incapacitating giddiness and vomiting, which may last for many hours. The attacks are best treated with chlorpromazine, but the cause of the complaint is unknown.

Streptomycin, especially if given over long periods, may damage the eighth nerve and give rise to deafness and giddiness.

Tumours of the eighth nerve may cause tinnitus and deafness and can be removed by operation.

THE TWELFTH NERVE (Hypoglossal)

The twelfth nerve supplies the muscles of the tongue. Paralysis of the tongue is generally seen as part of a hemiplegia. Here, when the tongue is protruded from the mouth, the unaffected half of the tongue pushes the tongue over to the paralysed side, e.g. in cases of paralysis of the right side of the tongue, the tongue is pushed over to the right side when it is protruded.

COMMON DISEASES OF THE NERVOUS SYSTEM

MULTIPLE SCLEROSIS (Disseminated sclerosis)

Multiple sclerosis is now the commonest major disorder of the nervous system in the Western world. Myelin is a fatty material which forms a sheath round nerve fibres and it is this material that is damaged and scarred in disseminated sclerosis. Patches or plaques of sclerosed (hardened), fibrous material are found disseminated through the nervous system replacing healthy white myelin. Hence disseminated sclerosis is known as a *demyelinating* disorder of the central nervous system.

It occurs in young adults and runs a prolonged course over many years. The most likely explanation is that it is due to a viral infection which settles in the nervous system in the second decade of life and leads to slow and patchy damage of myelin over the years. But so far no particular virus has been isolated or identified in man.

In the early stages, the myelin affected is inflamed and damaged but not destroyed. Impairment of function at this stage may only be temporary and apparent recovery occurs. As times goes on, fibrosis of the affected areas takes place with permanent destruction of nervous tissue.

Clinical features

Early symptoms:

1. Young adults in the twenties or thirties are most commonly affected.
2. Weakness of one or both legs is a common early symptom,

sometimes associated with numbness, tingling and altered sensation in the limbs. These symptoms vary in severity and often clear up completely for many years.

3. Ocular symptoms. The optic nerves are often involved leading in the early stages to temporary mistiness of vision or even temporary loss of vision in one or other eye. Attacks of double vision are common and sometimes nystagmus, a rapid jerky movements of the eyes, can be detected.

4. Unsteadiness of the arms may be noted on making purposeful movements such as reaching out to take a cup of tea.

Further symptoms appear as time goes on, improvement becomes less frequent and incapacity more permanent.

(a) The legs become more stiff (spastic) and the gait more unsteady so that walking becomes difficult or impossible.

(b) Unsteadiness becomes more pronounced making arm movement clumsy and inco-ordinated.

(c) Nystagmus becomes permanent and vision itself may be lost in either eye.

(d) The speech becomes stiff and the words disjointed (*dysarthria*).

(e) Disturbances of bladder function occur with lack of control and sometimes retention with inability to empty the bladder.

(f) Mental changes become evident, occasionally an inappropriate and fatuous cheerfulness (*euphoria*), but more often emotional instability with bouts of understandable depression.

In the later stages of disseminated sclerosis the patient may be confined to bed or a chair with incontinence of bladder and bowel.

Management

1. In the early stages, rest is advisable when symptoms appear. Experience has shown that physical activity prolongs symptoms and delays improvement.

2. ACTH (see p. 457). A course of ACTH is helpful in the relief of symptoms during an acute phase, probably by reducing inflammation of the affected areas in the nervous tissues.

3. Diet. There is no evidence that diet plays a part in disseminated sclerosis but various special diets are being tried, e.g. a gluten-free diet (see p. 235).

4. When the legs are stiff and spastic, drugs such as diazepam in large doses may be helpful.

5. Physiotherapy can help the patient make best use of what function he possesses. For example, trained use of the upper part of the body can enable a patient with spastic legs to transfer himself from bed to chair.

6. The occupational therapist may recommend the provision of ramps and rails at home to make it possible for the patient to get about. Walking appliances may be necessary and special utensils for eating.

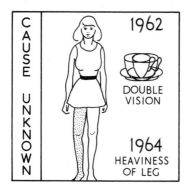

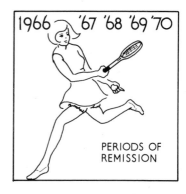

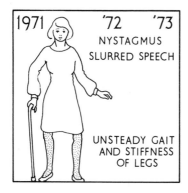

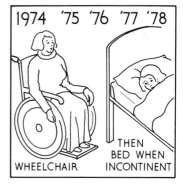

Fig. 9.17   Disseminated sclerosis.

7. Bladder symptoms of urgency and loss of control can be helped by drugs such as propantheline (probanthine) which relieve spasm. When retention occurs, an indwelling catheter may become obligatory.

The diagnosis of disseminated sclerosis is usually made on the clinical signs and symptoms. It is important to realise that after the initial occurrence of symptoms, many patients regain full physical capacity for 10 or 15 years. Hence although some cases run a down-hill course over a few years, it is wrong to take too gloomy a view. In most cases, doctors prefer not to tell patients the diagnosis in the early years since the diagnosis is not always certain and the course unsure.

CEREBRAL TUMOUR

Primary

Tumours of the brain are fairly common and often occur in people younger than those affected by tumours of other parts of the body. There are many types of primary tumours of the brain which include:

1. Glioma, which tends to be very malignant and rapidly fatal.
2. Meningioma. This is a tumour growing from the meninges on the surface of the brain and is not malignant.
3. Pituitary tumour. This grows from the pituitary gland and in many cases can be successfully removed. It causes endocrine disturbances as well as pressure changes.
4. Auditory nerve tumour, which is seen in older people and is of slow growth.

Secondary

Secondary cerebral tumours are due to spread from a primary growth somewhere else in the body, usually the bronchi or stomach. Secondary brain tumours are more common than primary.

Symptoms and signs

Tumours of the brain cause symptoms and signs in two main ways:

1. Symptoms and signs due to the increased intracranial pressure.
2. Symptoms and signs due to the local damage to the brain from the growth of the tumour—localising signs.

SYMPTOMS AND SIGNS DUE TO THE INCREASED INTRACRANIAL PRESSURE

The symptoms and signs of increased intracranial pressure are invariably the same whatever the cause (tumour, abscess or meningitis) producing the increased pressure within the skull.

1. *Headaches.* These are usually very persistent and severe and are characteristically associated with

2. *Vomiting.* The combination of headaches and vomiting should always lead to the suspicion of a brain lesion.

3. *Papilloedema.* This is oedema of the optic nerve. The pressure on the optic nerve causes a swelling of the nerve with blurring of the margins of the optic disc. The importance of this sign is that it can be seen clinically by examination of the fundus of the eye by means of an ophthalmoscope. Such an examination gives definite and visible proof that there is increased pressure within the skull.

4. *Drowsiness,* passing eventually into a state of coma. This is a comparatively late sign in tumours.

5. *Convulsions* or fits are frequent.

6. *Slow pulse.* The pulse is usually slow in cases of increased intracranial pressure and this is a helpful diagnostic sign.

7. *Mental changes,* such as slowness of action, deficient memory and personality changes, occur at some stage in most cases.

LOCALISING SIGNS

These depend on the area of the brain which is affected by the tumour. As has been seen earlier, different parts of the brain deal with different functions, and a lesion in a particular area will affect

the functions of that area, enabling the lesion to be localised. However, there are many areas in the brain which are known as silent
areas, i.e. as far as is known they have no definite functions. A lesion
in these areas tends to produce no definite localising sign. Some
common localising signs of tumours in the non-silent areas are:

    (a) In the motor cortex. Fits are very common and in many cases
         they tend to cause localising convulsive movements of the face,
         arm or leg. These fits are called *Jacksonian epilepsy*. In addition,
         a weakness or paralysis in the form of a monoplegia is common.

    (b) In the occipital cortex. A tumour in this area tends to cause
         early blindness as the sight centre is situated here.

    (c) Of the auditory nerve. Deafness, giddiness and vertigo are
         common and predominant.

    (d) In the pituitary gland. Disturbances in the endocrine function
         of the gland, leading to such conditions as Simmonds' disease
         or acromegaly, are often present (p. 432).

Diagnosis

    The diagnosis will be suspected from the signs and symptoms but
if treatment is to be considered investigations will be necessary to

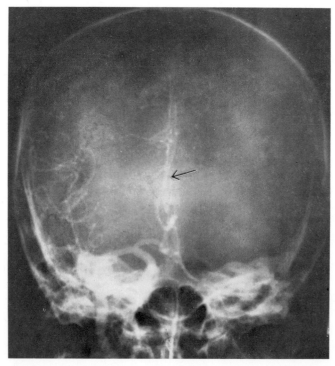

Fig. 9.18 Normal cerebral angiogram showing the normal pattern of the blood vessels.

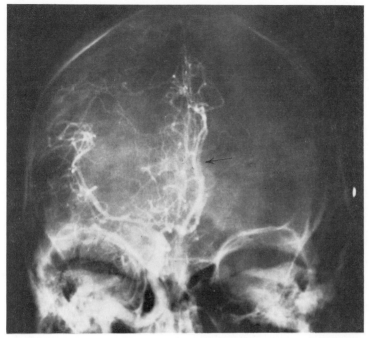

Fig. 9.19 Cerebral angiogram in a patient with a cerebral tumour. The anterior cerebral artery which should run exactly in the midline (see Fig. 9.18) is displaced from the midline by a large tumour.

provide more precise information as to the presence and location of any tumour. Several procedures are available to the neurosurgeon.

1. X-ray of the skull occasionally reveals erosion of the bone caused by a tumour. X-ray of the chest may reveal a carcinoma of the bronchus, a common cause of cerebral metastases (p. 190).

2. Electroencephalogram (EEG). This is a record of the electrical activity of the cerebrum, and shows a regular sequence of waves. The presence of a tumour will be revealed by an area of disturbed cerebral electrical activity.

3. Brain scan. Radioactive material (technetium 99m, ^{99}Tc) is preferentially taken up by a cerebral tumour and its presence detected and recorded by scanning techniques.

4. Cerebral angiography entails the injection of a radio-opaque dye into the carotid artery and X-rays then reveal displacement of arteries by the tumour or an abnormal circulation in the vicinity of the tumour.

5. Ventriculography. Air is injected into the ventricles of the brain and abnormalities in their shape or size can be detected on X-ray.

6. CAT scanner (computerised transverse axial tomography). The

scanner may ultimately replace X-ray techniques since it is capable of revealing with accuracy the presence, position and size of a cerebral tumour. Because it is a very expensive apparatus, it is available only in specialised neurosurgical units.

Treatment

Surgical removal of the tumour offers the best hope of a cure but this is usually only possible in benign tumours such as meningioma. Malignant tumours or secondary deposits are seldom amenable to total removal. In some cases, radiotherapy may be helpful in shrinking the size of the tumour with relief of headache and vomiting.

CEREBRAL ABSCESS

Cerebral abscess is usually caused by spread of infection from septic disease in the ears, mastoid cells or nasal sinuses. A cerebral abscess can also result from a septic embolus lodging in the brain, particularly in cases of bronchiectasis.

Symptoms and signs

These are essentially the same as for cerebral tumours. There will be the signs of increased pressure and also the localising signs according to the site of the abscess in the brain. Signs of infection, like fever and raised white cell count both in the blood and the cerebrospinal fluid, help to distinguish abscess from tumour. Evidence of septic ear disease or bronchiectasis also helps in the diagnosis.

Treatment

Antibiotics are of great value, but, in addition, operation to evacuate the abscess may be necessary. Penicillin and streptomycin may be injected locally into the abscess cavity after evacuation of the abscess. The primary focus of infection (ear, mastoid, etc.) must also be dealt with by the appropriate measures.

POLIOMYELITIS (Infantile paralysis)

Poliomyelitis is caused by a virus infection which specifically attacks the anterior (motor) horn cells in the spinal cord. It may also, however, affect the brain, especially the midbrain, producing what is called *encephalitis*. (An encephalitis is an inflammation of the cells in the brain and may arise from several causes, e.g. as a complication of certain infectious fevers, especially measles and whooping-cough. It may, in rarer instances, follow vaccination.) The encephalitis caused by the poliomyelitis virus is known as *polioencephalitis*. Acute anterior poliomyelitis tends to occur in epidemics in the autumn.

SPREAD OF INFECTION. The virus grows in the intestinal tract and is excreted in the faeces. It is more likely to spread where sanitation is neglected and where hygiene is poor. Transmission is by contamination of food and also by droplet infection.

INCUBATION PERIOD. Seven to 14 days.

Symptoms and signs

1. Children and young adults are most commonly affected, but the incidence of the disease varies in different epidemics; in recent years older patients have been affected. The onset is sudden, with fever, headache and the general feeling of malaise.

2. Stiffness of the neck with pain in the back are common early symptoms.

In some patients the disease may progress no further than this stage, which is known as the *preparalytic stage*. These abortive attacks are often suspected and diagnosed only during an epidemic.

3. Other cases go on to the stage of paralysis. Here one or more limbs or the trunk muscles may become paralysed. The areas most commonly affected are the legs, shoulder girdle muscles (especially the deltoid), intercostal muscles or diaphragm. Any part of the body may, however, be affected.

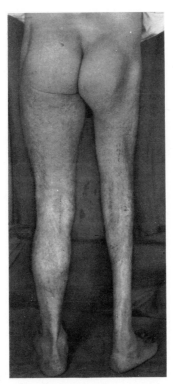

FIG. 9.20   Poliomyelitis, late stage of the disease, showing permanent wasting of the muscles of the right leg.

The paralysed part is limp and the deep tendon reflexes are lost. Wasting of the muscles is an early and prominent feature. This is, in fact, a typical example of a lower motor neurone paralysis.

4. Pain in the affected muscles is usually present and in some cases may be very pronounced. The muscles are usually tender to touch in the acute stage.

5. In cases where the brain cells are affected (polioencephalitis) paralysis of some of the cranial nerves, such as the seventh (facial) nerve, with a resulting weakness of one side of the face, occurs. More important, however, is the paralysis of the vital centres (*bulbar paralysis*) which may develop. Paralysis of the respiratory centre, with marked dyspnoea and cyanosis, is a common form of bulbar paralysis. Respiratory failure in poliomyelitis may, however, also be caused by paralysis of the intercostal muscles and diaphragm.

Pharyngeal paralysis is another most important result of bulbar paralysis. Pharyngeal paralysis causes difficulty in swallowing with consequential accumulation of secretions in the throat which may lead to choking and asphyxia.

Diagnosis and course

The sudden onset after a few days of fever, during an epidemic, of a flaccid paralysis of a limb or part of a limb allows the diagnosis to be readily made. The diagnosis may be confirmed by examination of the cerebrospinal fluid, which will show an increase in the number of the white cells.

The paralysis usually reaches its maximum in the first few days, after which it remains stationary. Paralysis is particularly likely to occur where strenuous physical exercise has been undertaken in the preceding few days. Slow gradual improvement usually takes place over the next few months, but it may take as long as a year before the maximum recovery has been effected. In some cases complete recovery may take place, but in others residual paralysis with severe wasting of the muscles remains.

Treatment of poliomyelitis

ACTIVE IMMUNISATION. After years of research an active and safe vaccine has been produced which offers good protection against paralytic poliomyelitis. This vaccine has already done much to eradicate the dreaded effects of a disease so long known as infantile paralysis. Today the vaccine most widely used throughout the world is an attenuated or weakened form of live virus. This vaccine can be taken by mouth and is usually administered as three drops of vaccine on a lump of sugar. The first dose can be given when the child is six months old and two further doses within the first year. A booster dose can be given at the age of 18. This virus, too weak to lead to

any ill effects, nevertheless causes the formation of sufficient antibodies to provide immunity for several years. All susceptible members of
the family should be immunised at the same time.

CURATIVE

The patient is nursed at complete rest and full isolation procedure
is carried out. Masks should be worn and the faeces must be handled
with care and disposed of promptly. It is essential to wash the hands
carefully after toileting.

The affected limbs must be placed in a position of optimum rest.
It is most important that paralysed muscles should not be stretched
as permanent damage may result. (See p. 281 for the proper care of
paralysed limbs and the prevention of pressure sores.)

Passive movements are started from the onset, and it is for this
reason that any splints used should be capable of easy removal.
Prolonged rigid fixation of a limb in heavy splints must at all cost
be avoided. As soon as the pains and the acute tenderness of the
muscles subside active exercises are started, preferably under the
supervision of a skilled physiotherapist. Baths are very useful in that
active exercises of the muscles are carried out with greater ease in
water. Physiotherapy may have to be continued for months or even
years to ensure the maximum degree of recovery possible.

Special orthopaedic appliances, like walking calipers, may be
necessary, and in some cases operations may be performed to aid
movement in the paralysed parts.

If the respiratory muscles (intercostals and diaphragm) are
affected respiratory failure may develop, and for these cases special

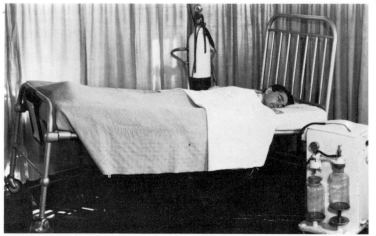

FIG. 9.21   The correct position for nursing a patient with pharyngeal paralysis. The
prone (or semiprone) position with the head on one side and elevation of the foot of
the bed allow the maximum drainage of the mouth secretions. The patient should be
turned frequently from side to side.

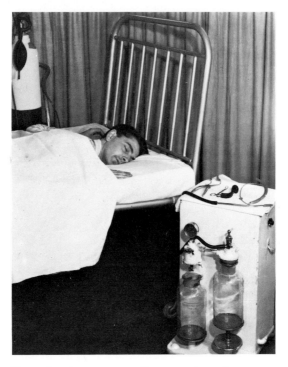

Fig. 9.22 The various instruments, suction apparatus and oxygen necessary for nursing a patient with pharyngeal paralysis. They must always be available at the bedside.

apparatus known as a respirator ('iron lung') is available to tide the patient over the acute phase. Several different types of respirator are used and all require the utmost skill in management. Patients who have to be placed in a respirator are naturally very apprehensive and often terrified. Constant reassurance and explanation of the benefits to be gained from the use of the respirator are therefore needed to allay this anxiety.

In the bulbar form of poliomyelitis pharyngeal paralysis may be present causing an inability to swallow which can lead to choking and asphyxia as a result of the accumulation of secretions in the throat. A suction apparatus must therefore always be available at the bedside to remove the mouth secretions. Postural drainage helps to prevent the accumulation of secretions in the throat and so these patients are best nursed in the prone or semiprone position with the foot of the bed elevated.

The bulbar form of poliomyelitis with its pharyngeal paralysis and also paralysis of the respiratory centre, calls for the greatest care and constant attention to ensure that a clear airway is at all times maintained. Tracheostomy is often needed in poliomyelitis to maintain a clear airway. Patients with respiratory and bulbar paralysis must never be left unattended.

Finally, it should be realised how apprehensive are patients suffering from poliomyelitis. Every encouragement must be given to them and they must be continually reassured that they will recover a great deal of the lost power in their limbs. As progress may be very slow and take many months or years the need for continued sympathy, understanding and encouragement for these patients must be stressed.

CONVULSIONS (Fits)

Convulsions or fits are commonly seen in a wide variety of diseases and tend to occur more frequently in infants and children than in adults; a fit or convulsion in an infant often takes the place of a rigor in an adult. On the other hand, epilepsy is a disorder characterised by repeated fits for which no cause can be found.

Symptomatic fits

Symptomatic fits are those in which there is some underlying discoverable cause. In contrast to symptomatic fits, idiopathic fits (or epilepsy) are those recurring fits without any obvious cause which are frequently seen in children and adults. Symptomatic fits are much more frequent than idiopathic epilepsy, so they will be described first. Again, for the sake of convenience, we can divide symptomatic fits into (1) in infants and children, and (2) in adults.

COMMON CAUSES OF FITS IN INFANTS AND CHILDREN. Fits or convulsions are very commonly seen in infants. Any severe general illness or fever in an infant may start with a convulsion. Rigors do not occur in young children, being replaced by a convulsion. Whooping-cough, measles, pneumonia and otitis media commonly cause convulsions in infants.

Gastrointestinal disturbances are another frequent cause of fits, especially in the first year of life; gastroenteritis and intestinal worms may be associated with convulsions. Simple digestive upsets, especially in the teething stage, may also cause fits.

Diseases of the central nervous system (such as meningitis, cerebral tumours, hydrocephalus and the various forms of paralyses due to maldevelopment or injury which are so often seen in infants) are especially liable to cause repeated fits.

COMMON CAUSES OF FITS IN ADULTS. The following is a brief list of the more common conditions in adults in which convulsions occur:

(a) Following severe head injury
(b) Uraemia (renal failure)
(c) Severe hypertension (hypertensive encephalopathy)
(d) Toxaemias of pregnancy (eclampsia)
(e) Cerebral tumours
(f) Neurosyphilis, especially general paralysis of the insane
(g) Hypoglycaemia
(h) Hysteria.

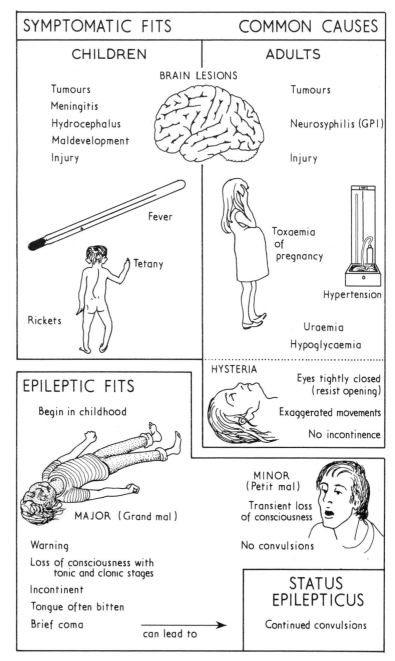

SYMPTOMATIC FITS   COMMON CAUSES

CHILDREN   ADULTS

BRAIN LESIONS

Tumours   Tumours
Meningitis
Hydrocephalus   Neurosyphilis (GPI)
Maldevelopment
Injury   Injury

Fever

Tetany   Toxaemia
                          of
                          pregnancy

                                  Hypertension

Rickets   Uraemia
                          Hypoglycaemia

HYSTERIA

EPILEPTIC FITS   Eyes tightly closed
                                  (resist opening)
Begin in childhood   Exaggerated movements
                                  No incontinence

                          MINOR
                          (Petit mal)
                          Transient loss
MAJOR (Grand mal)   of consciousness

Warning   No convulsions
Loss of consciousness with
   tonic and clonic stages
Incontinent   STATUS
Tongue often bitten   EPILEPTICUS
Brief coma   ⟶   Continued convulsions
         can lead to

Fig. 9.23   Some common causes of convulsions.

Epilepsy

Epilepsy is the term given to the frequently seen recurring fits without obvious underlying cause. Epilepsy usually begins in child-hood, rarely occurring for the first time in adult life. Fits which do start for the first time in adult life therefore usually have some definite underlying cause and so come into the category of symptomatic fits.

There are two main forms of idiopathic epilepsy, major epilepsy (grand mal) and petit mal.

Major epilepsy. In this form fits occur with loss of consciousness and usually in well-defined stages.

1. The warning. This takes different forms in different people, e.g. a peculiar sensation, an odd taste or smell, a sense of nausea, etc.
2. Tonic stage. In this stage the patient falls unconscious, often with an epileptic cry. All the muscles go rigid, the breathing ceases and the patient goes blue in the face. The tongue is frequently bitten.
3. Clonic stage. Spasms of the muscles occur, resulting in violent movements of the limbs. Frothing at the mouth and in-continence of urine and faeces are also usually present.
4. Stage of coma. After the clonic spasms the patient remains in a coma, which, however, quickly passes into a deep ordinary sleep if the patient is not awakened. The duration of the fit is hardly ever more than two minutes and may be much less. In severe cases, fit may succeed fit, causing the condition of *status epilepticus*. This may go on for hours and, if the fits are not controlled, death from exhaustion can occur.

Petit mal. Minor fits are much more common than major fits and may occur separately or in a patient also suffering from major fits. The attacks are much briefer and often more numerous. The fit consists of a transient loss of consciousness, perhaps lasting only for a second or two and sometimes known as 'absences'. This loss of consciousness may be so brief that the patient feels only 'dazed' and onlookers may not notice anything wrong. The patients often describe their attacks as 'blackouts'. No convulsions occur, the patient merely staying still with a vacant expression and ceasing any action he may be carrying out.

Post-epileptic automatism. Post-epileptic automatism is a peculiar state which may follow epileptic fits. It may last for several hours, and while in this state the patient appears normal even to carrying out any work. There is no recollection, however, on the part of the patient of what has been done. The importance of this state is that the patients may perform actions which can have serious legal consequences. The term *psychomotor epilepsy* is used to describe the disorders of behaviour often associated with loss of memory (amnesia) where this is due to epilepsy.

Course and diagnosis

The diagnosis of a single attack of loss of consciousness is often difficult if no reliable witness has observed the episode.

A fainting attack (*syncope*) is a common occurrence, especially in young people, and has to be differentiated from epilepsy. Syncope is due to a temporary deprivation of the blood supply to the brain and is associated with a slow pulse and a fall in blood pressure. It is liable to occur on standing too long in a warm room or in some susceptible people, at the sight of blood or even the mention of a medical matter. It is usually preceded by a swimmy feeling and sweating so that there is some warning that something is wrong. The face is pale, the pulse is slow and weak and the skin is moist. Convulsive movements rarely occur and are not sustained. Although the subject may sink to the floor, recovery soon takes place and there is no prolonged confusional state on recovery.

In an epileptic attack, there is no warning and usually no discernible precipitating factors. The convulsive movements may be strong and persistent and may be followed by a confusional state. The pulse is full and rapid and there is no sweating. The electroencephalogram (EEG) may be of help in confirming the diagnosis. This is a recording of the electrical activity of the brain and may reveal abnormalities when epilepsy is present. Where it is available, Computerised Axial Tomography (using the CAT scanner) provides a composite series of X-ray pictures of the brain and reveals the presence of any abnormal areas in the brain. Unfortunately, although the technique gives valuable information, it is very expensive.

Many cases of epilepsy tend to lessen in severity when adult life is reached, and in some patients the fits may cease completely. Some severe cases may, however, be associated with mental deterioration, and these patients are best treated in special epileptic colonies or homes.

Treatment of epilepsy

MANAGEMENT OF THE FIT

A major fit is often very alarming to the uninitiated onlooker and the nurse should remain calm and prevent others from acting rashly. It is usually not necessary to do anything more than to ensure that the person having the fit is out of harm's way, for example from traffic or from an electric fire. Obstruction to the patient's movements should be removed and something soft, such as a folded jacket, placed under the head. Tight clothing round the neck can be carefully loosened if this is not likely to frighten a semi-conscious patient. When the convulsions have ceased, the patient can be turned onto the side in a semi-prone position to aid breathing and for comfort. The patient is often confused for a time after a major fit and the nurse can offer reassurance and sympathy during this phase. It is never wise to restrain convulsive movements or to try to put anything between the teeth.

Especially in undiagnosed cases, the nurse may be a vital witness of the seizure and her observations may allow a firm diagnosis to be reached. A record should be made of onset of the attack, the nature of the convulsions, the recovery stage and the pulse rate.

In status epilepticus, consciousness does not recover between attacks. Here urgent measures to stop the recurring fits are necessary. Injections of diazepam intravenously or intramuscularly are valuable. If this is not successful phenobarbitone intramuscularly is usually tried.

PREVENTION OF THE FITS

The following drugs are in common use in the treatment of epilepsy, either alone or in combination:

1. Phenobarbitone. This drug is most frequently used and is given in doses of 60 to 90 mg three times a day, according to the patient's age and the severity of the fits. Primidone is an alternative to phenobarbitone and is sometimes more effective.

2. Phenytoin sodium (Epanutin) is given in capsules of 100 mg each, usually up to a maximum of three daily. It is often combined with phenobarbitone when phenobarbitone alone does not succeed in controlling the fits.

3. Ethosuxamide and sodium valproate are particularly successful in the treatment of petit mal.

Regular supervision of patients taking anti-epileptic drugs is necessary since side-effects are likely to occur after prolonged use. The level of the drug should be measured in the blood so that the dose can be monitored according to response.

LATER MANAGEMENT

In some children the attacks are so frequent despite all treatment that admission to special schools is necessary. Adults liable to epilepsy must find employment which would not involve danger if a fit occurred; they should not drive vehicles, work at heights or near machinery for example.

Operative measures may be carried out in some cases of severe epilepsy to remove a focal abnormality in the brain. Removal of part of the temporal lobe, in what is called temporal lobe epilepsy, is the most common operative treatment at present performed.

PARALYSIS AGITANS (Parkinson's disease)

CAUSE. Paralysis agitans was first described by Parkinson in 1817 and so bears his name. It is a degenerative disorder of the basal ganglia of the brain associated with a lack of dopamine. Dopamine is a neurotransmitter, one of a series of chemical substances (amines) which help transmit impulses through the brain tissue.

It usually comes on in later life and can become disabling. It can be induced by various drugs such as rauwolfia or haloperidol, but in this case the disorder is reversible and the symptoms clear when the drug responsible is discontinued.

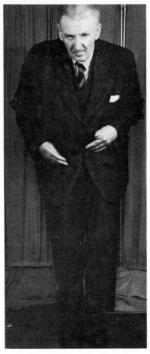

FIG. 9.24 Paralysis agitans. The fixed rigid attitude of the patient and lack of emotional expression are characteristic of the disease.

Symptoms

1. There is the characteristic rigidity of appearance and movement. The face tends to be mask-like, showing very little emotion. The patient walks in a characteristic manner with short shuffling steps; the arms are pressed to the sides and do not swing on walking.

2. Tremor. This is very common and is usually most marked in the hands. There is the constant movement of the fingers which has been given the name of 'pill-rolling'. The tremor may be very severe in some cases, affecting the arms and the head too. The tremor is usually made worse by emotion, but tends to stop when performing any definite action.

3. Speech becomes slurred and monotonous and movements slow.

DIAGNOSIS. The diagnosis is usually obvious on looking at the patient from his typical appearance, walk and tremor.

Treatment

Various drugs are now available which do much to ameliorate the stiffness and tremor.

1. L-dopa (levodopa) helps to form dopamine in the brain and leads to considerable improvement in the majority of patients, allowing them to get about more freely and with less tremor. Combined

with carbidopa, which can concentrate the action of L-dopa in the brain, it is given in the form of sinemet half a tablet three times a day. Nausea and loss of appetite can be troublesome side effects.

2. Benzhexol (Artane) 2 to 5 mg three times a day reduces the tremor and rigidity.

3. Amantadine (Symmetral) 100 mg twice a day has a good effect in the initial stages but the benefits tend to wear off after a time.

4. Drugs of the belladonna group (atropine, stramonium, hyoscine) when given in large doses help some patients while antihistamines such as benadryl may be effective in others.

In some patients who have failed to respond to medical treatment and who are seriously disabled, recourse to neurosurgery may be advised. An operation has been devised which cuts into the centre in the brain controlling muscle tone (globus pallidus), and this manoeuvre may be strikingly successful in reducing rigidity and tremor.

POST-ENCEPHALITIC PARKINSONISM

The picture of paralysis agitans, with some modifications, is sometimes seen in much younger patients. In these it is a late complication (often many years later) of a form of encephalitis known as *encephalitis lethargica*, or, as it is often called, sleepy sickness. This disease, now rare, occurred in an epidemic form in the 1920s.

Post-encephalitic Parkinsonism, in addition to the general picture of paralysis agitans, also produces a marked tremor of the eyes and tongue with excessive salivation. Mental retardation, which may necessitate treatment in a mental hospital, is also frequently present in these patients.

CHOREA

Chorea, which occurs in young children, causes irregular purposeless movements as the characteristic feature. It is allied to rheumatic fever, as many children who have suffered from chorea later on develop signs of rheumatic heart disease. For some unknown reason this form of chorea never occurs in adults except during pregnancy.

Symptoms and signs

1. There are the characteristic choreiform movements. These are sudden, changing, purposeless movements which occur in the face, arms and legs, so that the child appears to be continually fidgeting and grimacing. He tends to drop articles held in the hands.

2. There is a clumsiness of movement which is due to the involuntary movements described above and also to the general weakness of the muscles.

3. The child is often nervous and emotional.

4. There may be evidence of acute rheumatic heart disease, such as a rapid and perhaps irregular pulse.

5. Chorea, when it occurs in women during pregnancy, may take

a very severe course with violent movements and mental confusion often bordering on acute mania.

Treatment

The child must be nursed with absolute rest as in acute rheumatic fever, so as to avoid any strain on a possibly damaged heart. For the same reason the child must not do anything for itself, but must be fed and washed. As these patients are inclined to be nervous and emotional the carrying out of all the necessary details in these cases will call for the utmost patience and skill.

The clothing should be light and warm, and as the clothing may get thrown off during the choreiform movements a sleeping suit and bedsocks are useful in severe attacks. Care must be exercised in the choice of feeding utensils as these may get broken as a result of the violent movements. The child must be prevented from injuring itself in severe attacks by suitable padding of the bed.

There is no specific treatment as yet available. If the choreiform movements are severe, sedatives, such as phenobarbitone (30 mg two or three times a day), are useful.

When all active signs of the disease have gone, i.e. when the choreiform movements have ceased, or almost so, when the pulse rate is normal and there are no abnormal signs in the heart, the child is gradually allowed to get up. Convalescence, as in cases of acute rheumatic fever, must be prolonged. Constructive toys help the child to regain co-ordinated movements and, in addition, keep him amused.

HERPES ZOSTER

Herpes zoster is a common disease caused by the virus also responsible for chickenpox. It is often known as *shingles* and involves the posterior nerve roots. Any nerve can be affected.

Symptoms and signs

At first there is pain along the course of the affected nerve, which is followed soon after by the characteristic eruption. This takes the form of small blebs, or vesicles, scattered along the line of the nerve so that they map out the path of the affected nerve. The vesicles dry up to form crusts.

The pain, particularly in elderly patients, may be most severe and persistent, lasting perhaps for many weeks or months after all signs of the eruption have gone. The pain may be so severe as to lead to marked mental depression.

Two nerves are commonly the site of herpes zoster infections:

1. The ophthalmic division of the fifth cranial nerve with resultant pain and eruption above the affected eye. The cornea of the eye may also be affected, leading to corneal ulceration.

2. The intercostal nerves, when pain and the typical eruption occur in a girdle fashion around one side of the chest.

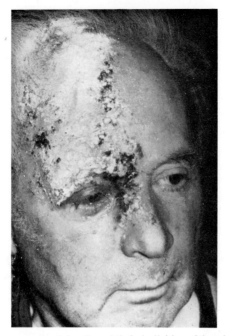

FIG. 9.25 Herpes zoster involving the ophthalmic division of the trigeminal nerve.

Treatment

In severe cases with a lot of pain the patient is best treated in bed. A light dusting powder, such as zinc oxide, is used for the eruption. Sedatives, e.g. aspirin, phenacetin or codeine, are usually needed to relieve the pain.

In the cases affecting the eye particular attention must be paid to prevent or minimise corneal ulceration. Hyoscine or atropine drops are instilled into the eye to dilate the pupil; hot bathing may also be useful.

SYPHILIS OF THE NERVOUS SYSTEM

Syphilitic disease of the central nervous system, often known as neurosyphilis, is now an uncommon disorder. There are three main types, meningovascular, tabes dorsalis and general paralysis of the insane (GPI).

MENINGOVASCULAR SYPHILIS

Particularly in the second stage of syphilis changes can occur in the meninges and the vessels of the brain. A rare cause of meningitis not previously mentioned is syphilis. The symptoms and signs of *syphilitic meningitis* are exactly the same as those in other acute forms.

In differentiating between syphilitic and other types of meningitis the Wassermann test is most helpful as it is usually strongly positive in syphilitic meningitis.

Cerebral thrombosis is the main syphilitic lesion of the blood vessels. Syphilitic cerebral thrombosis tends to occur in a younger age group than is affected by the common form of cerebral thrombosis due to cerebral arteriosclerosis. The signs and symptoms of cerebral thrombosis caused by syphilis are similar to those described under Strokes.

Treatment is given on page 281.

TABES DORSALIS

PATHOLOGY. The form of neurosyphilis known as tabes dorsalis occurs in the tertiary stage of syphilitic infection from five to 15 years after the primary stage. The main lesions are in the posterior columns of the spinal cord, and as these carry sensory impulses the early predominating symptoms tend to be sensory.

Symptoms and signs

Men are more commonly affected, usually in middle life. A juvenile form of tabes, however, is seen in congenital syphilis.

1. The earliest symptoms are the characteristic *lightning pains*, so called because they last for a few brief seconds, shooting up and down or through the legs. They are often likened to the effect of pins being stuck into the limb. The patients may refer to the pains as 'rheumatism'. The pains come on in periodic attacks which may last several hours.

2. Disturbances of bladder function occur early, usually consisting of difficulty in holding the urine or, in other cases, retention of urine.

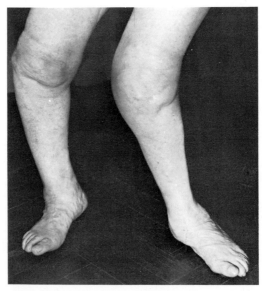

FIG. 9.26 Charcot's joints in a case of tabes. The knee joints are grossly swollen and deformed with painlessly abnormal mobility.

3. The gait is very typical, there being a well-marked ataxia present. This is often so predominant that the other name for tabes dorsalis is *locomotor ataxia*. The patient tends to fall about, especially when the eyes are closed or in a dark room. The patient characteristically walks with the feet wide apart and with marked stamping of the feet. The difficulty in walking gets progressively worse, and eventually getting about even with the aid of sticks is impossible and the patient becomes bed-ridden.

4. Owing to the loss of the sensation of pain, trophic changes in the joints, such as gross swelling, marked destruction and deformity, develop. Extreme abnormal mobility without pain is the typical result of these changes. Similar trophic joint changes, which are commonly known as *Charcot's joints*, can and do occur in any neurological disease where the sensation of pain in a joint is lost. The absence of the sensation of pain allows repeated trivial injuries to effect the destructive changes in the joints. Other frequently seen trophic lesions are perforating ulcers on the feet, especially on the ball of the big toe.

5. Sudden acute severe abdominal pain with vomiting may occur, which may give the appearance of an acute abdomen. This attack is known as a *gastric crisis* of tabes. Similar crises may affect other parts, e.g. the larynx, causing difficulty in breathing owing to spasm of the laryngeal muscles, or the rectum, causing pain and the constant desire to defaecate.

6. Characteristic eye changes, known as Argyll Robertson pupils, occur in tabes dorsalis as in all forms of neurosyphilis. These changes are absolutely diagnostic of syphilis and so form an extremely valuable sign. The complete eye changes as described by Argyll Robertson are:

(a) Unequal pupils.

(b) Very small pupils with irregularity of outline.

(c) Failure of the pupils to contract like normal pupils on exposure to light. The reaction to accommodation is, however, normal.

7. The deep tendon reflexes, especially the ankle and knee jerks, are absent from an early stage.

DIAGNOSIS. The lightning pains, marked ataxic gait and the presence of Argyll Robertson pupils are usually sufficient for diagnosis. A lumbar puncture is, however, usually done in most cases to confirm the diagnosis, when changes such as an increase in cells and in the protein in the cerebrospinal fluid are found to be present. The Wassermann test on the spinal fluid is usually but not always positive.

GENERAL PARALYSIS OF THE INSANE (GPI)

General paralysis of the insane, like tabes, arises in the tertiary stage of syphilis. It affects the higher centres of the brain and also the

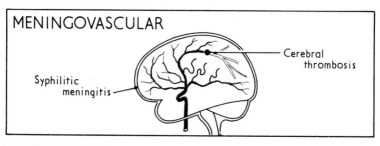

MENINGOVASCULAR

Cerebral thrombosis

Syphilitic meningitis

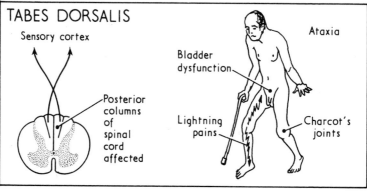

TABES DORSALIS

Sensory cortex

Ataxia

Bladder dysfunction

Posterior columns of spinal cord affected

Lightning pains

Charcot's joints

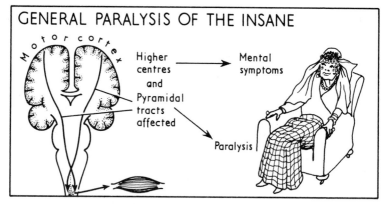

GENERAL PARALYSIS OF THE INSANE

Motor cortex

Higher centres and Pyramidal tracts affected

Mental symptoms

Paralysis

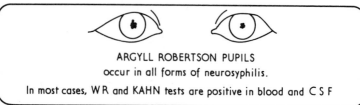

ARGYLL ROBERTSON PUPILS
occur in all forms of neurosyphilis.

In most cases, WR and KAHN tests are positive in blood and CSF

FIG. 9.27   Syphilis affecting the nervous system.

pyramidal motor tracts. The name is descriptive, emphasising the predominant changes, i.e. a paralysis associated with insanity.

Symptoms and signs

1. Mental changes. The earliest symptoms are usually a deterioration of intellect and abnormal behaviour on the part of the patient, particularly as regards personal appearance and moral conduct. Eventually complete dementia sets in. The grandiose form, with ideas of grandeur and delusions of power and wealth, is nowadays much less frequently seen.

2. Paralysis. This mainly affects the legs, causing a paraplegia (paralysis of both lower limbs). This paralysis may progress so that getting about becomes so difficult that the patient becomes bedridden and incontinent.

3. Convulsions or fits are frequent.

4. Well-marked fine tremors of the lips and tongue are a feature of this disease.

5. Argyll Robertson pupils are often present, as in other types of neurosyphilis.

6. Lastly, tabes dorsalis and general paralysis of the insane may occur in the same patient (*Tabo-paresis*).

DIAGNOSIS. The mental changes combined with paralysis and often with fits, together with the Argyll Robertson pupils, give a characteristic picture. Lumbar puncture to obtain a specimen of the cerebrospinal fluid is usually performed, and the fluid always shows a positive Wassermann reaction. A Wassermann test of the blood will also be positive.

Treatment of neurosyphilis

1. The specific treatment for neurosyphilis, as for all types of syphilitic infection, is large doses of penicillin. At least 10 million units are given over a period of approximately 14 days. A second course may be necessary.

2. Tabes dorsalis. Re-educational exercises to improve the walking are extremely useful and may enablé a patient to get about who otherwise would be bedridden. As with patients with disseminated sclerosis, the tabetic patient must be encouraged to keep up and about as much as possible.

Sedatives and analgesics, such as aspirin or codeine, are necessary for the lightning pains. Phenobarbitone and chlorpromazine are the most useful drugs for the crises.

For a Charcot's joint supportive splints will be needed.

Occlusive dressings should be applied to any ulcer present.

Finally, a careful watch on the urine for any sign of infection of the urinary tract is essential, and if infection develops it should be treated with sulphonamides or suitable antibiotics.

DISEASES OF THE NERVOUS SYSTEM IN INFANTS AND CHILDREN

BIRTH INJURIES

Facial paralysis

A facial paralysis, usually due to forceps delivery, often occurs, but is of little importance as it always clears up completely.

Brachial plexus injuries

The brachial plexus is the main network of nerves which supplies the upper limb. This plexus may be injured at birth in cases of difficult labour.

Two main forms of paralysis occur: *Erb's palsy*, where the shoulder girdle muscles are particularly involved, and the upper limb takes up a characteristic attitude known as the 'porter's tip' position, with the palm of the hand facing backwards and outwards; and *Klumpke's palsy*, where the hand and forearm are mainly involved, giving rise to marked wasting and the typical 'claw hand'.

Treatment

Treatment consists of applying light splints to relax the affected muscles and massage is started early. Active movements are encouraged as far as possible and it is important to gain the understanding and cooperation of the parents. Operative measures may have to be undertaken if the paralysis has not improved after six months.

Intracranial haemorrhage

In cases of difficult labour, such as may result from disproportion or a difficult forceps delivery, trauma to the brain may lead to cerebral haemorrhage which if severe is usually fatal. In some cases the meninges may be torn and adhesions may then form which block the flow of the cerebrospinal fluid. This leads to the development of hydrocephalus, which in infancy is accompanied by gross enlargement of the head.

Severe birth injury, such as intracranial haemorrhage, may also give rise to paralysis, e.g. a hemiplegia, and, in addition, may be responsible for the development of epileptic fits and mental deficiency.

SPASTIC PARALYSIS IN CHILDREN

Owing to failure of the brain to develop properly in the womb, children may be born with various forms of paralysis. Damage to the cortex of the brain involves the upper motor neurones and leads to a form of spastic diplegia known as Little's disease, in which paralysis occurs on both sides of the body. The legs are so stiff and rigid that the child has great difficulty in walking and does so with the legs crossed over each other—'scissors gait'. Damage of the deeper brain centres may lead to frequent jerky involuntary movements (athetoid type) while involvement of the cerebellum causes an unsteady gait and difficulty in balancing (ataxic type). Seriously handicapped spastics may have a combination of these disabilities

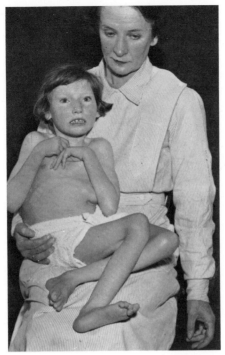

FIG. 9.28 Spastic diplegia (Little's disease) showing the characteristic position of the spastic limbs. The child was mentally defective and suffered from fits.

which may be associated with mental subnormality and a tendency to convulsions.

What must be emphasised strongly is that many spastic children are both intelligent and capable of training to lead a useful life. Some 1000 cerebral palsied babies are born every year in Great Britain and offer a challenge in education and training to enable them to fulfil their potential abilities.

HYDROCEPHALUS

Interference with the circulation of the cerebrospinal fluid leads to distension of the brain, and in children this is also accompanied by enlargement of the skull itself. The enlarged head of a hydrocephalic infant or child is at once apparent. It is globular or rounded in outline and the forehead bulges forward over the eyes.

Causes

1. CONGENITAL. Failure of the brain to develop properly is a frequent cause of hydrocephalus. Congenital hydrocephalus is often associated with other abnormal developmental changes such as hare-lip, cleft palate and spina bifida.

2. BIRTH INJURIES. Intracranial haemorrhage is another common

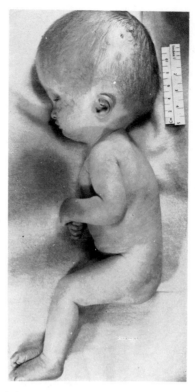

FIG. 9.29   Hydrocephalus.

cause of hydrocephalus. Difficult labour, especially with forceps delivery, may give rise to intracranial haemorrhage.

3. MENINGITIS. Adhesions resulting from meningitis may block the circulation of the cerebrospinal fluid and so lead to hydrocephalus.

4. CEREBRAL TUMOURS. A short-lived hydrocephalus is often seen as a result of a cerebral tumour.

As with many serious intracranial diseases in early childhood, convulsions and mental deficiency are often present with hydrocephalus.

In some cases where the circulation of the cerebrospinal fluid is blocked, surgical intervention may be needed. Insertion of a plastic tube with a one-way valve in it allows the cerebrospinal fluid to drain away from the distended cerebral ventricles into the left atrium of the heart, thus relieving the pressure causing the hydrocephalus.

MENTAL SUBNORMALITY

Mental disorder can be associated with a wide variety of diseases. It is proposed to give here a brief list of the more common forms of mental subnormality.

Many mentally subnormal cases can be improved by medical treatment or by special training, but severely subnormal patients are incapable of ever leading an independent life.

1. Failure of the central nervous system to develop properly during foetal life results in mental subnormality, and usually physical defects like an abnormally small skull (microcephaly), hydrocephalus or various types of paralysis, e.g. spastic diplegia of Little's disease, are also present. Birth injuries may cause brain haemorrhage and subsequent mental or physical disorders.

2. *Phenylketonuria.* This is an inherited disorder occurring in families. The baby may be abnormal from birth with vomiting and convulsions and the diagnosis can be confirmed by testing the urine and the blood. This is a rare cause of mental retardation but its importance lies in the fact that the mental changes are preventible if the condition is diagnosed and treated early enough.

The inherited defect is a missing enzyme which normally converts phenylalanine into a harmless protein. Phenylalanine is present in milk

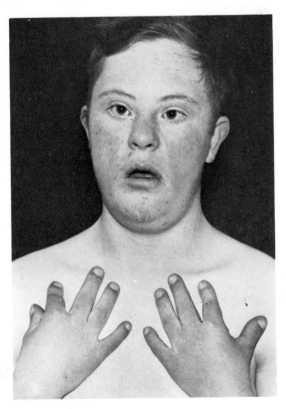

FIG. 9.30   Down's syndrome (mongolism), showing characteristic features and broad fingers.

feeds and in this condition it accumulates in the blood and causes damage to the brain. The missing enzyme cannot be supplied so the baby must be reared on a special synthetic milk which does not contain phenylalanine. Providing this is begun early enough before brain damage has occurred, the child can develop normally.

The diagnosis can be confirmed by testing the urine for phenylketonuria with Phenistix and examination of the blood for phenylalanine (Guthrie test). The baby's progress can also be monitored by these tests.

3. *Down's syndrome* (mongolism) is due to a chromosomal defect at the time of conception (p. 14). This common and tragic disorder places a great strain on the family, particularly where there are other normal children. The characteristic features can be detected at birth. The eye-slits are narrowed and slanting with an epicanthic fold across the inner aspect, the tongue is thick and fissured and the nose is stubby and depressed. The hands are broad and clumsy, with a single crease across the palm. There is often an associated congenital heart lesion. Mental subnormality may be severe and although sometimes the temperament may be sunny, more often there is apathy and disordered behaviour.

4. *Cretinism* is due to diminished function of the thyroid gland and unless diagnosed and treated in infancy, leads to stunting of growth and mental development (see p. 445).

Many cases of mental disorder, especially where there is some physical defect as well, are accompanied by convulsions. Another feature is the occasional presence of peculiar writhing snake-like movements of the limbs, to which the name *athetosis* is given.

Severe cases of mental subnormality have to be looked after in a suitable institution, but less severe cases can often be trained to some useful occupation and even become self-supporting.

MYOPATHIES (Muscular dystrophies)

Diseases which primarily affect the muscles, leading to profound weakness and wasting, are called myopathies. They usually occur, or start, in childhood and differ in type according to the particular muscles affected. For example, in the *facio-scapulo-humeral* form the face, shoulder girdle and upper arms are mainly involved, with marked wasting (atrophy) and weakness of power in these parts. The child has a vacant look, the normal facial expression being absent, and there is inability to raise the arms above the head. If the distal parts of the arms and legs are mainly affected it is often known as the *distal type* of myopathy.

One striking form does occur which differs from the others in that the wasted muscles are replaced by fat, and so look larger than normal instead of wasted. This form is known as the *pseudo-hypertrophic type*. It usually affects boys, and starts about the age of 4 or 5. The shoulder and pelvic girdle muscles are particularly involved, and these muscles become enlarged. In addition, the calf muscles too are enlarged. The child has difficulty in getting about and has a waddling gait. One characteristic feature is the peculiar way in which the child rises from the lying-down position. The child has to roll over on to his face, and then on to his hands and knees, and gradually 'works up' the legs with the hands—the so-called 'climbing up his knees' position. Many of these children become bedridden in later childhood. Mild cases, however, may live in fair health for many years. So far no treatment is of any real benefit.

SOME RARER CENTRAL NERVOUS SYSTEM DISEASES

Apart from the many different diseases of the central nervous system so far discussed, there remain many more which, however, are less common and so of less importance to the nurse. These rarer neurological diseases are mostly seen in special neurological hospitals or centres.

SUBACUTE COMBINED DEGENERATION OF THE CORD

This disease is associated with pernicious anaemia, and early cases respond to treatment with vitamin B_{12} given by injection in large doses. It causes a spastic weakness of both lower limbs with sensory disturbances such as numbness, pins and needles and sensory loss in the legs; the gait is usually ataxic.

SYRINGOMYELIA

This malady is due to defective drainage of the cerebrospinal fluid. This leads to distension of the central canal in the spinal cord, which becomes progressively larger and presses on the various tracts in the spinal cord. It usually starts in early adult life and slowly progresses.

The main distinguishing features of syringomyelia are a slow paralysis starting usually in the arms and spreading to the lower limbs, with profound wasting of the hands. There is also the characteristic *dissociated anaesthesia* where pain, heat and cold sensations are lost, but touch sensation is retained. This is due to the crossing of the sensory tracts in the spinal cord which allows the touch sensory tracts to escape damage in syringomyelia. These patients frequently burn themselves from holding cigarettes or matches and also develop ulcers from injuries which they do not feel. Charcot's joints are frequently present.

In some cases, if the diagnosis is made before widespread irreparable damage has occurred, surgical intervention can be undertaken to improve the flow of the cerebrospinal fluid.

PROGRESSIVE MUSCULAR ATROPHY (Motor neurone disease)

Slow progressive degeneration of the anterior (motor) horn cells in the grey matter of the spinal cord, the cause of which is unknown, leads to profound wasting and paralysis of the affected limbs. The disease usually occurs in adults and often starts in the anterior horn cells supplying the muscles of the hands, causing severe wasting of the hands—'claw hands'. Eventually most of the muscles of all limbs become affected, resulting in complete paralysis, by which time the patient has a skeleton appearance.

The wasting muscles show typical twitchings or tremors known as *fasciculation*. The pyramidal tracts may be affected in some cases, leading to a spastic paralysis, usually of the legs. It is characteristic of this disease that no sensory changes develop because only the motor tract or anterior motor horn cells are damaged.

All treatment so far used is of little avail, and ultimately the patients become bedridden and incontinent.

TRANSVERSE MYELITIS (Compression of the spinal cord)

The term transverse myelitis is often used to describe severe damage to the spinal cord, usually caused by lesions pressing on the cord. The term myelitis is therefore in most cases a misnomer as inflammatory lesions are seldom responsible for the disease.

Compression of the spinal cord leads to marked motor and sensory disturbances below the level of the lesion, which is usually in the lumbar region of the cord. There is complete loss of sensation in the legs and in part of the trunk, associated with a paralysis of the affected area. Incontinence or retention of urine is present. Trophic ulcers and pressure sores are very prone to develop, due to the sensory loss.

The causes of compression of the cord can be conveniently divided into the acute (sudden) and the slow and progressive. In the acute forms the sensory loss and degree of paralysis are much more complete and severe than in the slow onset types. Fracture-dislocations of the spine, usually in the cervical region, account for most of the acute cases. Haemorrhage and thrombosis in the spinal cord, due to hypertension or syphilis, are more rarely responsible.

Slow compression of the cord is usually due to one of two main causes: firstly, to tuberculous disease of the spine seen in young people, and secondly, to malignant tumours of the spine in older people.

In all cases nursing calls for a great deal of skill to prevent pressure sores and urinary infections. Most patients are treated by immobilising the spine in a plaster-bed for many months. Suitable cases may be operated on, as in tuberculous caries when a bone graft is done. Cases due to malignant tumours are hopeless and only palliative treatment can be given.

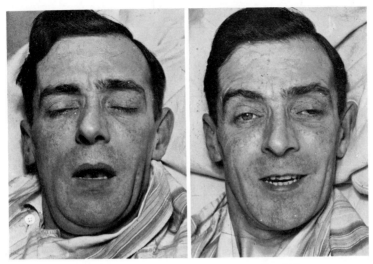

FIG. 9.31   FIG. 9.32

FIG. 9.31   Myasthenia gravis, patient cannot open his eyes or fully close his mouth.

FIG. 9.32   Myasthenia gravis after an injection of Prostigmin showing a marked improvement. The typical 'snarling' smile still remains, however.

MYASTHENIA GRAVIS

Myasthenia gravis is a slow progressive disease usually met with in adults and rare before the age of puberty. It causes a most peculiar form of paralysis, which tends to get worse with fatigue or use of the affected muscles and to improve with rest. Characteristically, therefore, the paralysis is minimal in the morning and worst at night. The disease most often affects the eye, facial and shoulder girdle muscles and, less often, the legs. Paralysis of the eye muscles (ophthalmoplegia), leading to squints and double vision, is present. Drooping of the eyelids (ptosis) and weakness of the face muscles cause the peculiar lack of expression and typical myasthenic (snarling) smile. Gradual loss of voice with prolonged speech or difficulty in chewing during the course of a meal are also frequent complaints. Weakness of the arms, especially in combing the hair or lifting anything, may be complained of.

Myasthenia responds to the drugs neostigmine (Prostigmin) and pyridostigmine (Mestinon) and a profoundly weak patient may be dramatically improved on taking these drugs. Nevertheless, in many cases the disease gradually progresses, and after many years death may occur owing to involvement of the respiratory muscles. Some cases have been greatly improved by removal of the thymus gland (thymectomy) which for some unknown reason tends to be enlarged in most cases of myasthenia.

COMA

When an individual is unconscious for any length of time he is said to be in coma. Coma can be caused by very many different conditions, most of which are both extremely important in medicine and of common occurrence.

COMMON CAUSES OF COMA

1. Drug overdosage

This is the commonest cause of coma in young people today. It should be realised that hypnotics and tranquillisers are prescribed for those who are anxious, harassed or depressed and this is the sort of person most likely to attempt suicide. Not all cases of deliberate overdosage really mean to commit suicide. More often, the taking of too many tablets is a gesture to demonstrate to others the depth of misery or despair that is being experienced. The tablets most commonly used are aspirins, barbiturates and various anti-depressants.

2. Injury, especially head injury

In most severe cases there is a fracture of the skull and laceration of the brain (contusion). The term *concussion* is often used to describe a transitory loss of consciousness due to head injury.

3. Cerebro-vascular accident (see p. 278) which includes cerebral haemorrhage, thrombosis or embolism.

4. Diabetic coma (see p. 426)

The onset is gradual, usually ushered in by vomiting. There is deep sighing respiration with breath smelling of acetone and the urine containing sugar and acetone.

5. Hypoglycaemia (see p. 423)

Liable to occur in any diabetic taking insulin.

6. Alcoholic coma

The breath smells strongly of alcohol. Alcohol can induce hypoglycaemia even with moderate intake.

7. Hepatic coma (see p. 257)

The end stage of severe liver destruction.

8. Uraemia (see p. 374)

The end stage of kidney failure.

9. Myxoedema (see p. 444)

If undiagnosed and untreated, coma may ensue.

10. Hypothermia (see p. 24)

In the elderly if neglected and undernourished without adequate heating in winter time.

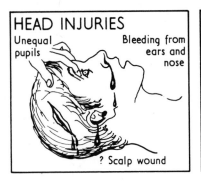

HEAD INJURIES

Unequal pupils

Bleeding from ears and nose

? Scalp wound

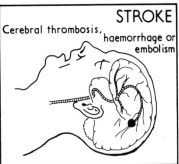

STROKE

Cerebral thrombosis, haemorrhage or embolism

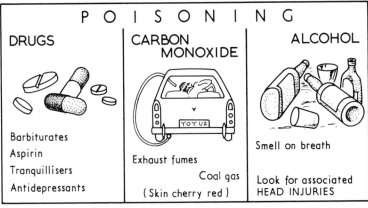

P O I S O N I N G

DRUGS

Barbiturates
Aspirin
Tranquillisers
Antidepressants

CARBON MONOXIDE

Exhaust fumes

Coal gas

(Skin cherry red)

ALCOHOL

Smell on breath

Look for associated HEAD INJURIES

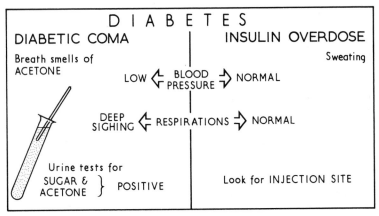

D I A B E T E S

DIABETIC COMA

Breath smells of ACETONE

INSULIN OVERDOSE

Sweating

LOW ← BLOOD PRESSURE → NORMAL

DEEP SIGHING ← RESPIRATIONS → NORMAL

Urine tests for
SUGAR & ACETONE } POSITIVE

Look for INJECTION SITE

| URAEMIA | ENCEPHALITIS | HYSTERIA |

FIG. 9.33   Some common causes of coma.

DIAGNOSIS AND MANAGEMENT OF A CASE OF COMA

When a patient is admitted to hospital in coma certain routine examinations and investigations are carried out in all cases. The nurse should be fully aware of the importance of all the following points, as when she is undressing the patient she will be able to verify the presence or absence of important details which can help to indicate the treatment of the patient.

1. The history of the case leading up to the coma is most important. The presence or otherwise of any *injury*, any past history of disease, such as hypertension, diabetes or kidney disease, and whether or not the patient has been taking drugs, especially sleeping drugs, are all significant factors. The relatives will be interviewed by the doctor to find if there has been any emotional crisis likely to lead to a suicidal attempt.

2. Careful examination of the head to find any scalp wounds or *bleeding* from the ears or nose is necessary. A fractured base of the skull often causes bleeding from the ear, which can be missed unless the ears are carefully looked at.

3. The size and shape of the *pupils* are important, especially any inequality of the pupils. The latter immediately points to local damage in the brain, as from injury or apoplexy. The very small pinpoint pupils of morphine poisoning should be looked for. The pupils in hysteria are often widely dilated.

4. The *breath* should be smelt, the typical sour smell of the alcoholic being easily recognised. The diagnosis of alcoholic coma, however, solely on the evidence of the smell of alcohol from the breath is most dangerous. A drunken person is very liable to sustain an injury which may well be the real cause of the coma. Indeed, the combination of alcohol and head injury is most common. Therefore in all cases of seemingly alcoholic coma the scalp and ears must be carefully examined for signs of injury and bleeding.

A sweet sickly smell, often likened to sweet pears or apples, is due to acetone in the breath and is characteristic, in particular, of diabetic coma.

5. The character of the *respirations* is important in diagnosis. Deep stertorous respirations are common in apoplexy and in diabetic coma. In insulin coma and in cases of severe injury and haemorrhage the respirations are shallow. In morphine poisoning the respiration rate is markedly depressed and may be as slow as 8 to 10 a minute. The peculiar waxing and waning respirations of Cheyne-Stokes frequently occur in apoplexy.

6. The *skin* is cold and clammy in shock, which would be present in coma due to severe injuries. A moist skin, often with marked sweating, is met with in insulin coma whilst, on the other hand, in diabetic coma the skin is extremely dry. The skin in diabetic coma

remains in a fold when it is pinched owing to the dehydration which is always present.

7. The limbs and trunk will be examined by the doctor for any injury, and the utmost care and gentleness used to ensure that any injury present is not made worse by handling the patient. Apart from locating an injury, it is also possible sometimes, even with the patient in coma, to discern a *paralysis* of one side of the body. This would of course lead to a diagnosis of hemiplegia, probably due to cerebral haemorrhage.

8. Examination of the *urine* is done as a routine in all cases of coma. If the cause of the coma is obvious, e.g. a head injury or carbon monoxide poisoning, then the examination of the urine can be delayed till the first convenient moment. In cases of suspected diabetes or poisoning, such as barbiturate or aspirin, or in uraemia, and in all cases where the diagnosis of the coma is not immediately obvious, examination of the urine is carried out immediately, and for this catheterisation will be necessary.

The urine is tested at once for sugar, acetone and albumin, and the remainder is saved and sent to the laboratory for further detailed examination. This will include tests for barbiturates and aspirin. The importance of saving all the urine for laboratory examination cannot be too forcibly stressed.

The presence of a heavy glycosuria and acetone immediately gives a diagnosis of diabetic coma in nearly all cases. A urine loaded with albumin would point to a possible uraemia.

By this stage the cause of the coma will be apparent in most cases. In a small number of cases, however, further immediate examinations, such as a lumbar puncture (to reveal blood in the cerebrospinal fluid or a possible meningitis) and blood urea and blood-sugar estimations, may be necessary to establish the diagnosis of the cause of the coma.

Treatment

The treatment of coma varies according to the cause and is therefore dealt with in the sections devoted to the causative conditions. The nursing of a patient in coma, whatever the cause, is of particular importance, and the general nursing care of a comatose patient is described under Strokes (p. 278).

10 Diseases of the Blood

PHYSIOLOGY

In an adult, about five litres of blood are present in the circulation. Blood withdrawn from the body and prevented from clotting separates into two parts, plasma and cells.

1. Plasma

Plasma is the clear yellow-coloured fluid in which the cells are suspended. It contains in solution many important substances derived from the food we eat, from the liver and from other organs. These are transported to various parts of the body. Amongst other substances, plasma contains:

    (a) The plasma proteins, albumin and globulin. These proteins are a reserve supply of nourishment and become depleted in times of illness or starvation.

    (b) Prothrombin and fibrinogen. As will be seen, these substances play an essential role in the clotting of blood to prevent undue bleeding after cuts or wounds.

    (c) Electrolytes. Sodium chloride (salt) and sodium bicarbonate are the principal electrolytes in plasma which also contains potassium, calcium, iodine, fluorine, and iron.

    (d) Nutrients such as glucose, aminoacids and fatty acids.

    (e) Vitamins and medicaments absorbed from the bowel.

    (f) Hormones derived from the endocrine system.

    (g) Waste products of metabolism, such as urea and creatinine, for excretion by the kidneys.

2. Cells

There are three types of cells in the blood: red blood cells (erythrocytes), white blood cells (leucocytes) and platelets (thrombocytes).

    (a) Red blood cells (erythrocytes) are flat cells containing haemoglobin. Haemoglobin is a pigment formed from protein and iron. When haemoglobin combines with oxygen, and it does so very readily, it becomes bright red thus imparting to blood its usual red colour. When oxygen is deficient, haemoglobin is blue and blood is said to be cyanosed.

    The main purpose of the red cells is to take up oxygen from the air in the alveoli of the lungs and to carry this oxygen to the tissues in all parts of the body. Waste carbon dioxide from the tissues is taken up by the red cells in exchange for oxygen and this carbon dioxide is breathed out when the red cells in the blood reach the lungs. Thus the red cells bring fresh oxygen to all parts of the body and get rid of waste carbon dioxide. This is part of the metabolic process of burning up fuel, just as a coal fire needs oxygen to burn and gives off carbon dioxide.

(b) White blood cells (leucocytes). There are three main types of leucocytes (see page 356), all concerned with overcoming infection.

(c) Platelets (thrombocytes) are small round bodies (see page 351) which are able to clump together. If there is any damage to the wall of a blood vessel, the platelets form a plug to seal off any leaks. Platelets also release a substance called thromboplastin important in the clotting of blood.

Normal blood formation

Before discussing the diseases that may affect the blood we must first see how blood is normally formed and what constitutes a normal blood count.

1. RED BLOOD CELLS

These are formed in the red marrow which in adults is found in the flat bones, such as the sternum and skull, and in the ends of the long bones. The red cells in the marrow are all in different stages of formation, from the early immature cells to the completely developed mature red cells such as are found in the peripheral blood. Normally only the completely mature red cells pass into the circulation, all the immature cells remaining in the marrow. In certain diseases, however, these immature red cells may pass out into the circulation.

FACTORS NECESSARY FOR THE NORMAL FORMATION OF RED CELLS. In order that the red cells may become completely mature and adequate in number various factors are necessary, of which the following are the most important:

(a) *Vitamin B_{12}* (cyanocobalamin). This substance is present in various foods, especially liver, meat, milk, eggs and cheese.

(b) *The intrinsic factor*. This is an enzyme normally formed by certain cells in the stomach. The intrinsic factor is essential for the proper absorption of vitamin B_{12}.

Vitamin B_{12}, which is absorbed into the body when the intrinsic factor is present, is stored in the liver and released to the bone marrow as required. Vitamin B_{12} is essential for the production of adequate numbers of fully mature red cells. If vitamin B_{12} is missing, the bone marrow will not produce sufficient numbers of red cells and, moreover, many of the red cells produced will be immature. They will tend to be larger than normal (macrocytes) and many of them will contain a nucleus (megaloblasts).

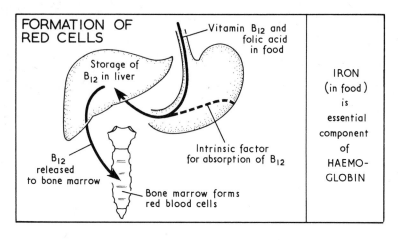

FORMATION OF RED CELLS

Vitamin B₁₂ and folic acid in food

Storage of B₁₂ in liver

B₁₂ released to bone marrow

Intrinsic factor for absorption of B₁₂

Bone marrow forms red blood cells

IRON (in food) is essential component of HAEMO-GLOBIN

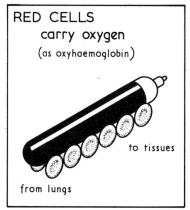

RED CELLS
carry oxygen
(as oxyhaemoglobin)

to tissues

from lungs

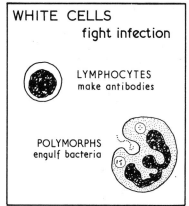

WHITE CELLS
fight infection

LYMPHOCYTES
make antibodies

POLYMORPHS
engulf bacteria

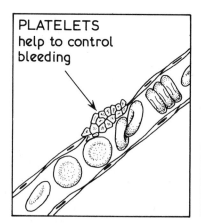

PLATELETS
help to control bleeding

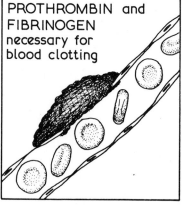

PROTHROMBIN and FIBRINOGEN necessary for blood clotting

Fig. 10.1   The formation and function of various components of the blood.

(c) *Folic acid.* Folic acid is part of the vitamin B complex. It has an action very similar to that of vitamin B_{12}, i.e. it is essential for the development of adequate numbers of fully mature red cells. In the absence of folic acid a macrocytic anaemia will develop.

2. HAEMOGLOBIN

Haemoglobin is the essential component of the red cells and it is by means of this that oxygen is carried in the red cells. Haemoglobin is mainly composed of iron, and if for any reason iron is not available there will be a reduction in the amount of haemoglobin in each red cell, and, as we shall see later, this is one cause of anaemia. This lack of iron can be caused in several different ways:

(a) By insufficient iron in the diet. For instance, the diet of normal infants is mainly composed of milk, which contains little iron, with the result that infants commonly suffer from an iron deficiency anaemia in the first year of life.

(b) Diseases of the stomach and intestines may prevent the proper absorption of iron from the intestinal tract. We shall see later that there are several diseases which are associated with a deficient absorption of iron and so cause anaemia.

3. WHITE BLOOD CELLS and PLATELETS (see later).

The normal blood count

The normal blood count in an adult is:
Red blood cells: 5,000,000 per mm^3.
Haemoglobin: 12·8 g per 100 ml of blood.
White blood cells: 5000 to 10,000 per mm^3.
Platelets: 200,000 per mm^3 approximately.

Erythrocyte sedimentation rate (ESR)

Blood is drawn from the patient's vein and sodium citrate is added to keep it fluid. This citrated blood is now drawn up into a long narrow graduated glass tube up to the 100 mm mark. The tube is held upright in a special container and allowed to stand. The corpuscles gradually settle, leaving clear plasma above. At the end of an hour, the height of the clear plasma is measured off on the tube, and this is known as the ESR. In good health, the corpuscles settle very slowly, so that the ESR is normally less than 10 mm after 1 hour. In various constitutional diseases the corpuscles settle more quickly and the ESR is at a higher level. Thus in rheumatic fever, for example, the ESR may be 40 mm in 1 hour but as the patient improves the ESR may return to normal. Thus the ESR is a valuable indication of disease, and a useful guide to progress.

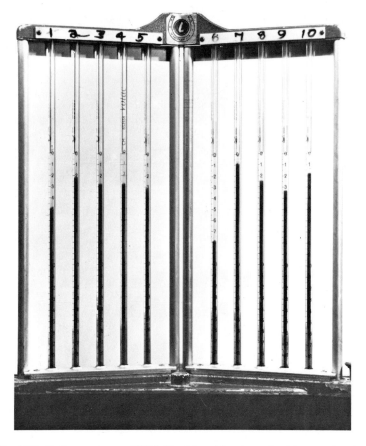

FIG. 10.2 Sedimentation rate (ESR). Blood from 10 patients after 1 hour: patient 1—ESR 50 mm/1 hour; patient 2—ESR 22 mm/1 hour, etc.

DISEASES AFFECTING THE RED CELLS

Anaemia is the term used for a reduction in the amount of available haemoglobin. Anaemia may be due to a number of different causes and often the diagnosis can be suspected by examining a smear of blood suitably stained (blood film) under the microscope. If the red cells are normal in size (normocytic) but reduced in number, this suggests blood loss from haemorrhage. If the red cells are small in size (microcytic) and pale in colour (hypochromic), the anaemia probably is caused by lack of iron. When anaemia is due to a deficiency of vitamin B_{12} or folic acid, the red cells are greatly reduced in number but are bigger than normal (macrocytic) and full of haemoglobin (hyperchromic) (See Table VIII). Measurement of the number of red cells, the size of the red

TABLE VIII

Type of anaemia	Number of red cells	Size of red cells	Haemoglobin content of red cell	Cause
Hyperchromic macrocytic	Reduced	Larger than normal (macrocytes)	Full (hyperchromic)	Lack of vitamin B_{12} or folic acid
Hypochromic microcytic	May be normal	Small (microcytes)	Very reduced (hypochromic)	Iron deficient
Normocytic	Reduced	Normal (hormocytic)	Normal	Acute haemorrhage

cells and the amount of haemoglobin each cell contains will complete the picture and offers a good idea as to the type of anaemia and its likely cause. Whatever the origin of the anaemia, lack of available haemoglobin causes various signs and symptoms.

GENERAL EFFECTS (SYMPTOMS AND SIGNS) OF ANAEMIA

Many of the symptoms and signs of anaemia are brought about by the deficiency in oxygen supply caused by shortage of the red cells and haemoglobin. The red cells and haemoglobin are the vital agents in the transport of oxygen throughout the body for the supply of all tissues and organs.

1. Pallor of the skin and mucous membranes. This is especially seen in the mucous membranes of the lower eyelid and the lips.

2. Weakness, giddiness and fainting. In women, amenorrhoea is commonly present.

3. Increased heart rate (tachycardia). To compensate for the deficiency in the amount of oxygen transported, which is caused by the reduction in the red cells and haemoglobin, the heart quickens its rate. This, by making the existing red cells and haemoglobin do more work, may overcome the oxygen deficiency in the tissues and organs in the less severe degrees of anaemia.

4. Dyspnoea and oedema of the ankles. These important signs are seen in severe cases where the heart fails to compensate for the reduction in the carriage of oxygen and so, as a result, heart failure develops. As in all cases of heart failure, from whatever cause, dyspnoea is the earliest symptom and is most marked on exertion.

5. If the anaemia is both rapid in onset and also severe, all the above symptoms (pallor, weakness, fainting and dyspnoea) will be very pronounced. In addition, the condition of shock may be present (p. 114). On the other hand, if the anaemia is more gradual in

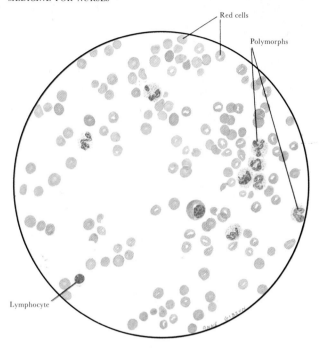

Fig. 10.3 Blood film showing the appearance of the normal red blood cells and the polymorphonuclear and lymphocytic white blood cells.

onset, symptoms may continue to be slight (mainly fatigue and loss of energy) until a profound degree of anaemia is present.

6. Blood examination. This will naturally reveal reductions both in the number of red cells and in the amount of haemoglobin to varying extents according to the particular type of anaemia present. Furthermore, in addition to the reduction in the number of the red cells and the amount of haemoglobin the size, shape and colour of the red cells are in most cases altered. Either macrocytic (large) or microcytic (small) cells may be present, according to the type of anaemia, whilst the cells may be highly coloured (hyperchromic) or pale (hypochromic).

Classification of the anaemias

Since treatment of anaemia depends very much on its cause, accurate diagnosis is essential. There are three main causes of anaemia.

1. Anaemia due to blood loss.
2. Anaemia due to decreased or abnormal blood formation.
3. Haemolytic anaemia due to increased blood destruction.

ANAEMIA DUE TO BLOOD LOSS

Haemorrhagic anaemias are probably those most frequently encountered in clinical practice. As can be readily appreciated, any sudden *acute* loss of blood is likely to result in a reduction in the red cells and haemoglobin. According to the size of the haemorrhage, it may take several weeks or more before the body can replace this loss in both red cells and haemoglobin. In medical diseases acute haemorrhage is most frequently seen as a haematemesis due to peptic ulcers, and as a haemoptysis from chronic chest conditions, especially tuberculosis and carcinoma. Acute haemorrhage is also commonly seen in maternity and surgical diseases such as post-partum haemorrhage, abortions, injuries, etc.

It is only when a sufficient quantity of blood, usually over half a litre, has been lost that any appreciable anaemia occurs. In most cases of acute sudden loss of large quantities of blood there is also an associated condition of *shock* which calls for proper treatment. The exact causes producing the clinical symptoms and signs associated with shock are not fully appreciated, but they are certainly in some way caused by actual loss of fluid from the circulation, which leads to failure of the peripheral circulation. When the blood volume is severely reduced the blood pressure falls, and if the fall is too great the vital centres are affected and shock results.

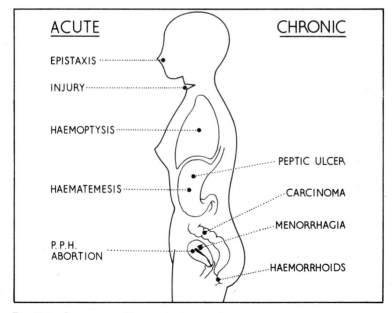

Fig. 10.4   Some causes of haemorrhagic anaemias.

Therefore in severe acute haemorrhage fluid is vitally needed to restore the blood volume and raise the blood pressure. In addition, it is also essential to replace the severe deficiency in the red cells and haemoglobin as otherwise the tissues will lack oxygen. The fluid lost to the circulation and the red cells and haemoglobin can all be replaced by transfusions of whole blood, which is the ideal therapy. Blood transfusions are indeed essential in all cases of severe acute haemorrhage. A fall in systolic blood pressure to below 100 mm. of mercury is a definite indication that a blood transfusion is required in acute haemorrhage. In these cases the patient is restless, with marked pallor and a cold clammy skin. The pulse is very rapid, usually in the region of 110, and it may be difficult to feel owing to the low pressure. There is also a marked reduction in output of urine.

It might be convenient at this stage to mention that the condition of shock with a low blood pressure may occur owing to severe injuries without actual haemorrhage. In these cases, too, it is essential to correct the low blood pressure by transfusions, but here transfusions with plasma instead of with whole blood may be sufficient. Transfusions with saline are useless to restore the blood pressure in severe acute haemorrhage and shock as saline is rapidly poured out of the circulation.

Chronic blood loss also leads to anaemia, and in these cases the haemoglobin is reduced more than the red cells because the red cells can be replaced much more quickly than the haemoglobin. The conditions which most commonly give rise to anaemia due to chronic blood loss are chronic haemorrhoids, severe menorrhagia, chronic peptic ulcer and carcinoma. The anaemia is treated by clearing up the cause of the chronic blood loss and by giving iron to manufacture haemoglobin. The red marrow usually replaces the red cells without special treatment.

ANAEMIAS DUE TO DECREASED BLOOD FORMATION

This second group of anaemias includes some very common and important types. In our earlier discussion on the red cells and the haemoglobin it was seen that several factors were essential for their proper formation, vitamin B_{12} and folic acid in food and the intrinsic factor in the stomach being necessary for the formation of the red cells, and iron being the essential component of haemoglobin. It can therefore be realised that either lack of or deficient absorption of any of these factors could lead to deficient blood formation.

Again, from the earlier statements on normal blood formation, it was seen that the blood is formed in the red bone marrow. Diseases of the bones, therefore, could interfere with the formation of the blood in the marrow, and in clinical practice we meet with several forms of anaemia due to bone diseases.

On the basis of the above remarks we can classify the more important types of anaemia due to decreased blood formation as follows:

1. Pernicious anaemia. Lack of the intrinsic factor.
2. Iron-deficiency anaemia. Deficient intake and absorption of iron, with lack of hydrochloric acid in the stomach.
3. Nutritional anaemia of infants. Lack of iron in the diet.
4. Anaemias of pregnancy. Increased demands for iron and deficiency of folic acid.
5. Anaemias associated with diseases of the gastrointestinal tract:
   (a) Malabsorption syndrome. Deficient absorption of folic acid, vitamin B_{12} and iron.
   (b) Carcinoma of the stomach.
6. Anaemias due to interference with the red marrow in the bones.

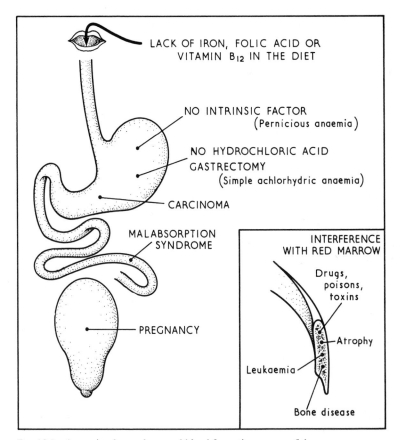

LACK OF IRON, FOLIC ACID OR VITAMIN B_{12} IN THE DIET

NO INTRINSIC FACTOR
(Pernicious anaemia)

NO HYDROCHLORIC ACID
GASTRECTOMY
(Simple achlorhydric anaemia)

CARCINOMA

MALABSORPTION SYNDROME

PREGNANCY

INTERFERENCE WITH RED MARROW

Drugs, poisons, toxins

Atrophy

Leukaemia

Bone disease

FIG. 10.5   Anaemias due to decreased blood formation—some of the causes.

(a) Drugs and toxic poisons (gold, chloramphenicol, benzol, chronic infections, X-rays and radioactive substances).

(b) Mechanical interference (anaemias of leukaemia and carcinomatosis of bones).

(c) Primary failure of the marrow (aplastic anaemia).

Some of the more important of these forms of anaemia will now be discussed in more detail.

PERNICIOUS ANAEMIA

Pernicious anaemia is the commonest form of anaemia caused by lack of vitamin B_{12}. As mentioned earlier (p. 338), vitamin B_{12} is necessary both for the formation of adequate numbers of red blood cells and also for the red cells to become fully mature. In pernicious anaemia, the intrinsic factor normally secreted by the stomach is blocked by antibodies with the result that vitamin B_{12} is not absorbed from the gastrointestinal tract.

Symptoms and signs

1. This anaemia is commonest after the age of 40 and affects both sexes equally. The onset is gradual and typical remissions occur when the anaemia improves of its own accord.

2. General symptoms and signs of anaemia, as outlined earlier, are present, including pallor and weakness. Their severity naturally varies with the degree of anaemia, but usually they are marked.

3. The patient often complains of soreness of the tongue, which is smooth and inflamed (glossitis).

4. The skin may have a slightly yellowish tint due to a mild degree of jaundice (of the haemolytic type) which, combined with the pallor, gives the pale lemon-yellow colour of pernicious anaemia.

5. Symptoms and signs of involvement of the nervous system may be present, including difficulty in walking (ataxia) and pins and needles in the hands and feet. These are due to the characteristic neurological complication of *subacute combined degeneration of the cord* met with only in pernicious anaemia.

6. Examination of the patient will often reveal an enlarged spleen.

Laboratory tests

1. There is a characteristic blood picture in pernicious anaemia which is always a hyperchromic macrocytic (large cell) anaemia.

Immature cells often appear in the peripheral blood and the white cells are reduced in number (leucopenia).

2. If the blood picture is not absolutely typical, examination of the red marrow is carried out, when in all cases a characteristic picture with numerous megaloblasts is obtained, thus giving a definite diagnosis. (Megaloblasts are abnormal immature red cells.) This

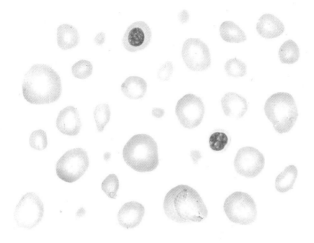

FIG. 10.6   Blood film from a case of pernicious anaemia showing the characteristic larger red cells (macrocytes) and one immature nucleated red cell (megaloblast)

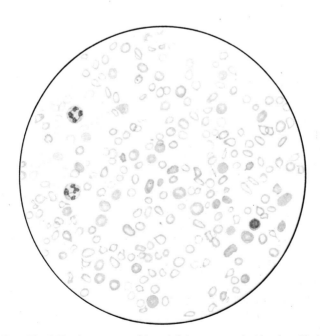

FIG. 10.7   Blood film from a case of iron deficiency anaemia (simple achlorhydric anaemia) showing the characteristic small pale red cells.

examination is known as a marrow puncture. As it is often performed from the marrow of the sternum it is also called a *sternal puncture*. A special needle (Salah's) is needed.

3. Vitamin B_{12} can be measured in the blood. The level in pernicious anaemia is very low.

4. Antibodies to the intrinsic factor can be detected in the blood.

5. Radio-active B_{12} can be administered by mouth and the amount excreted in the urine can be measured (Schilling test). In pernicious anaemia the body is greedy for B_{12} and very little appears in the urine.

6. Achlorhydria. An injection of pentagastrin normally stimulates a flow of hydrochloric acid from the stomach. In pernicious anaemia, analysis of the stomach contents withdrawn by a stomach tube shows no hydrochloric acid (achlorhydria) even after an injection of pentagastrin.

DIAGNOSIS. The diagnosis of anaemia is readily made on the pallor, fatigue and other general signs of anaemia. The diagnosis of pernicious anaemia is made from the typical blood picture, the special tests mentioned and, if necessary, by a sternal puncture.

Carcinoma of the stomach or intestinal tract often gives rise to effects similar to those of pernicious anaemia, so that careful examination of the gastrointestinal tract by barium X-rays and examination of the faeces for occult blood are necessary in any doubtful case.

Treatment of pernicious anaemia

The essential aim in treatment is to supply the missing vitamin B_{12} (hydroxocobalamin). In the early stages of treatment when there is severe anaemia, 1000 micrograms (μg) of vitamin B_{12} are injected intramuscularly once or twice a week until the number of red blood cells and the amount of haemoglobin return to normal. Thereafter a maintenance dose of vitamin B_{12} of 500 μg every three months is given as the patient will relapse if vitamin B_{12} is stopped. The patient must be warned that vitamin B_{12} will be necessary for the rest of his life. This point is of importance. At periodic intervals a blood count is done to ensure that adequate vitamin B_{12} therapy is being given.

If subacute degeneration of the spinal cord is present much larger doses of vitamin B_{12} are necessary; usually 1000 μg are given weekly for at least six to 12 months and then followed by the usual maintenance doses mentioned above.

IRON-DEFICIENCY ANAEMIA

This is the commonest type of anaemia seen in Great Britain and it usually occurs in women in the child-bearing age. It is due to a combination of causes. The diet is often deficient in iron-containing foods, especially meat, and absorption of iron is inadequate because of lack of hydrochloric acid in the stomach (achlorhydria). Loss of blood at menstruation and the increased nutritional demands during pregnancy further exacerbate the anaemia.

In addition to the general signs and symptoms of anaemia already

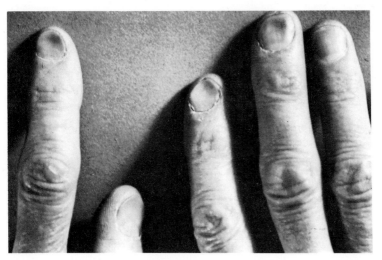

FIG. 10.8 Spoon-shaped nails (koilonychia) from a case of simple achlorhydric anaemia.

discussed (pallor, weakness, tachycardia, dyspnoea and oedema), these patients have dry skin and hair, the nails are cracked and spoon-shaped (koilonychia) and the tongue is sore and smooth. Examination of the blood shows a severe reduction in the haemoglobin content (often about 9 g per 100 ml) and the red cells are small and hypochromic.

Treatment

The diet should contain adequate quantities of meat and other iron-containing foods. Iron must be taken regularly until the anaemia is fully corrected and is best given as tablets by mouth. There are many satisfactory preparations of iron mixtures and tablets. Ferrous sulphate tablets (200 to 400 mg) can be taken three times a day after meals. They are usually well tolerated but occasionally give rise to nausea or diarrhoea. The stools are always stained black when iron is taken, and this should be explained to patients to avoid unnecessary anxiety.

In exceptional cases where iron cannot be tolerated by mouth, parenteral preparations are available. For intravenous iron therapy, saccharated iron oxide (Ferrivenin) is used, the initial dose being 1 to 2 ml (20 to 40 mg). If there are no unpleasant reactions (nausea or faintness), the dose is increased to 5 ml on alternate days until the anaemia is corrected. An iron-sorbitol compound (Jectofer) is available for intramuscular injection. An intramuscular injection of 2 ml (100 mg) should raise the haemoglobin level about 4 per cent.

NUTRITIONAL ANAEMIA OF INFANTS

Milk, which is relatively poor in iron content, forms practically the entire diet during the first months of life. An iron-deficiency anaemia, therefore, frequently occurs in infants and is called the nutritional anaemia of infants. Premature infants are particularly likely to suffer from anaemia.

In the milder cases the anaemia usually corrects itself at the end of the first year. In more severe cases, however, iron is needed.

ANAEMIAS OF PREGNANCY

During pregnancy an iron-deficiency anaemia is often seen. Various factors combine to bring about this anaemia, including the demands of the foetus for iron and also a deficiency of iron in the diet.

Less frequently an anaemia similar in type to that of pernicious anaemia (the macrocytic anaemia of pregnancy) is met with. The exact cause of this form of anaemia is unknown, but the anaemia seems to respond best to folic acid therapy.

ANAEMIAS ASSOCIATED WITH DISEASES OF THE GASTROINTESTINAL TRACT

In discussing the anaemias due to blood loss it was seen that a common cause of anaemia was haemorrhage from a bleeding peptic ulcer or from a carcinoma. Apart from these causes there are various other gastrointestinal conditions which may be accompanied by anaemia.

1. In the malabsorption syndrome, in which chronic diarrhoea is a feature, lack of absorption of vitamin B_{12} or folic acid may lead to a macrocytic anaemia similar to that of pernicious anaemia. Alternatively an iron deficiency anaemia may develop from deficient absorption of iron.

2. Carcinoma of the stomach usually causes an iron-deficiency anaemia due to chronic bleeding, but sometimes it also causes a macrocytic anaemia similar to pernicious anaemia owing to interference with the formation of the intrinsic factor in the stomach. A similar anaemia may also arise after the stomach has been removed (gastrectomy) in the treatment of carcinoma or a large gastric ulcer.

Again, removal of large portions of the intestines (colectomy), as carried out for carcinoma or chronic ulcerative colitis, may interfere with the absorption either of iron or of vitamin B_{12} to cause anaemia.

ANAEMIAS DUE TO INTERFERENCE WITH THE RED MARROW IN THE BONES

Many different diseases have as a predominant feature an anaemia which in all cases has the same underlying cause, i.e. interference with the formation of blood in the red bone marrow. Blood formation may be depressed by chemical poisons like benzol or arsenic or by drugs such as chloramphenicol, phenylbutazone or gold salts. In addition such conditions as chronic sepsis, rheumatoid arthritis, chronic nephritis and uraemia are often accompanied by an anaemia due to depression of blood formation.

Overexposure to X-rays, radium and some radioactive substances may cause a very severe anaemia. This is so important that people like radiologists and radiographers, who are constantly in contact with X-rays, have a blood examination at periodic intervals. The anaemia due to X-rays and radioactive substances is typically associated with a depression of the white cells. This fact is often made use of in treating such conditions as leukaemia, where there is a great increase in the white cells. Here deep X-rays are often of value.

Extensive bone disease may interfere with the marrow and so depress blood formation. Thus widespread carcinomatous deposits in the bones may cause anaemia. In leukaemia vast numbers of abnormal white cells crowd the marrow to such an extent that red cell formation is greatly reduced. Leukaemia always leads to anaemia for this reason.

In some cases the marrow may become atrophied (*aplastic*) and a very severe and often fatal anaemia may result. This form of anaemia, known as aplastic anaemia, may be secondary to any of the above poisons (drugs, infections or X-rays), but a primary type of unknown cause also occurs.

HAEMOLYTIC ANAEMIAS

The third main group of anaemias is that due to an increased destruction of the red cells. Normally a red cell has a life of about 120 days, after which it is worn out and destroyed by certain types of cells present in the spleen, liver and the connective tissues, known as the reticuloendothelial system of cells. The haemoglobin is broken down into the pigment bilirubin, which is then excreted by the liver through the biliary passages into the intestines.

In some diseases an overdestruction of the red cells takes place with the result that an anaemia occurs, known as haemolytic anaemia. One of the features of a haemolytic anaemia, in contrast to the other types, is that it is usually associated with a form of jaundice called *haemolytic jaundice*. It has just been stated that the haemoglobin of the broken-down red cell is turned into bile pigment, bilirubin. Excess of bile pigment accumulating in the blood stream causes jaundice. Therefore in haemolytic anaemias, where there is an excess of bile pigment owing to the excessive breakdown of the red cells, haemolytic jaundice often occurs. In mild haemolytic anaemias, however, the jaundice may be slight or even absent as the body is able to deal with a small excess of bile pigment without jaundice developing.

Some causes of haemolytic anaemias
1. Severe infections, especially septicaemias.
2. Toxic chemicals and drugs.
3. Incompatible blood transfusions.
4. Haemolytic disease and the Rhesus Factor.
5. Congenital Haemolytic Anaemias (Acholuric Jaundice).

1. Severe infections

Some infectious diseases, especially where the organisms actually grow in the blood stream, cause a haemolytic anaemia. Such diseases are streptococcal septicaemias, malaria and also gas gangrene infection.

2. Toxic chemicals and drugs

Certain chemicals, e.g. lead, cause haemolysis of the red cells. The poisonous venom of some snakes also has this effect. Again, some drugs such as sulphonamides or methyldopa occasionally produce this form of anaemia.

3. Incompatible blood transfusions

Whilst anaemia is not commonly caused by incompatible blood transfusions, there are other important reactions from giving a patient the wrong blood group and it is convenient to discuss the subject here.

When a transfusion is given, blood from one person (the donor) is transfused into the blood stream of the patient (the recipient). Unless precautions are taken, the donor's red cells could clump together (agglutinate) and cause serious harm to the recipient. Agglutination of the red cells is due to the presence of certain factors (agglutinogens) present in the donor's red cells which are reacted upon by antibodies in the recipient's serum. Not all donors have these

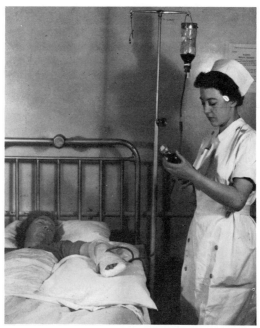

FIG. 10.9   The nurse is checking the particulars on the bottle of blood to make sure that it is the correct blood to give to the patient.

factors in the red cells, and in fact blood can be divided into four main groups. Group O blood does not contain any of the main agglutinogens, and so can usually be transfused without risk of reaction. Group A blood contains agglutinogen A, group B contains agglutinogen B, while group AB contains both agglutinogens A and B. Naturally, blood containing the agglutinogen A in the red cells does not contain the A antibody in the serum, since this would lead to agglutination of one's own red cells. Hence it is usually safe to give group A blood to a group A recipient or to a group AB recipient. Similarly, group B blood can be given to patients who are group B or group AB. Group AB blood can only be given to group AB patients: on the other hand, group AB patients can usually receive blood from any group without danger of agglutination.

Hence, before a transfusion is given, the blood group of both donor and recipient must be known. This is known as *blood grouping*. Unfortunately, this is not enough since other less common factors may be present which also could cause agglutination. Therefore, having tested the blood group before a blood transfusion is given a second check must be made. Some of the recipient's blood is withdrawn and allowed to clot. The serum (clotted plasma) thus obtained is mixed with a small amount of the proposed donor's blood, and if the donor's blood is suitable, i.e. of the right group, no agglutination or clotting should occur. This is known as *direct cross-matching*.

If, through some mistake or failure to carry out these essential preliminaries, the wrong blood is given, the result is agglutination and destruction (haemolysis) of the transfused red cells with jaundice. This is often spoken of as an incompatible or *mismatched transfusion*. Another effect seen in mismatched transfusions is that the clumped red cells may block the kidneys, when renal failure (uraemia) may result, which is often fatal.

In incompatible blood transfusions the patient becomes restless and has a severe rigor, whilst there is a rise in pulse rate and temperature. There is usually pain in the chest and back. In severe cases anuria and jaundice develop after a few hours. The nurse must keep a close watch on all patients having a blood transfusion, particularly at the start of each new bottle of blood, so that the transfusion can be immediately stopped if any untoward reactions (severe rigor, pain in the back and rise in temperature) occur.

After all blood transfusions, the transfusion bottle must not be washed out but returned (with the small drop of blood remaining in the bottle) to the laboratory. This is so that further compatibility tests may be done if any adverse reactions have occurred.

4. Haemolytic disease and the rhesus (Rh) factor

In addition to the four blood groups mentioned above there is another factor present in the blood of some people which can also cause serious haemolysis and jaundice. This is known as the Rh factor.

Eighty-five per cent of people are supposed to have this factor and are said to be *Rh-positive*; the remaining 15 per cent of people lack this factor and are *Rh-negative*. If Rh-positive blood is given to an Rh-negative person, even though it may be the right blood group (that is, O or A, etc.), Rh antibodies are produced in the Rh-negative person which may destroy the Rh-positive blood. It is necessary, therefore, in giving transfusions to ascertain not only the normal blood group of the person but also the Rh factor, and if this is Rh-negative to give only Rh-negative blood.

At this point it is convenient to discuss the diseases seen in infants due to this Rh factor.

Even though a pregnant woman may be Rh-negative the foetus's blood may be Rh-positive because it may have inherited this Rh-positive factor from the father. The Rh-positive factor of the child can give rise to antibodies (agglutinins) in the mother's blood, and in the course of time sufficient antibodies may be produced in the mother's blood to destroy the baby's red cells. In severe cases the child may be born dead with severe anaemia and jaundice. In many cases, however, for some unknown reason the crisis develops only as the child is born. As a result, as soon as it is born the baby may become jaundiced and anaemic owing to the destruction of its blood by the Rh antibodies produced in the mother's blood. In mild cases the effect may not be too serious, but in severe cases it can lead to rapid death, or after a few months may give rise to serious changes in the brain with mental deficiency (*kernicterus*).

Various names are used to describe the effects on infants of the Rh factor. In the most severe cases the infant is born dead, and is also usually macerated and very oedematous; the condition of *hydrops foetalis* is then said to be present. In the most common cases, where the infant becomes deeply jaundiced immediately after birth, the name *icterus gravis* is used. Lastly, where the main effect is a severe anaemia with slight jaundice the term *congenital haemolytic anaemia* is used. All these effects are different degrees of the same underlying condition, i.e. haemolytic disease due to the Rh factor. The name *erythroblastosis foetalis* is also used as well as haemolytic disease of the newborn.

Treatment of haemolytic disease of the newborn

Nowadays it is the commonly accepted practice to blood-group all women during pregnancy and also ascertain their Rh factor. If it is found that they are Rh-negative and that antibodies have already developed in their blood premature labour is induced and a replacement transfusion of the child's blood may be done. Here as much of the infant's blood as possible is taken off and replaced by Rh-negative blood. In many cases this leads to a complete cure. In milder cases a simple transfusion with Rh-negative blood instead of a replacement transfusion is sufficient.

As has been seen, the stimulus to the formation of anti-Rh factor in the mother is provided by the action of the Rh factor from the foetus on the mother's antibody-forming lymphocytes. Once stimulated, these cells go on forming more and more anti-Rh factor. Hence if the Rh factor from the foetus could be neutralised before it had the chance to stimulate the antibody-forming cells, no excessive anti-Rh factor production could occur. In fact, this can be done by obtaining anti-Rh factor from the blood of women already sensitised, known as anti-D gamma globulin. If this is injected into the Rh-negative mothers with Rh-positive babies, the Rh factor is neutralised before it can stimulate the antibody-forming lymphocytes to produce more and more anti-Rh factor. This technique has been used with

RHESUS-NEGATIVE MOTHER   RHESUS-POSITIVE FATHER
RHESUS-POSITIVE BABIES

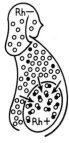

FIRST PREGNANCY

Rhesus Positive Antigens cross the placental barrier and provoke maternal lymphocytes to produce Antibodies. ooooo

Baby is usually unaffected but Mother goes on and on producing Anti-Rh +ve Antibodies after delivery.

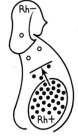

SECOND AND SUBSEQUENT PREGNANCIES

Anti-Rh +ve Antibodies are now present in Mother and production is boosted by Rh +ve Antigens from new Baby.

Anti-Rh +ve Antibodies cross the placental barrier and react with Rh +ve Antigens in Baby.

Baby is affected. (Haemolytic Disease of the Newborn)

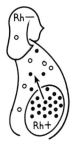

PROTECTION

Mother is given Anti-Rh +ve Serum (Anti-D gamma globulin) which depresses her production of Antibodies.

Baby is protected.

Fig. 10.10.

considerable success though supplies of anti-D gamma globulin are limited (Fig. 10.10).

Finally, it must again be stressed that when blood transfusions are necessary, especially in women, the Rh factor must be determined. If the patients are Rh-negative then only Rh-negative blood must be used. If not, antibodies may be produced in the woman's blood, and if at a later date (even after several years) she becomes pregnant these antibodies can destroy her infant's blood if the latter is Rh-positive.

5. Congenital haemolytic anaemias (acholuric jaundice)

This form of haemolytic anaemia is due to a congenital defect in the red cells which makes them more fragile than normal and so more easily destroyed. The disease is chronic and usually recognised in childhood, although mild cases may be missed for many years. Recurrent attacks of jaundice of the haemolytic type, with anaemia, are the main features. The spleen is usually enlarged.

The diagnosis of the disease can be confirmed by performing a fragility test, when the abnormally increased fragility of the red cells will be evident.

The only effective remedy is to remove the spleen. This increases the life of the red cells and so decreases the amount of red cell destruction. (The function of the spleen as one of the main parts of the reticulo-endothelial system is normally to destroy damaged or worn-out red cells.)

THE HAEMORRHAGIC DISEASES

We saw earlier, in the discussion on the functions of the various components making up human blood, that there were several factors present which had to do with controlling haemorrhage. We saw that the platelets were concerned with this and that the substances prothrombin and fibrinogen were important in causing blood to clot and so controlling haemorrhage. The blood vessels themselves also play an important role in controlling haemorrhage, and contraction of the blood vessel (vasoconstriction) usually takes place when a blood vessel is injured.

The haemorrhagic diseases are a large group which have as a predominating feature the presence of haemorrhages. These haemorrhages may occur into the skin to give rise to purple spots which do not fade on pressure and are called purpura (small purpuric haemorrhages are usually known as petechiae). In addition to purpuric haemorrhages into the skin, bleeding may occur from the mucous membranes, e.g. from the nose (epistaxis), from the bowels (melaena), or from the kidneys (haematuria).

The commoner haemorrhagic diseases can be roughly classified according to the type of underlying interference with the normal mechanism for the control of bleeding:

Damage to the wall of the blood vessels.

Diminished platelets (thrombocytopenic purpura).
Prothrombin deficiency.
Haemophilia.

DAMAGE TO THE WALLS OF THE BLOOD VESSELS

This group comprises by far the most common causes of purpura, and can be divided into the following types.

1. Infections

Many infections are associated with purpuric haemorrhages caused by damage to the vessel wall. In some cases small emboli actually containing bacteria cause the purpuric or petechial spots. This is seen in *meningococcal meningitis* (also called *spotted fever* owing to the occurrence of purpuric spots) and *bacterial endocarditis*, another cause of embolic purpura, where the petechial spots occur in the skin and also under the nails.

In the severe haemorrhagic forms of such acute infectious fevers as measles, scarlet fever or smallpox the purpuric spots are caused by damage to the walls of the blood vessels.

2. Drugs

Many drugs such as isoniazid, quinine and sulphonamides may cause purpura; also the heavy metals used in medicine, e.g. gold.

3. Vitamin C deficiency

The classical sign of vitamin C deficiency is haemorrhage due to alteration in the vascular wall.

4. Allergic diseases

Purpura is sometimes associated with various allergic manifestations, such as urticaria, oedema of the skin and joint pains. The underlying factor is damage to the lining of the vascular wall which allows leakage of blood and fluid. Henoch-Schönlein's purpura occurs in young adults and the purpura may be associated with abdominal pain, joint swellings and nephritis.

5. Senile purpura

This is the commonest type of purpura and is found most often in elderly people, recurrent purpuric spots appearing in the skin. There is little or no upset in the general health and the purpura is of little significance.

DIMINISHED PLATELETS (Thrombocytopenic purpura)

One of the functions of the small round bodies known as the platelets (or thrombocytes) is to seal off any lesions or openings in the small blood vessels (capillaries) and so prevent undue loss of blood from a slight injury. The platelets are formed in the bone marrow and, like the red cells, are destroyed by the spleen. Most of the causes, therefore, of this group of haemorrhagic diseases (purpura) are diseases affecting the blood, the bone marrow and the spleen.

1. *Leukaemia*, by crowding the marrow with abnormal white cells, may depress the formation of platelets in exactly the same way as it may cause anaemia. Purpura, including bleeding from the mucous membranes, may be a feature of some severe cases of leukaemia.

2. *Secondary carcinomatosis of the bones* acts like leukaemia in causing purpura in that the widespread invasion of the bone marrow by the malignant cells decreases the formation of the platelets. We have already seen that carcinomatosis of the bones causes an anaemia in the same fashion.

3. *Aplastic anaemia* is due to atrophy of the marrow by poisons, toxins, drugs or unknown causes. Severe purpura with bleeding from the mucous membranes caused by depression of the platelets is often a feature of aplastic anaemia.

4. *Drugs*, such as quinine, phenylbutazone, sulphonamides and carbimazole, may cause purpura associated with a deficiency of platelets.

5. *Thrombocytopenic purpura.* Often the cause of the diminished platelets is not known. This is seen most commonly in women and gives rise to severe bleeding from the mucous membranes (nose, bowel, kidneys) and into the skin. Anaemia is present, and the spleen is nearly always enlarged. Careful search for any of the causes mentioned above must be made and also for systemic lupus erythematosis (p. 471) in which thrombocytopenia occurs. The treatment depends on the severity of the conditions, and in mild cases treating the anaemia only may suffice. In cases of severity, however, the spleen is usually removed since the spleen may be responsible for excessive platelet destruction. Blood transfusions to control any severe haemorrhage may be necessary. Cortisone or allied steroids have also proved of value in bringing about either a complete remission or a temporary improvement and so making the patient fit for splenectomy.

PROTHROMBIN DEFICIENCY

Coagulation of blood

At the begining of this chapter the roles of various components of the blood were discussed. It was stated that the substances prothrombin and fibrinogen were concerned with the coagulation of blood. Blood coagulation or clotting plays a major part in the control of haemorrhage, and although the actual mechanism of blood coagulation is, indeed, very complex and not yet fully understood a simple version should enable the nurse to understand the various diseases which involve blood coagulation. The process of blood clotting can most easily be described as follows:

1. Prothrombin + Thromboplastin + Calcium = Thrombin.
2. Thrombin + Fibrinogen = Fibrin (clot).

The substance thromboplastin is liberated from injured tissues and also from platelets to convert the prothrombin in the blood into thrombin. Calcium, normally present in the blood, assists in this process. The thrombin thus formed quickly acts on the fibrinogen (which is also normally present in blood) to form fibrin. Fibrin is a solid tough fibre network which is the actual basis of the blood clot.

A deficiency in prothrombin is the only condition which commonly arises as a result of interference with this clotting mechanism of the blood. (The disease haemophilia, which is also associated with a prolonged clotting time, is much rarer. It is discussed later.)

Prothrombin is produced in the liver by utilisation of vitamin K. This vitamin is present in certain foods, such as spinach, cabbage and egg yolk. Those bacteria which are normally present in the bowel can also manufacture vitamin K. For the proper absorption of vitamin K bile salts are necessary.

Causes of prothrombin deficiency

1. *Obstructive jaundice.* Here the absence of bile salts leads to deficient absorption of vitamin K and so, after a matter of six to eight weeks, to a fall in the prothrombin level in the blood. When this is severe, haemorrhages occur. Jaundiced patients are often known to bleed very readily at an operation, and in former years this was supposed to be due to lack of calcium. It is now known that it is not the calcium but vitamin K that is lacking.

In any operation on a patient with obstructive jaundice the prothrombin level should be estimated, and if below normal, vitamin K must be given.

2. *Haemorrhagic disease of the newborn.* Occasionally during the first week of life haemorrhages, such as epistaxis or melaena, may occur giving rise to the condition known as haemorrhagic disease of the newborn. The cause is prothrombin deficiency brought about by a shortage of vitamin K received from the mother, combined with the inability of the infant during the first week to manufacture vitamin K itself. The newborn infant's bowel is sterile, and the absence of bacteria is thus the cause of the infant's inability to form vitamin K.

Premature infants are especially lacking in prothrombin and should be given vitamin K after birth as a routine.

3. *Diseases of the liver.* Diseases of the liver may be associated with prothrombin deficiency as prothrombin is manufactured and stored in the liver. Prothrombin deficiency with its resulting haemorrhages is mainly seen in cases of acute liver damage such as occurs in acute yellow atrophy, and less often in chronic conditions such as cirrhosis of the liver.

4. *Chronic diseases of the gastrointestinal tract.* Those chronic intestinal diseases which cause severe and persistent diarrhoea may lead to a deficiency in vitamin K absorption, resulting in some cases in so

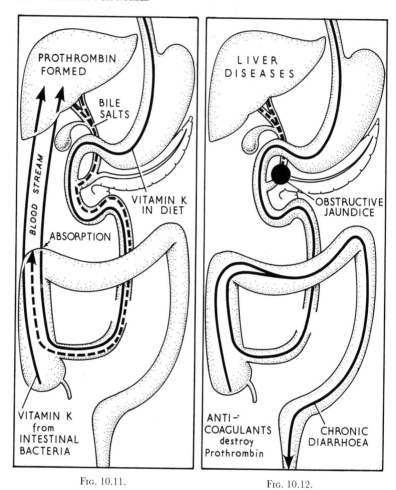

Fig. 10.11.   Fig. 10.12.

Fig. 10.11   The formation of prothrombin.
Fig. 10.12   The causes of prothrombin deficiency.

severe a prothrombin deficiency that actual haemorrhages may occur. Such intestinal diseases include chronic ulcerative colitis and sprue.

    5. *Anticoagulant drugs.* Anticoagulant drugs are used in the prevention and treatment of thrombosis and embolism, especially thrombosis of the veins. Anticoagulant drugs destroy the prothrombin and thus cause a prolonged blood-clotting time. The aim in treatment is to prolong the clotting time of the blood so that thrombosis does not occur or, if already present, does not spread; the risk of a complicating embolism is thus greatly reduced.

An overdosage of anticoagulant drugs may cause too great a prolongation of the clotting time so that haemorrhages occur. Haematuria, epistaxis and severe bruising of the skin are those most frequently seen.

In all patients on anticoagulant drugs (such as Dindevan) frequent estimation of the prothrombin time is essential to control the treatment. Daily routine examination of the urine for red cells, whose presence may give forewarning of a more massive haematuria, is also valuable.

Treatment of prothrombin deficiency

In all cases of prothrombin deficiency, except those due to liver disease and to overdosage with anticoagulant drugs, treatment with injections of vitamin K (menaphthone or Synkavit), 10 to 15 mg, leads to a rapid and complete cure. In infants with haemorrhagic disease of the newborn, only 1 mg of Synkavit is necessary, as larger doses may cause a toxic haemolytic anaemia. In liver disease there is usually only a partial response. In overdosage with anticoagulant drugs, vitamin K_1 (5 to 20 mg) is needed to restore the prothrombin level to normal. If any appreciable haemorrhage is present transfusions with fresh blood, 1 to 2 units, are needed.

HAEMOPHILIA

Haemophilia is a rare disease in which severe haemorrhages into the joints are the predominant feature. The haemorrhages are usually brought on by some injury which may be no more than trivial, such as the patient knocking himself. Haemophilia is seen only in men and is a hereditary disease passed down in certain families from generation to generation. It is passed on through the females who are, however, never themselves affected by the disease. Haemophilia is caused by the lack of a factor which is essential for the proper clotting of blood, namely antihaemophilic globulin. Consequently, there is in haemophilia a markedly prolonged blood clotting time leading to haemorrhages.

Treatment

The missing factor, antihaemophilic globulin (AHG), has now been isolated and is available for intravenous injection as soon as bleeding starts. Haemophilics must be admitted to hospital for dental extractions and must be given AHG injections before and after the operation. In severe cases major operations are very hazardous even with frequent blood transfusions and AHG injections since neither may be totally successful in stemming the bleeding.

POLYCYTHAEMIA

Polycythaemia is an uncommon disorder of the blood wherein there is a marked increase in the number of red blood cells and in the volume of the blood. Instead of the normal count of approximately five million red cells per mm³, the number of red cells may be as high as seven million or more per mm³. The condition may arise as a compensatory mechanism in diseases where there is incomplete oxygenation of the blood, e.g. severe chronic diseases of the heart and lungs, especially congenital heart diseases. Certain drugs may also produce this condition.

A primary form of the disease, of unknown cause, *polycythaemia vera*, is more rarely seen. This form is usually treated with radio-active phosphorus (^{32}P), which diminishes the number of red cells. Regular venesection, in which 500 ml of blood is withdrawn, may be undertaken at monthly intervals.

THE WHITE BLOOD CELLS

There are three main types of white cell in the blood:
1. Polymorphonuclear white cells or granulocytes (so-called because they have granules present). There are three forms of polymorphonuclear white cells—neutrophils, eosinophils and basophils.
2. Lymphocytes.
3. Monocytes.

The polymorphonuclear cells and the monocytes (like the red cells) are formed in the red marrow of the bones, while lymphocytes are produced in the spleen and the lymph glands. The main function of the white cells is to help defend the body against infection. The polymorphs and the monocytes move towards the site of infection and engulf the bacteria.

The lymphocytes act in two ways. B-lymphocytes produce antibodies to counteract bacterial toxins and T-lymphocytes destroy foreign cells by direct contact.

The normal total white cell count varies between 5000 and 10,000 per mm³ in an adult. The polymorphonuclear cells form 65 per cent of this total, the lymphocytes 30 per cent and the monocytes 5 per cent. In most bacterial infections, the white cell count increases, sometimes to more than 20,000. This is known as a *leucocytosis* and shows that the body is responding to overcome the infection.

A reduction of white cells below normal is called a *leucopenia* and occurs in certain infections such as typhoid fever or tuberculosis, probably due to a toxic effect on the marrow itself. When the number of polymorphs is greatly or even completely suppressed, the condition is known as *agranulocytosis*. This is usually due to the toxic effect of certain drugs and is described later.

DISEASES OF THE WHITE BLOOD CELLS

LEUKAEMIA

Leukaemia is a disease in which the white cells of the blood are not properly formed and start to increase in numbers in a malignant way.

They crowd out the bone marrow and interfere with the formation of the red cells and platelets. This leads to anaemia and haemorrhages. Leukaemia can be classified according to the type of white cell involved. Myeloid leukaemia is a disease of the polymorphs while lymphatic leukaemia affects the lymphocytes. Monocytic leukaemia, involving the monocytes, is the least common. The type of leukaemia is identified by examining the blood and the marrow obtained from a sternal biopsy.

It should be emphasised again that leukaemia is actually a malignant disease of the cells, of unknown cause, which leads to a great increase in the number of cells. Leucocytosis is an increase in the number of white cells as the result usually of infection by organisms such as bacteria. It is the natural response of the body to overcome the infection.

Leukaemia can be acute or chronic, the acute form being commonest in children.

Acute leukaemia

Acute leukaemia is commonest in children but can occur at any age. The onset is usually sudden with fever, pallor and purpura. There may be bleeding from the nose or from the mouth and general symptoms of severe anaemia with fatigue and loss of strength. When the blood is examined under the microscope, the total white count is usually vastly increased and the cells are immature and abnormal.

The treatment of acute leukaemia has become more successful but more complex, so that children with leukaemia are best treated in special units expert in the latest forms of treatment and the complications arising from them.

The aim of treatment is to use drugs which destroy all abnormal cells in the blood and bone marrow, without proving too toxic to healthy tissues and cells. In acute lymphatic leukaemia this can be achieved in the majority of cases by using intravenous injections of vincristine with prednisone tablets taken by mouth. Further courses of cytotoxic drugs such as methotrexate or cyclophosphamide are then given, sometimes with the additional use of radiotherapy. This treatment has greatly improved the outlook in acute lymphatic leukaemia; many patients are still healthy more than 10 years after the start of the illness and there is hope of achieving a complete cure. The outlook is less favourable for acute myeloid or acute monocytic leukaemia.

Chronic leukaemia

Chronic myeloid leukaemia usually comes on in middle age with gradually increasing tiredness and anaemia. The spleen becomes so greatly enlarged that it may give rise to dragging abdominal discomfort and indigestion. There may be troublesome irritation of the skin.

The diagnosis is confirmed by examination of the blood. The white count may be more than 200,000, the majority of the cells being abnormal polymorphonuclears.

Treatment may make the patient more comfortable and prolongs life. Busulphan is a drug which delays proliferation of the white cells and has to be taken regularly, the dose being adjusted according to the white count. When the spleen is very enlarged, deep X-ray therapy may be applied to reduce its size.

Chronic lymphatic leukaemia occurs mainly in men and may run a mild course over many years with few symptoms. The spleen is not greatly enlarged but the lymph glands increase in size. Chlorambucil is the most useful drug to keep down the white count and has to be taken regularly under medical supervision.

MYELOMATOSIS

This ailment is caused by a malignant proliferation of special cells called plasma cells in the bone marrow. Plasma cells normally produce protein antibodies and in myelomatosis large quantities of abnormal protein can be detected in the blood and urine. The cells invade the bones themselves, leading to erosion and spontaneous fractures.

Myelomatosis is commonest in the elderly and is characterised by bone pains, malaise, anaemia and pyrexia. The sedimentation rate is very high and excessive numbers of plasma cells can be seen in the marrow.

There is no curative treatment, but the drug melphelan helps to suppress plasma cell activity. Radiotherapy may relieve the pain of local bone involvement.

AGRANULOCYTOSIS

The term *agranulocytosis* is used to denote either the complete absence of the granular cells (or polymorphonuclear cells as they are more often called) or a severe reduction in their number, combined with clinical symptoms and signs due to this deficiency. It must be stressed that a leucopenia means a reduction in the white cells which does not necessarily cause harmful results and is not the same condition as agranulocytosis.

Causes

The usual cause of agranulocytosis is some toxic depression of the bone marrow, as a result of which the polymorphs are not formed in adequate numbers. Drugs are the commonest cause of this toxic depression, especially the sulphonamides, antithyroid drugs (thiouracil and carbimazole), phenylbutazone, chloramphenicol and gold salts.

In view of the frequent use of phenylbutazone and antithyroid drugs, with their special liability to give rise to agranulocytosis, it is absolutely essential that the early symptoms and signs of this condition should be watched for. The lack of white cells means that there is a lowered resistance to bacteria, so that infection is liable to occur, especially in the throat.

Symptoms and signs

1. The commonest early symptom is one of sore throat, which may be very severe, with marked oedema and exudate in the throat. The sore throat is so invariable that the disease is often given the name *agranulocytic angina*.

2. The temperature rises, and if it is already above normal it usually rises further.

3. The patient becomes toxic and lethargic. The pulse is rapid.

DIAGNOSIS. The complaint of a sore throat with fever in a patient on phenylbutazone or antithyroid drugs should immediately raise the suspicion of agranulocytosis. The drugs must at once be stopped until a white cell count is done and the presence of agranulocytosis confirmed or not.

Treatment

Penicillin is given by injection, perhaps a million units every four hours. This is to combat any infection that is present or likely to arise. Penicillin is non-toxic to the white cells so that it can be given with safety.

THE SPLEEN AND LYMPH GLANDS

The spleen and the lymph glands play an important part in protecting the body against infection and are the main sites of production of lymphocytes, which manufacture antibodies. The spleen also filters out damaged red cells, bacteria and parasites which pass through it, and then destroys them. This explains why it enlarges in such diseases as typhoid fever and malaria. Sometimes it becomes too active and destroys healthy cells, as in thrombocytopenic purpura, when the platelets are destroyed. Removal of the spleen (splenectomy) then becomes necessary. The lymph glands, with their lymphatic ducts, also form a drainage system and act as a local filter to prevent bacteria and malignant cells from entering the general circulation.

SPLENOMEGALY (Enlargement of the spleen)

As has just been mentioned, the spleen is often affected in the course of a wide variety of ailments, including acute and chronic infective diseases and also blood diseases.

An enlarged spleen is a most important finding in medicine for the diagnosis of many diseases. A brief list of the more important causes of an enlarged spleen is therefore given.

1. *Acute infections.* The acute infective diseases which in Great Britain most commonly give rise to an enlarged spleen are enteric fever, subacute bacterial endocarditis and miliary tuberculosis. In tropical countries an enlarged spleen is a most frequent finding, usually as a result of acute and chronic malarial infection. Typhus fever and undulant fever (brucellosis) are also common causes of splenomegaly in the tropics.

2. *Chronic infections.* Malaria is by far the commonest cause of splenomegaly due to chronic infection. Other causes include syphilis and tuberculosis.

3. *Blood diseases.* It is in this group of diseases that greatly enlarged spleens are met with. Leukaemia, especially the myeloid type, is one of the commonest causes. Congenital haemolytic anaemia (acholuric jaundice) and thrombocytopenic purpura are often associated with enlargement of the spleen.

4. *Cirrhosis of the liver.* Since blood from the spleen drains into the liver via the portal vein, chronic obstruction of the liver occurring in cirrhosis sometimes leads to engorgement and enlargement of the spleen. Distended veins in the oesophagus often bleed, with resultant haematemesis and anaemia. This is sometimes known as splenic anaemia, or Banti's disease.

LYMPHADENOPATHY (Enlargement of the lymph glands)

Generally, when disease affects the lymph glands the glands become enlarged. For the sake of convenience we can divide such enlargement into local and general.

1. Local

Localised enlargement of one group of lymph glands is commonly due to septic inflammation of the tissues drained by those lymph glands. For instance, a septic finger often causes an enlarged axillary gland, while inflammation of the throat may give rise to enlarged cervical glands.

Apart from inflammatory lesions, tumour cells often spread along the lymphatics to cause enlargement of the lymph glands draining the area, e.g. carcinoma of the breast giving rise to enlarged axillary glands.

Another frequent cause of localised lymph gland enlargement is tuberculosis, which very commonly affects the cervical glands.

2. General

The most common causes of a generalised enlargement of the lymph glands include:
(a) Lymphatic leukaemia
(b) Glandular fever

(c) Hodgkin's disease

(d) Syphilis (secondary stage).

HODGKIN'S DISEASE

CAUSE. Unknown.

Symptoms and signs

1. The disease is commonest in the 20 to 40 age group, but it may arise at any age. The first sign of the disease is often an enlargement of one group of lymph glands.

2. Any group (or groups) of lymph glands may be affected. Usually the cervical glands in the neck or the axillary or inguinal glands are involved. In some cases, however, the deep internal lymph glands in the thorax or abdomen may be the first to be affected, and here the diagnosis of the condition is often difficult till the superficial palpable lymph glands also become enlarged.

3. The general health may be little affected at first, but as the disease advances weakness, anaemia and loss of weight develop. A characteristic feature of many cases is the recurrent pyrexia, which typically comes in waves lasting 10 to 14 days and then subsides only to rise again. This undulating type of fever is called the Pel-Ebstein fever.

4. Enlargement of the thoracic lymph glands can give rise to the pressure symptoms of cough and dyspnoea, while the enlarged abdominal glands may cause abdominal distension or ascites.

DIAGNOSIS. The disease has to be distinguished from the other causes of enlargement of the lymph glands. Lymphatic leukaemia, which also causes a generalised enlargement of the lymph glands, is

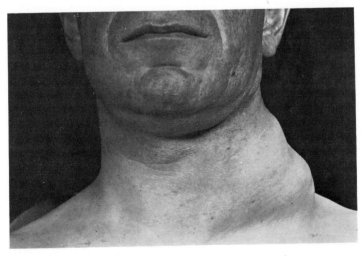

FIG. 10.13 Hodgkin's disease showing enlarged glands in the neck.

differentiated by the diagnostic gross increase in the white cells accompanied by the presence of abnormal types of white cells. Tuberculosis of the lymph glands remains confined to one group only, and the affected glands become matted together and may break down to form a chronic sinus. Hodgkin's glands remain mobile and do not adhere to the skin or break down. Malignant disease of the lymph glands, which is usually due to secondary invasion, gives rise to very hard fixed glands and the primary growth is usually easily found.

The diagnosis of Hodgkin's disease rests on removal (biopsy) of an enlarged lymph gland, usually from the neck, and histological examination under the microscope. The presence in the gland of abnormal cells typical of Hodgkin's disease confirms the diagnosis. The extent to which the glands and the spleen are involved is of first importance from the view point of treatment.

LYMPHANGIOGRAPH involves the injection of a dye into the lymphatic system and this shows up enlarged glands on X-ray, especially glands in the abdomen alongside the aorta and in the pelvis. Sometimes laparotomy is necessary to establish an exact diagnosis.

Treatment

This will depend on the degree of glandular and splenic enlargement. In the early stages, particularly when the glands involved are not widespread, radiotherapy is the treatment of choice and offers good opportunities for complete cure.

Chemotherapy with cytotoxic drugs and steroids may be given in addition to deep X-ray treatment in early cases. In patients where the involvement of the lymph glands is too widespread to warrant radiotherapy, chemotherapy is used as the sole treatment.

The cytotoxic drugs commonly used are vincristine and mustine, given intravenously, with procarbazine in tablet form by mouth. Prednisone is given as well, and helps to suppress the toxic effects of the cytotoxic drugs.

The treatment of Hodgkin's disease demands considerable expertise and is best carried out in special units.

11 Diseases of the Urinary System

ANATOMY AND PHYSIOLOGY

The urinary system consists of two *kidneys*, each of which secretes urine. The urine is conveyed from each kidney by a long narrow tube, the *ureter*, into the bladder. The *bladder* stores urine until ready for evacuation. The bladder then contracts and the urine is expelled through the *urethra*.

The kidneys lie behind the peritoneum on either side of the

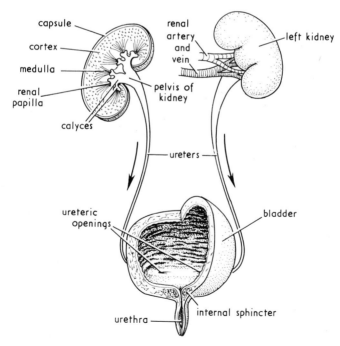

capsule

renal artery and vein

left kidney

cortex

medulla

renal papilla

pelvis of kidney

calyces

ureters

ureteric openings

bladder

urethra

internal sphincter

Fig. 11.1 The kidneys and bladder.

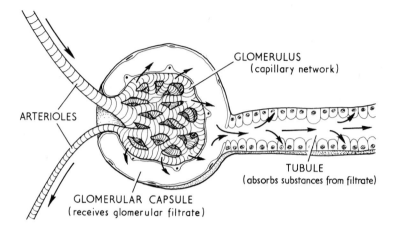

GLOMERULUS
(capillary network)

ARTERIOLES

TUBULE
(absorbs substances from filtrate)

GLOMERULAR CAPSULE
(receives glomerular filtrate)

FIG. 11.2   A close-up diagram of glomerulus and tubule.

vertebral column. The kidney substance is composed of large numbers of microscopic structures known as glomeruli and tubules.

The *glomerulus* is a network of arterial capillaries with walls so thin that fluid and waste products can filter through them into the glomerular capsule. The glomerular capsule surrounds the glomerulus and leads by a system of *tubules* into the pelvis of the kidney for passage of urine down the ureter. The fluid that filters through the glomerulus (glomerular filtrate) is not urine because it contains many substances that the body needs. The function of the tubules is to absorb back into the blood from the glomerular filtrate important materials and fluid that should not be excreted. Many litres of fluid pass through the glomeruli and much of this has to be re-absorbed back into the circulation. Urine is what is finally excreted after the tubules have absorbed necessary materials and fluid back into the circulation from the glomerular filtrate.

The essential function of the kidney is to remove the waste products of metabolism from the body in the urine. For example, urea is a waste product of protein metabolism excreted in the urine.

In addition to this function, by excreting certain minerals and retaining others, the kidneys maintain the acid–alkali reaction of the blood at a constant level. The kidneys also regulate fluid balance. If a great amount of fluid is taken, the kidneys excrete more. In very hot weather when a lot of fluid is lost in perspiration, the kidneys excrete less urine.

Normally, the protein molecules present in the blood are too large to pass through the glomerular filter. Thus with healthy kidneys, no protein (mainly albumin) appears in the urine. But if the glomerular filter is damaged as in chronic nephritis, protein passes through and appears in the urine.

Other substances only appear in the urine if they exceed the normal level in the blood. Although there is always some glucose in the blood, glucose only appears in the urine if there is an excessive amount in the blood as in diabetes or if there is some abnormality of the tubules (low renal threshold).

EXAMINATION OF KIDNEY FUNCTION

1. The urine

The most important index of kidney function is provided by examination of the urine (p. 9).

(a) The volume of urine excreted in 24 hours in a healthy subject depends on the amount of fluid ingested and the amount of fluid lost in sweat, in the stools and in respiration—exhaled breath contains moisture. The kidney maintains the balance so that the total body fluid remains steady. Kidney disease causes an upset in this balance. In acute nephritis, the output of urine may be seriously diminished (*oliguria*) or may even cease (*anuria*). In some forms of chronic nephritis, the kidneys are unable to concentrate waste products in the urine and to compensate for this, large quantities of dilute urine are passed.

The absorption of fluid from the glomerular filtrate by the tubules is controlled by a hormone (antidiuretic hormone, or ADH). In diabetes insipidus (p. 437), this hormone is deficient and this leads to the loss of large quantities of urine (*polyuria*).

Polyuria is also a feature of diabetes mellitus (p. 411). Excessive amounts of glucose appear in the blood and the kidneys try to excrete this excess in the urine by forming large quantities of urine.

A fluid balance chart is a record of all the fluid taken by mouth or administered by intravenous drip, and of all the fluid lost in the urine, vomit or by aspiration. It enables the physician to see if the kidneys are maintaining a proper fluid balance.

(b) *Proteinuria.* Protein (albumin) in the urine usually indicates leakage through a damaged glomerular filter and is present in almost every type of renal disease. Occasionally, healthy young adults show protein in the urine after exercise or prolonged standing (*orthostatic proteinuria*). The simplest method of testing the urine for protein is to dip a stick of Albustix in the urine (p. 10); the colour changes to green if protein is present.

(c) *Haematuria.* Blood in the urine can arise from the kidney, the ureters, the bladder or the urethra. Heavy bleeding may occur in haemorrhagic diseases (p. 337), carcinoma of the kidney, a stone in the ureter or papilloma of the bladder. In these cases, blood in the urine may be apparent to the naked eye: the urine appears red or smoky. Lesser amounts of blood in the urine may be due to conditions such as acute nephritis, bacterial endocarditis, pyelitis or cystitis. In healthy women, blood from menstruation may appear in the urine.

Two tests are available for haematuria. The first is a ward test, simple and accurate, using the test strip (Hemastix). This is dipped into urine and the conversion of the off-white colour to blue within 30 seconds means haemoglobin is present. Comparison with the colour chart gives an indication of the amount of blood present. The second test is performed in the laboratory. The urine is centrifuged or spun round to make all the cells settle at the bottom of the tube: the deposit is then examined under the microscope and red cells identified and counted.

(d) *Pyuria* (pus cells in the urine). Pus cells are best examined in a fresh unspun sample of urine placed in a special chamber under the microscope, but sometimes centrifuging is necessary if not many cells are present. When pyuria is severe, the urine may be cloudy and have a fishy smell. Pyuria is due to infection of the renal tract, pyelitis (infection in the pelvis of the kidney), cystitis (infection of the bladder) or urethritis (infection in the urethra).

(e) *Casts.* These are small solid protein bodies in the urine visible under the microscope. They are formed in the tubules and if they contain cells (cellular or granular casts) they are an indication of renal disease.

2. Blood urea and creatinine

These are two products of protein metabolism present in the blood and although variations occur with the amount of protein taken in the diet, the kidneys excrete excess of these products and the levels in the blood remain remarkably constant. When the kidney is not functioning properly, as in nephritis for example, the amount of urea and of creatinine in the blood increases because the kidney is incapable of excreting adequate amounts.

In good health, the urea level does not exceed 6·6 mmol per litre (40 mg/100 ml) and creatinine is below 124 μmol per litre (1·4 mg/ 100 ml). Levels in excess of these figures suggest inadequate excretion due to renal impairment.

3. Creatinine clearance test

This is a more exact measure of kidney function and depends on the *rate* at which the kidney can excrete creatinine. The urine excreted over 24 hours is collected and a blood sample taken. By measuring the amount of creatinine excreted in the urine and the amount present in the blood, the rate at which creatinine is cleared from the blood can be calculated and compared with normal. The worse this is, the worse the outlook from the view of renal function.

4. Intravenous pyelography (IVP)

This is an X-ray of the kidneys after the intravenous injection of an iodised oil. This dye is concentrated by the kidney and is opaque to X-ray. Consequently, the X-rays reveal details of the kidneys, the ureters and the bladder and expose any anatomical defects in the

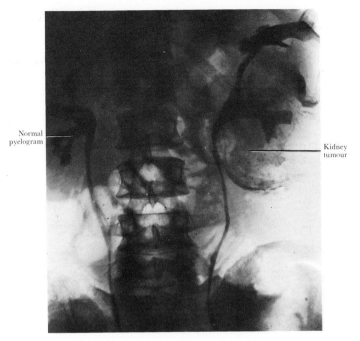

Normal
pyelogram

Kidney
tumour

Fig. 11.3   Retrograde pyelography. The calyces and pelvis of the right kidney are normal. In the left kidney a large tumour has caused marked distortion of the calyces and pelvis.

renal tract. An aperient should be given 36 hours before if the bowels have not been opened and the patient should be on a light diet the day before. No fluids should be allowed for 6 hours before the IVP is performed.

When the IVP does not yield adequate information, a *retrograde pyelogram* can be undertaken by a surgeon. This is done in the operating theatre since it requires cystoscopy and the introduction of fine catheters into the ureters from the bladder. Dye is then injected into these catheters and X-rays taken of the kidney.

5. Renal biopsy

A special needle can be inserted through the skin and directly into the kidney, allowing a small piece of kidney to be withdrawn. This biopsy is then suitably stained and examined under the microscope. Renal biopsy yields valuable information in some cases where the nature of the renal disorder is in doubt, since it shows the microscopic structure of the glomerulus and the capsule. This information provides a guide to treatment and to the outlook for the patient. But renal biopsy is a procedure that can lead to haematuria and so is only reserved for exceptional cases.

NEPHRITIS

Nephritis can be defined as a diffuse inflammatory disorder affecting both kidneys, especially the glomeruli.

Acute nephritis can occur for no obvious reason, but sometimes in association with a bacterial or virus infection. It may be part of a constitutional ailment such as polyarteritis nodosa (p. 472), or subacute bacterial endocarditis (p. 126). The commonest cause of acute nephritis is following a streptococcal infection of the throat. The majority of such cases get better completely in a short space of time.

Chronic nephritis is a progressive disorder of kidney function. It sometimes follows acute nephritis but more often is due to other causes.

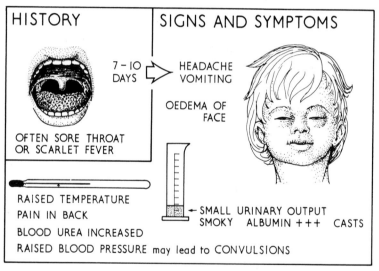

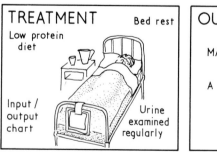

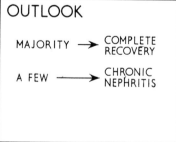

FIG. 11.4   Acute nephritis.

Acute nephritis

Symptoms and signs

1. The patient is generally a child or young adult, and quite often has had a sore throat or an attack of scarlet fever about seven to 10 days before. The onset is fairly sudden with:
   (a) Fever
   (b) Headache
   (c) Pain in the back
   (d) Vomiting.

2. The presence of *oedema* is typical, particularly in the face (especially around the eyes) and in the ankles. It tends to be worse in the morning and better in the evening. (This oedema should be contrasted with the oedema of heart failure, which never occurs in the face and is worse in the evening and better in the morning.) The oedema gives the patient a characteristic bloated appearance. In severe cases fluid may accumulate in the pleural cavity (pleural effusion) or the peritoneal cavity (ascites).

3. URINARY CHANGES. These are fairly constant, and are most important as they denote the degree and severity of the kidney damage.
   (a) There is diminished output of urine (oliguria). In very severe cases very little urine may be passed.
   (b) The urine is dark, concentrated and often smoky in colour from the presence of blood (haematuria).
   (c) Albumin is always present, usually in very heavy amounts.
   (d) Casts (which can be seen under the microscope) are present. Red blood cells and granular casts are the types of cast most frequently present in the acute stage of nephritis. Casts, when present in any number, are always evidence of severe kidney disease, particularly nephritis.

4. The blood pressure is usually raised, and in severe cases may be extremely high, with severe headaches, vomiting and perhaps convulsions (*hypertensive encephalopathy*).

COURSE. Most patients with acute nephritis recover completely, but a small percentage become chronic. In the majority of cases of chronic nephritis, however, there is no history of an acute attack, the cases presenting themselves as chronic from the start.

Treatment of acute nephritis

1. REST. The patient is nursed at complete rest in a warm well-ventilated room. Bed rest is continued until all the symptoms have gone and the urine is free of red blood cells and, if possible, of albumin also. As, however, in some patients the albumin persists indefinitely in the urine (the acute nephritis going on into the chronic stage) it may not be possible to keep all patients in bed till the urine is completely normal.

2. DIET. Because of the need to rest the diseased kidneys as much as

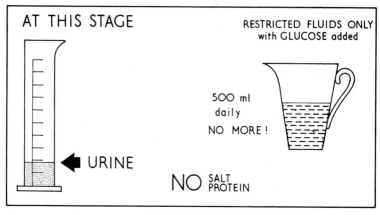

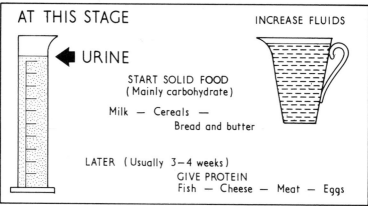

FIG. 11.5   Stages in acute nephritis.

possible, perhaps the most important item in the treatment of acute nephritis is the diet. As most of the work of the kidneys consists of excreting the waste products of protein, as little protein as possible is given in the vital early days. In addition, owing to the presence of oedema, fluids and salt are restricted.

To carry out these principles of diet an initial period of starvation is necessary, when only 1 pint a day of sweetened orange juice, lemon juice or barley water is given, with perhaps some coffee. Nothing else is given until the kidneys begin to recover, the signs of this being an increased output of urine and the lessening or disappearance of blood from the urine. In most cases a *diuresis* sets in after a few days and the diet can then be increased by the addition of bread, butter, cereals, milk and puddings. Eggs, fish, cheese and meat are gradually added later with the continued improvement of the patient.

It is important to realise that an initial starvation period followed

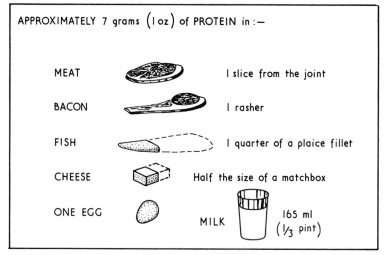

APPROXIMATELY 7 grams $\left(1\,oz\right)$ of PROTEIN in :—

MEAT   1 slice from the joint

BACON   1 rasher

FISH   1 quarter of a plaice fillet

CHEESE   Half the size of a matchbox

ONE EGG   MILK   165 ml
                                    $\left(\frac{1}{3}\,\text{pint}\right)$

FIG. 11.6   Protein foods.

by a very limited protein diet (usually in the region of 40 g) is of the utmost value in resting the kidneys; if, however, there is no improvement in the urinary findings after two or three weeks this low protein diet must be increased in order to supply sufficient protein (70 to 90 g) to build up the patient's general nutritional state.

An *intake and output chart* must be kept for all patients, and the urine examined daily for albumin, red cells and casts. The bowels are kept open by means of a suitable aperient, but excessive purgation does no good and only distresses the patient.

3. COMPLICATIONS. The convulsions seen in severe cases are treated by sedatives such as chloral hydrate, paraldehyde or barbiturates. If the blood pressure is very high the rapid withdrawal of a pint of blood is often very useful in relieving the strain on the heart.

4. INFECTIVE FOCI. As stated earlier, acute nephritis often follows a streptococcal infection (tonsillitis, scarlet fever, otitis media, etc.) and therefore penicillin may be given to treat the infection.

Chronic nephritis

Sometimes chronic nephritis follows an attack of acute nephritis but more often it is found to exist without evidence of any antecedent cause. Chronic nephritis may be associated with other systemic disorders, especially diabetes, and can be brought about by certain drugs, for example phenacetin or gold.

Symptoms and signs

The course of chronic nephritis is extremely variable as the disease may show itself in various ways.

1. THE LATENT STAGE. In this type the presence of chronic nephritis may be discovered by a routine examination of the urine, which reveals the presence of albumin and casts. There may be no symptoms or merely a general feeling of being run down. Anaemia is a fairly constant feature, and in many cases the blood pressure is raised.

2. OEDEMATOUS STAGE. Many cases of chronic nephritis have oedema at some stage or other. In some patients the oedema may be very mild and escape notice, while in others the oedema is a predominating feature (nephrotic form of chronic nephritis). The oedema occurs in the face and legs, and in very severe cases a pleural effusion and ascites may also be present. In addition, very heavy albuminuria is a constant finding in the oedematous stage of chronic nephritis, and it is this continued loss of protein from the blood that mainly accounts for the massive oedema.

3. STAGE OF RENAL FAILURE. Here the symptoms are those of chronic uraemia, with weakness, vomiting, drowsiness and eventually coma. The blood urea is extremely high as is also the blood pressure. Uraemia is more fully described later (p. 374).

Treatment

1. IN THE LATENT STAGE. Here, where there are few or no symptoms and there is no evidence of renal failure, e.g. the blood urea is normal, no very active measures are called for. The patient is encouraged to carry on with his normal work as far as possible, although excessive fatigue and exposure must be avoided. A normal well-balanced diet is given, with perhaps a restriction in the amount of protein. Fruit and vegetables should be taken in sufficient quantities to supply the necessary vitamins and minerals. The anaemia must be treated with iron.

2. IN THE OEDEMATOUS STAGE. If this is at all severe the patient is best nursed in bed until the oedema has completely or almost completely disappeared. The diet in this stage is important.

(a) Salt must be curtailed as much as possible as salt tends to retain water in the body and thus to increase the oedema.

(b) In the oedematous stage there is a continued loss of protein in the urine, which plays a large part in causing the oedema. For this reason a moderately high (100 to 125 g) protein diet is often given. It is possible to give a high protein diet in most cases in the oedematous stage of chronic nephritis because the blood urea is normal, showing that there is no gross evidence of renal failure.

(c) Diuretics are the most effective method of reducing oedema and the dose can be increased if the initial response is inadequate. Bendrofluazide 5 mg or frusemide 40 mg daily may be given, and spironolactone 25 mg four times a day can be added if the oedema still persists. A careful watch must be kept for signs of the salt depletion syndrome (p. 389) and for potassium deficiency (p. 390).

3. STAGE OF RENAL FAILURE. At this stage palliative treatment to relieve the symptoms (headache, vomiting, convulsions) only is possible. As the blood urea is high the protein in the diet must be restricted (40 g daily), but since there is usually little or no oedema fluids are not limited.

Chronic nephritis usually runs a prolonged course. The most essential factors in the treatment are, therefore, provision of a suitable diet varying, as described above, according to the stage of nephritis present; the avoidance, as far as possible, of intercurrent infections which may cause an acute exacerbation of the nephritis and appropriate modification of the patient's daily work to suit his state of health.

The nephrotic syndrome

This is a condition occurring particularly in children, but also in adults. It is characterised by generalised oedema and by heavy albuminuria. The oedema is usually most marked in the legs to begin with, but this may be followed by ascites, pleural effusion and oedema of the face and arms. So much albumin is lost in the urine that the plasma protein is seriously depleted.

These features may be due to chronic nephritis or to a form of subacute nephritis. Often the cause of the nephrotic syndrome is unknown though it might be due to abnormal antibodies and, especially in children, the outlook for recovery may be good. Sometimes a kidney biopsy is performed to help decide the diagnosis. A fragment of kidney is removed by a special needle and examined under the microscope.

Treatment

In children particularly, cortisone and its derivatives (steroids) are often successful in reducing the oedema and albuminuria. A high dose of prednisolone, perhaps 60 mg a day, must be given in the initial stages, but this is reduced when a satisfactory response occurs. Salt restriction and diuretics may also be used, as in chronic nephritis.

Where steroids are ineffective, cyclophosphamide may be prescribed. This drug suppresses antibody formation but must be carefully supervised to avoid toxic effects on the bone marrow.

Hypertensive kidney disease

In discussing hypertension (p. 101) it was noted that while the majority of cases of hypertension end in congestive heart failure or cerebral haemorrhage a small number develop uraemia. Severe kidney damage, ending in uraemia, is particularly common in the very severe and rapidly progressive form of essential hypertension known as *malignant* hypertension (to distinguish it from the more common form called *benign* hypertension). The treatment of renal failure due to hypertension is as outlined under Uraemia.

URAEMIA

Uraemia is the term used to describe the condition of renal failure and may be chronic or acute.

Chronic renal failure

Causes

Chronic renal failure is the end stage of many forms of renal disorders including the following:

1. Chronic nephritis.
2. Chronic pyelonephritis.
3. Hypertensive kidney disease.
4. Chronic obstruction of the renal tract (hydronephrosis) due to such causes as enlarged prostate, or renal stones.
5. Polycystic kidneys. This is a congenital renal disorder with cyst formation in the kidneys and poor renal function.
6. Kidney disease due to constitutional disorders such as diabetes, gout, myelomatosis or polyarteritis nodosum.

Symptoms and signs

1. The onset of symptoms in chronic uraemia is usually very gradual, and in the early stages the main features are a general fatigue and exhaustion usually accompanied by anaemia. As the renal failure progresses the patient becomes increasingly and excessively drowsy and more acute symptoms develop.

2. Vomiting and diarrhoea are frequently present and *hiccoughing* is often a predominant feature.

3. The drowsiness lapses into a coma in the terminal stages, and twitchings developing into convulsions may occur.

4. The breathing is usually laboured, and in the late stages the waxing and waning type of respiration (Cheyne-Stokes) is usually present.

5. The total output of urine is usually normal or even increased. Albumin is usually present to some extent, thus denoting the presence of a kidney lesion, but in some cases the amount may be small.

6. Well-marked changes in the retina of the eye (*retinitis*) are present in most cases of uraemia, and the patients usually complain of dimness of vision. White patches (exudates), haemorrhages and swelling of the optic disc are the common findings when the retina is examined by an ophthalmoscope.

7. In most cases the blood pressure is raised.

8. The blood urea is markedly elevated and the presence of a high blood urea in conjunction with the above symptoms confirms the diagnosis.

Treatment

As there is no cure for chronic kidney disease, treatment is directed towards alleviating the effects. Since urea is derived from protein, the patient must follow a diet with a very low content of protein, perhaps only 40 g a day. This will help to prevent the urea from rising too rapidly. If the blood pressure is raised, hypotensive drugs (p. 104) should be given. A high blood pressure leads to further renal damage. Blood transfusions may be necessary when anaemia is severe.

In some cases of chronic renal disease, recourse may be made to the artificial kidney (extracorporeal dialysis), and patients have to be moved to special hospitals for this purpose. The patient's blood is anticoagulated with heparin to prevent clotting and is passed through the artificial kidney apparatus. Urea, potassium and other toxic substances are removed from the blood by a process of dialysis before its return to the patient. This treatment soon leads to a considerable improvement in the patient's condition and the process can be repeated at regular intervals. The patient can return to his home and his work and need only attend hospital for dialysis.

Renal transplantation offers the best hope for patients with chronic kidney disease. The diseased kidneys can be replaced by healthy kidneys taken from patients who have recently died. Many difficulties have to be overcome before this can be done on a wide scale. There is a limited supply of suitable kidneys and methods for preserving such kidneys for more than a few hours have not been successful. Rejection of the implanted kidney is likely to occur unless it is of the right type (see p. 47). Nevertheless, growing experience in this field has led to many patients with hopeless kidney disease enjoying a new lease of life.

Acute renal failure (acute anuria)

Although the outlook in most cases of established chronic renal failure is extremely bad and any treatment is merely palliative, this is far from being the case with acute renal failure.

Causes

1. Severe toxic poisons causing acute intense damage to the kidneys. Mercurial poisons are especially prone to cause severe kidney damage.

2. Acute obstruction within the kidney tubules resulting from the deposit of crystals during sulphonamide therapy.

3. Mismatched blood transfusions. The agglutinated (clumped) red cells obstruct the kidney tubules.

4. Severe shock. Here the blood pressure may fall so low that the blood flow through the kidneys practically ceases, and as a result little or no urine is formed. The severe shock may be caused by injury (serious crushing injuries are for some reason especially liable to cause acute renal failure), by severe haemorrhage or by overwhelming toxic infections.

5. Severe dehydration, with its excessive loss of fluid from the body, may result in markedly reduced blood circulation through the kidneys, with a consequential cessation of urinary secretion.

The fundamental change resulting from all the causes of acute

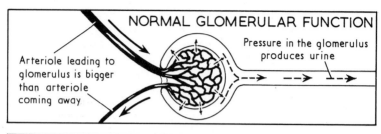

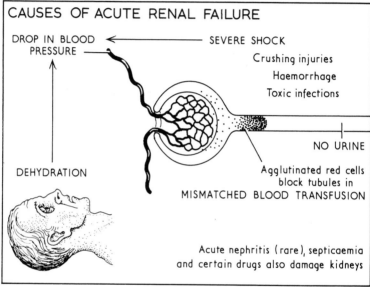

Fig. 11.7   The causes of acute renal failure (acute anuria).

renal failure is a sudden cessation of urinary output. In all cases the kidneys, previously normal, are suddenly prevented from performing their prime function of secreting urine in order to excrete the waste products of metabolism.

Symptoms and signs

The cardinal sign of acute renal failure is thus the complete, or almost complete, suppression of urine—*anuria*. In the early stages the few ounces of urine passed may contain frank blood, especially in the cases caused by mismatched transfusions and sulphonamides. In the severe cases complete anuria develops and may last for as long as seven to 10 days, after which time the kidneys in many cases recover and begin to secrete urine. If after 10 to 14 days urinary secretion does not recommence death is likely to occur.

In the first few days of the anuria the patient may have few symptoms and the general condition may remain good. After five or six days, however, vomiting usually starts and the patient's general condition slowly deteriorates, with perhaps increasing drowsiness and in some cases twitching and convulsions. With the sudden onset of diuresis the patient will make a rapid recovery or, alternatively, with no diuresis may die.

Treatment of acute anuria
PREVENTION

1. *Mismatched transfusions.* The carrying out of all the essential preliminaries before giving a blood transfusion will prevent these cases. Blood grouping, giving blood of the same group and, in addition, cross-matching the patient's serum against the donor's red cells are the essential preliminaries to all blood transfusions. Before giving a blood transfusion, the patient's name, hospital number, the number of the unit of blood, its group and evidence of compatibility on cross matching all should be checked by two nurses.

- BEFORE <u>ALL</u> BLOOD TRANSFUSIONS

<u>ALWAYS</u>   1 Group patient
  2 Cross-match patient's serum against donor's red cells
- GIVE BLOOD OF THE SAME GROUP
- WATCH PATIENT CLOSELY FOR REACTION

EARLY AND PROMPT TREATMENT FOR SHOCK AND HAEMORRHAGE

Frequent BP readings

Serum or blood of the same group

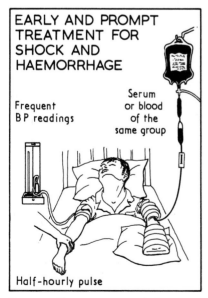

Half-hourly pulse

IN ALL ILLNESSES watch for signs of DEHYDRATION

Sunken eyes

Dry tongue and lips

Pinched skin

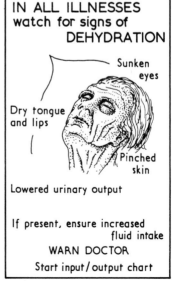

Lowered urinary output

If present, ensure increased fluid intake
WARN DOCTOR
Start input/output chart

FIG. 11.8   The prevention of acute anuria.

When a blood transfusion is started a very close watch must be kept on the patient to make sure that there are no severe reactions. If by mistake incompatible blood is given, as little as an ounce of such blood may be enough to make the patient complain of severe shivering, restlessness, nausea and pain in the back. The skin is cold, the pulse and temperature rise and the patient becomes shocked. In the presence of any of these symptoms, the transfusion must immediately be stopped and the doctor notified.

It must be stressed that giving correctly matched blood to every patient is the only way to prevent transfusion reactions (p. 346).

2. *Shock*. In all cases of shock, with its low blood pressure and diminished blood circulation to the organs and tissues, early and adequate transfusions with blood (or serum) will prevent acute renal failure. The essential aim in cases of shock is to raise the blood pressure enough (at least above a systolic reading of 100 mmHg) to ensure an adequate circulation of blood to all organs and tissues.

3. *Dehydration*. The provision of an adequate fluid intake in all illness has been repeatedly mentioned. With severely ill patients, especially children and elderly people, the nurse must not only provide adequate fluids but see that the patient takes them. Accurate measurement of the urinary output, which should reach 1·2 to 1·5 litres a day, will enable the nurse to see whether sufficient fluids are, in fact, being taken. In addition, the presence of a dry tongue and pinched skin (in infants the sunken fontanelle and sunken eyes are further signs) means that sufficient fluids are not being taken.

CURATIVE

Once anuria has developed it means that the kidneys are severely damaged and the aim in treatment is to rest the kidneys as much as possible until recovery begins. As there is no chronic damage to the kidneys, if the patient can be tided over the acute phase the outlook is good.

DIET AND FLUIDS. To rest the kidneys as completely as possible protein is reduced to an absolute minimum whilst the fluid intake too is kept at the lowest level necessary for metabolism. Sufficient fluid is given to counterbalance the loss from the skin and lungs (about 500 to 800 ml) with, in addition, a further amount of fluid equal in quantity to any urine passed.

Nutrition can be maintained by artificial carbohydrates such as Caloreen or flavoured Hycal given by mouth. However, in most cases intravenous therapy becomes necessary if nausea or vomiting is to be avoided. Fat emulsions (Intralipid or Lipiphysan) can be given intravenously and supply the necessary energy.

Frequent estimations of blood potassium and other electrolytes are necessary throughout the course of the illness. In the anuric stage, potassium may accumulate in the blood, giving rise to signs of potassium intoxication (marked lethargy, weakness and heart

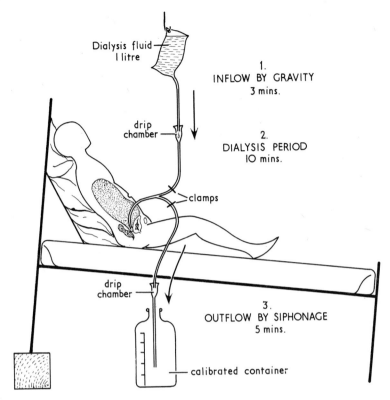

Dialysis fluid
l litre

1.
INFLOW BY GRAVITY
3 mins.

drip
chamber

2.
DIALYSIS PERIOD
10 mins.

clamps

drip
chamber

3.
OUTFLOW BY SIPHONAGE
5 mins.

calibrated container

FIG. 11.9 Peritoneal dialysis.

damage as revealed by a slow and irregular pulse; a careful watch
must always therefore be kept on the pulse).

In patients not responding to this treatment, hiccough, lethargy,
vomiting and even convulsions are ominous signs of uraemia.
Recourse may now be made to peritoneal dialysis. A special solution
is allowed to flow into the peritoneal cavity and remain there for
about ten minutes. The peritoneum acts as a membrane through
which potassium and other waste products are extracted by the
dialysing fluid. The process can be repeated for several hours until
the blood urea shows a return to near normal, and soon leads to an
obvious improvement in the patient's well-being. However, this
treatment can only be regarded as a temporary expedient and
ultimately the patient's recovery depends on a return of kidney
function with normal output of urine.

URINARY TRACT INFECTION

Infections in the urinary tract can occur in the urethra (urethritis), in
the bladder (cystitis), in the pelvis of the kidney (pyelitis), or in the
kidney substance (pyelonephritis). There is nothing to suggest that

infection usually progresses from one part of the urinary tract to another although in debilitated patients cystitis can lead to pyelo-nephritis.

Cystitis

Inflammation of the bladder is called cystitis, and is frequently due to organisms similar to those causing pyelitis. Cystitis is more frequently seen in females (where the infection often spreads from inflammation of the vulval region). Cystitis is also especially likely to arise where there is any obstruction or other disease in the bladder, such as stones, tumours or enlarged prostate. In diseases of the central nervous system, paralysis, causing incontinence or retention of urine, is very prone to set up infection in the bladder. Repeated catheterisa-tion, necessary in cases of retention, is particularly liable to cause cystitis. Finally, such specific diseases as gonorrhoea and tuberculosis may cause a cystitis.

The symptoms of cystitis are chiefly pain and frequency of micturition; the urine contains albumin, pus and the infecting organisms. In the acute stage fever and rigors may be present.

The treatment is similar to that of pyelitis with sulphonamides or antibiotics. In addition, any primary disease predisposing to cystitis must be dealt with. The need for the utmost care in achieving adequate asepsis in carrying out all catheterisations must be stressed.

Patients who are paralysed often develop retention of urine with subsequent bladder infection. This infection can spread to the kidneys (*pyelonephritis*) with a fatal outcome.

Pyelitis

This is a common and troublesome disorder occurring in women. As a rule, the onset is sudden and characterised by frequency and dysuria. It may be necessary to pass water every few hours although the volume of urine passed may be small. Micturition is painful or burning in character. The temperature may be raised a little above normal and there may be a feeling of malaise, but often constitutional symptoms are not marked.

Examination of the urine shows the presence of white cells and culture of the urine often shows a significant growth of bacteria, usually e. coli.

Although an attack of pyelitis usually subsides without treatment, usually a course of co-trimoxazole is prescribed.

In many women, attacks of pyelitis may recur and prove a troublesome disability. In view of the danger that pyelonephritis may develop, it is often wise in such cases to give courses of alternating treatment, each course lasting for several weeks. Thus a course of co-trimoxazole can alternate with a course of other chemotherapeutic agents. These include ampicillin, nalidixic acid and nitrofurantoin, the choice of the particular drug depending on the sensitivity of the organism on culture to its action.

Acute pyelonephritis

The symptoms of frequency and dysuria are associated with pyrexia, sweating, general malaise and pain in the loins. The onset may be abrupt and rigors may occur. The white count may be high, a sign of a systemic bacterial infection. The urine shows a quantity of pus (pyuria) and culture yields a heavy growth of bacteria, usually e. coli.

The patient must be nursed in bed and given large quantities of fluid to drink, up to three litres a day. A course of co-trimoxazole is started but may be changed to another drug if necessary when the results of culture sensitivity are obtained.

Chronic pyelonephritis

This serious renal disorder is a common cause of renal failure. One or both kidneys may be affected. The evidence of infection is that the kidneys are scarred and renal biopsy confirms signs of infection and inflammation.

Clinical features and diagnosis

1. There may be constitutional symptoms of fever, malaise and aching in the loins associated with frequency and dysuria.

2. Quite often the first symptoms are those of chronic renal failure (p. 374) and the diagnosis depends on the result of the investigations.

3. The urine shows pus and bacteria on culture.

4. The blood urea may be raised and the creatinine clearance test may be depressed (p. 366).

5. An IVP (p. 366) shows irregularly shaped kidneys due to scarring and damage of kidney structures by chronic infection.

Treatment

If an infecting organism can be identified, appropriate chemo-therapy must be instituted and maintained continuously for many months. Alternate courses of different agents may be used, as described with recurrent pyelitis. If renal failure supervenes, treatment will be necessary in this respect (p. 374).

TUBERCULOSIS OF THE URINARY SYSTEM

Tuberculosis may affect one or both kidneys and the infection may spread to involve the bladder. In advanced cases of renal tuberculosis large, multiple, tuberculous abscess cavities develop.

Symptoms and signs

The most common symptom is frequency of micturition, which is usually very severe and persistent. The patients pass urine in very small amounts throughout the day and night. Haematuria is also commonly present. Pain in the loins and on micturition is often

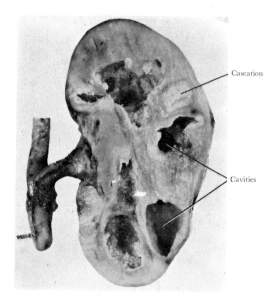

Caseation

Cavities

FIG. 11.10 Tuberculosis of the kidney. The progressive caseation has produced widespread cavitation.

complained of. There are usually general symptoms, including malaise, loss of appetite and fever.

The diagnosis is usually made by finding the tubercle bacilli in the urine. For this, a 24-hour specimen of urine must be collected as the organisms are present in very scanty numbers. X-ray examination (*pyelography*) may show some deformity of the kidneys, such as distortion of the outline of the calyces.

Treatment

When the disease is localised in one kidney surgical removal of the affected organ is usually carried out. Before and after operation chemotherapy such as streptomycin, isoniazid and para-aminosalicylic acid is given. In bilateral renal tuberculosis, surgery is not usually possible, and for these patients only chemotherapy and the usual general measures to build up the patient's resistance are possible.

RENAL CALCULI

Renal calculi, or stones, are very common, but as they are usually fully described in surgical textbooks only a brief mention is necessary here.

Renal calculi may remain silent in the kidney and cause no symptoms; on the other hand, they may move and give rise to *renal*

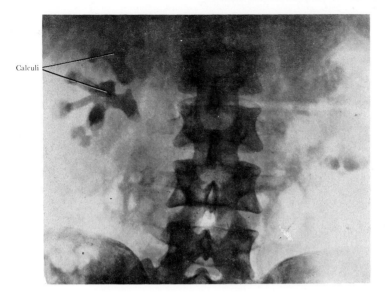

Calculi

FIG. 11.11   Renal calculus. Typical staghorn stone in the right kidney.

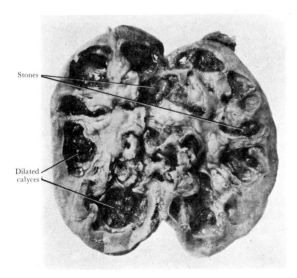

Stones

Dilated
calyces

FIG. 11.12   Hydronephrosis of the kidney showing the dilatation of the pelvis and calyces. The multiple stones causing the obstruction and consequent dilatation can be seen.

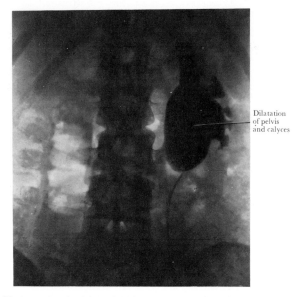

Dilatation
of pelvis
and calyces

FIG. 11.13   Hydronephrosis of the left kidney, outlined by retrograde pyelography.

colic. Here severe pain occurs causing restlessness, sweating and vomiting. The pain characteristically starts in the loin and radiates downwards and forwards to the groin. The urine usually contains albumin and blood.

Renal calculi in addition to causing colic can obstruct the kidney and so lead to dilatation and distension (*hydronephrosis*). If the hydronephrosis is severe the kidney loses its power to function properly. (Not only calculi but also any obstruction, such as an enlarged prostate, can cause hydronephrosis.)

X-ray examination after administration of an opaque dye (pyelography) usually reveals the dilated hydronephrotic kidney.

The treatment of renal calculi, where these are causing symptoms, is operative removal. Small stones, however, are frequently passed in the urine. In cases where there is a severe hydronephrosis with a poorly functioning kidney the affected kidney is usually removed (nephrectomy), the fact that the opposite kidney is normal having first been established.

12 Metabolism and Vitamins

Before considering the specific diseases which affect the metabolism of the body it is first necessary to understand a little about normal metabolism and how it can be upset.

The term *metabolism* is used to define the various changes which continuously take place in the body in everyday life. An example of these changes is the breakdown of foods into suitable substances which can be used by the body for the provision of energy and the repair of tissues. The metabolism of the body requires very many different factors if normal health is to be maintained.

THE ESSENTIALS OF NORMAL METABOLISM

1. Carbohydrates and fibre
2. Fats
3. Proteins
4. Mineral salts
5. Vitamins
6. Hormones
7. Water
8. Normal gastrointestinal tract
9. Normal liver and bile.

CARBOHYDRATES

Carbohydrates are the least expensive and most freely available type of food. Bread, cereals, rice, potatoes and farinaceous foods such as spaghetti form the bulk of the diet in most parts of the world. Sugar is also a carbohydrate and is obtained from cane and from beet. It is a highly concentrated form of carbohydrate, very quickly absorbed from the bowel into the blood stream as glucose. Sugar is not only used as a sweetener in tea, coffee and fruit drinks but it is also present in jams, sweets, chocolates, biscuits and cakes. In this country, the average consumption of sugar is about 120 lb (55 kg) per person annually. Fruit and milk also contain natural sugar.

The carbohydrates are digested to glucose by the various juices in the saliva, stomach and intestines, and it is in the form of glucose that carbohydrates are absorbed into the blood. Glucose is stored in the liver and muscles in the form of glycogen, and is reconverted into glucose when needed to supply fuel and energy for the body.

Dietary fibre

Fibre is the term used for the supporting structure of plants and is present in all parts of the plant, the leaves, flowers, seeds, fruit, stem roots, bulb and tuber. Consequently fibre is present in vegetables, fruit and the grain of wheat and rye. For the most part, fibre is not digested in the gastrointestinal tract and, since it is not absorbed, it has no energy value. Nevertheless, it plays an important part in the proper functioning of the bowel. Fibre enmeshes bile and many food products in its substance, and so delays absorption of products such as glucose and cholesterol.

Modern dietary habits have greatly reduced the intake of fibre in our food. The outer layers of the wheat grain (bran) are discarded in order to produce white flour and white bread. White bread, biscuits, pastry, cakes and puddings made from white flour contain very little fibre or roughage. Sugar is particularly bad in this respect. White sugar is refined from beet and cane and is quickly absorbed into the blood stream. It is a concentrated and unnatural food, high in energy value but lacking in fibre and vitamins.

Sugar disposes to tooth decay (*caries*), since it encourages the growth of bacteria at the gum margins. Because sugar is concentrated food and can be taken to excess in beverages, chocolates and biscuits, it increases the energy intake and leads to obesity. Excess sugar in middle age may dispose to diabetes by throwing a strain on the insulin mechanism: the more sugar absorbed, the more insulin has to be produced.

A healthy diet should contain adequate fibre or roughage. Wholemeal bread contains the husk of the wheat germ as well as the germ itself and is preferable to white bread. Plenty of fruit and lightly cooked vegetables should be eaten. Wholemeal cereals should be taken at breakfast and, where constipation is troublesome, bran itself can be added to the food. It is best to avoid sugar and foods made from white flour.

Control of carbohydrate metabolism

In health the level of blood sugar is kept fairly constant. The control of carbohydrate metabolism depends on various factors, including:

1. INSULIN. Insulin, which is a secretion of the islets of Langerhans of the pancreas, plays a most important part in ensuring the proper use of glucose in the body. Insulin enables the glucose both to be stored in the liver and muscles in the form of glycogen and also to be utilised as necessary.

With a deficiency of insulin, such as is met with in the disease *diabetes mellitus*, glucose is neither utilised nor stored, so that it accumulates in the blood and is excreted in the urine (glycosuria). On the other hand, too much insulin causes a fall in blood sugar, which, if severe, produces coma (hypoglycaemia).

2. Normal liver function is essential for the proper storage of glucose (as glycogen). In some diseases of the liver the metabolism of glucose is upset.

3. Certain of the endocrine glands, especially the thyroid and adrenals, play a part in glucose metabolism. Thus with overactivity of the thyroid gland, e.g. in thyrotoxicosis, an excess of glucose may occur in the blood, to be excreted in the urine. The adrenals secrete cortisone which can convert protein into carbohydrate. If excessive cortisone is produced, the blood sugar may be permanently elevated and diabetes mellitus results.

FATS

The fats, next to the carbohydrates, form the chief energy foods. The principal fats eaten in the average diet are:

1. Butter and margarine
2. Cream
3. Oils and lard, as used in cooking
4. Bacon and the fat in meat.

The diet in Western countries tends to be rich in fat and this may be a contributory factor in the causation of coronary thrombosis. Fat in the diet is composed of glycerol and different types of fatty acids, some with compact structures (*saturated*) and others with looser structures (*polyunsaturated*). Saturated fats are chiefly solid fats of animal origin such as lard, butter and milk. Polyunsaturated fats are those in many vegetable oils, such as corn oil and sunflower oil. Saturated fats are a source of cholesterol and so a diet rich in animal fats leads to a rise in blood cholesterol. This cholesterol contributes to thickening of the coronary arteries. Hence it has been recommended that the diet should be adjusted so that it contains less saturated fats and more polyunsaturated fats. Corn oil can replace lard for frying food and vegetable margarine can replace butter, for example.

The fats after digestion by the intestinal and pancreatic juices are absorbed into the body, which they supply with energy and heat. Fat is stored in the subcutaneous tissues, which are almost all fat, thus providing a large reserve for future energy requirements.

Factors affecting control of fat metabolism

1. Bile is necessary for the digestion and absorption of fat, and in obstructive jaundice (in which bile is absent from the intestinal tract) there is improper absorption of fat. The faeces then become bulky and pale from excess of fat.

2. If the intestinal juices, especially the pancreatic juices, are absent the fat will not be split up into a form suitable for absorption and an excess of fat will therefore be excreted in the faeces. Absence of the pancreatic juice is sometimes seen in infants with disease of the pancreas.

3. In the malabsorption syndrome deficient absorption of fat from the bowel leads to an excess of fat in the stools, which become pale and bulky. In this syndrome poor absorption of fat and other food substances leads to wasting and deficient growth.

4. In a normal diet carbohydrates and fats are the chief foods supplying energy. If the carbohydrates are not being utilised properly, e.g. as in diabetes mellitus, an excessive use is made of the fats instead. Some of the final end-products of fat metabolism are, however, the poisonous acids *diacetic acid* and *acetone,* which normally are burnt down very rapidly. When, however, an excess of fats is being burnt (as in diabetes) diacetic acid and acetone accumulate in the body and the condition known as *acidosis* develops. (These acids are also known as ketone bodies, so the term *ketosis* is also used.) Ketosis (or acidosis) is commonly seen in diabetes and is the cause of diabetic coma. Ketosis is discussed further under Diabetes.

PROTEINS

Protein foods are primarily of value for the replacement of the normal wear and tear of tissues and for the growth of new tissues. Apart from this first essential function they can also be utilised, like carbohydrates and fats, as a source of energy. The main sources of proteins in a normal diet are:

1. Meat and fish   ⎫
2. Cheese and milk ⎬ Animal proteins
3. Eggs   ⎭
4. Peas, beans and flour. Vegetable proteins.

Proteins are made up of many different types of amino acids, many of which are essential for the proper building up of the tissues of the body.

Proteins are broken down into the constituent amino acids in the process of digestion by the pepsin and hydrochloric acid of the stomach and by the intestinal juices. The various amino acids are then absorbed into the blood stream and distributed to the tissues.

The amino acids which are not used for repair and building up of tissues are broken down by the liver into urea, which is excreted in the urine. The proteins, unlike the carbohydrates and fats, cannot be stored for future use.

ELECTROLYTES (Mineral salts)

To maintain good health many different electrolytes are essential, of which the following are some of the more important:

1. Sodium
2. Potassium
3. Calcium
4. Iodine
5. Fluorine
6. Iron.

1. Sodium

Salt contains sodium and chlorine, which are essential constituents of all the fluids of the body. Water is not retained in the body without salt. This is clearly seen in the case of heavy manual workers who sweat a good deal, e.g. miners, stokers, and as a result lose both salt and water in the sweat. Drinking ordinary water does not, without salt, replace the lost fluid and they consequently suffer from cramps caused by the lack of fluid. Taking extra salt with water, however, overcomes the cramps.

Oedema is accumulation of water in the tissues and commonly occurs in congestive heart failure and in the nephrotic stage of chronic nephritis. Diuretics cause excretion of salt in the urine and fluid is therefore excreted as well.

Cortisone (p. 456) is one of the hormones responsible for retaining sodium in the blood. When this is deficient, as in Addison's disease, the loss of sodium leads to loss of fluid. The body becomes dehydrated. The dehydration can be corrected by giving saline and cortisone.

Excessive vomiting, such as may occur in *pyloric stenosis* or *intestinal obstruction*, leads to a loss of chlorides in the vomit (gastric juice contains a large amount of chlorides), and in these conditions it is usually necessary to replace the lost chlorides as well as the fluid. In these cases saline is usually given.

Salt depletion syndrome. As mentioned earlier, salt restriction is most important in the treatment of oedema, especially in cardiac and renal oedema. The present-day therapy of oedema with potent diuretics can, however, lead to a severe fall in the body salt with serious results. The early recognition of salt depletion in all patients on a rigid salt-free diet, especially where diuretics and ion-exchange resins are also used, is most important. The signs are:

  (a) The patient becomes lethargic and drowsy and complains of marked weakness.
  (b) Appetite is lost and nausea and vomiting may be present.
  (c) There is severe reduction in urinary output and in the excretion of urinary chlorides.
  (d) Abdominal and muscular cramps are sometimes present.
  (e) Oedema may be, and often is, present.
  (f) The blood pressure falls.
  (g) The blood sodium is severely reduced. The blood urea is raised.

2. Potassium

Potassium is an important constituent of all tissue cells. Disturbances in potassium metabolism have been increasingly recognised in recent years. Excess of potassium in the blood (hyperkalaemia) occurs to any significant degree only in conditions associated with severe oliguria or anuria (p. 365) and in the crises of Addison's disease. Symptoms of potassium excess include marked weakness and mental confusion, numbness and tingling of the extremities. Heart block develops with a slow and irregular pulse and finally cardiac arrest occurs.

Potassium depletion (hypokalaemia) is more commonly met with than potassium excess. The causes of potassium depletion are:

(a) The prolonged use of diuretics in large doses.

(b) It may develop in any disease or condition with a prolonged low food intake and especially when there is, in addition, excessive intake of sodium. Thus, after major operations, prolonged intravenous saline therapy combined with diminished food intake, is very liable to cause potassium deficiency. Similarly, this deficiency may arise in the recovery stage of diabetic coma, owing to the diminished food intake, intravenous saline therapy and, in addition, the excessive loss of potassium in the urine.

(c) Excessive vomiting and diarrhoea, especially where there is an inadequate diet.

(d) Ion-exchange therapy, by absorbing the potassium in the intestines, can lead to severe potassium depletion.

The symptoms of potassium depletion include severe lethargy and weakness, mental confusion, abdominal distension and finally respiratory and cardiac failure. Potassium depletion is corrected by giving potassium chloride, 8 g in divided doses by mouth. In very severe cases intravenous potassium may be necessary.

In prolonged treatment with such potent oral diuretics as the chlorothiazide group of drugs, especially when large doses are given, potassium supplements may be prescribed as a routine to prevent potassium depletion. A most careful watch must be kept on all patients, particularly elderly patients on prolonged therapy with chlorothiazide or similar diuretics and not eating, as it is in these circumstances that potassium (and sodium) depletion may easily develop.

Potassium deficiency greatly enhances the action of digitalis. Digitalis overdosage is therefore very liable to occur in patients being treated with digitalis and chlorothiazide at the same time. Particular care must therefore be taken to note any signs of digitalis overdosage, and if seen, the dose of digitalis must be reduced.

3. Calcium

Calcium, which is mainly present in milk and cheese, is essential for health, especially for:

(a) Formation of the bones
(b) Formation of the teeth
(c) Proper functioning of nerves and muscles.

It can be seen, therefore, that the requirements for calcium are likely to be greatest in childhood (the period of growth), and for adults during pregnancy and lactation. For this reason disturbances in calcium metabolism are most often seen during these times of extra need.

Control of calcium metabolism

VITAMIN D

Vitamin D is necessary for the proper absorption of calcium from the bowel, so that lack of this vitamin causes a deficiency of calcium in the body with consequential effects on the bones. In infancy and early childhood, when there is a great demand for vitamin D, a lack of this vitamin causes the disease known as *rickets*, of which predominant signs are changes and deformities of the bones. In adults a lack of vitamin D is seldom seen except in pregnant women in tropical countries. Here the poor diet and social customs may cause a marked deficiency of vitamin D leading to the disease *osteomalacia*. Osteomalacia causes bone changes similar to those seen in rickets.

In some cases of rickets the lack of calcium may be so great as to lead to a fall in the level of calcium in the blood. Low blood calcium causes the condition known as *tetany* with its irritability of the nerves and muscles.

PARATHORMONE

Disturbances of the normal hormone secreted by the parathyroid glands (parathormone) have a marked effect on calcium metabolism. Excess of parathyroid hormone, which occurs in tumours of the glands, causes the calcium to leave the bones. The calcium in the blood rises and an excess of calcium is excreted in the urine.

On the other hand, lack of parathyroid hormone causes a fall in blood calcium and is therefore another cause of tetany. Lack of parathormone leading to tetany is occasionally seen after thyroid-ectomy if the parathyroid glands have been accidentally damaged or removed during the operation.

Calcitonin is a hormone produced by special cells in the thyroid gland. It has an opposite effect to parathormone since it causes calcium to leave the blood and enter the bones. It is used in the treatment of Paget's disease.

4. Iodine

Iodine is essential for the formation of thyroxine, the hormone of the thyroid gland. It is normally found in many foodstuffs, but the amount depends on the soil and water. Soil and water in areas far from the sea, especially hilly areas, may lack iodine, and thus the inhabitants of such areas often suffer from iodine deficiency. Iodine deficiency causes one form of *goitre*.

5. Fluorine

Fluorine is necessary for the proper function and maintenance of teeth enamel. There is usually sufficient fluorine in drinking water for this purpose, but in areas where the water contains too little fluorine the teeth of growing children are unable to resist dental infection and caries develops. The addition of fluorine to the water supply in these areas has yielded encouraging results in reducing the incidence of dental decay in school children.

6. Iron

Haemoglobin, which is present in the red blood cells and which is essential for the carriage of oxygen throughout the body, is partly made up of iron. Therefore, in the absence of sufficient iron there is a deficiency of haemoglobin resulting in an iron-deficiency anaemia.

Deficiency of iron is usually due to insufficient intake, excessive bleeding or inadequate absorption. Iron is mainly found in meat, liver, eggs, peas and beans, and a diet which does not contain enough of these foods will lead to an iron-deficiency anaemia.

In infants whose sole diet is milk, which has a poor iron content, anaemia is common. In women continued heavy loss of blood in the menstrual flow frequently results in an iron-deficiency anaemia.

The absorption of iron depends on, amongst other things, the presence of hydrochloric acid in the stomach. If there is no acid in the gastric juice (achlorhydria) this predisposes to an iron-deficiency anaemia. In women with achlorhydria, the additional factor of blood loss from menstruation makes the anaemia more pronounced.

In addition to the above mineral salts many others are essential for health, but as these others are very rarely lacking, and therefore are not associated with disease, they will not be discussed here.

VITAMINS

Vitamins are certain factors present in various foods which are essential for the proper maintenance of health. There are many different vitamins, all of which tend to have some specific action on some part of the body's metabolism. Lack of a vitamin usually leads to certain well-recognised changes in the body.

Deficiency of a vitamin may arise in several ways. *Inadequate diet* is a frequent cause of vitamin deficiency. Again, even if the diet is entirely adequate, *deficient absorption* from the gastrointestinal tract, because of some disease in the tract, may lead to vitamin deficiency. Finally, at certain times there may be an *increased demand* for vitamins, which if not met may give rise to vitamin deficiency. It is for this reason that vitamin deficiencies are most frequent during the periods of active growth, during pregnancy, in the course of severe prolonged illnesses and after major operations.

VITAMIN A

ACTION. Vitamin A is necessary for the proper growth of certain epithelial cells of the body, especially those of the eyes, respiratory tract and skin.

SOURCES. Animal fats, butter, cream, eggs, milk and cod-liver oil.

DISEASES DUE TO LACK OF VITAMIN A

1. Eye diseases

(a) *Conjunctivitis* and *corneal ulceration*, due to improper development of the epithelium of the eye.

(b) *Night blindness*, i.e. great difficulty in seeing in the dark. Here the pigment in the eyes (visual purple) which is necessary for proper vision is not adequately formed.

2. Respiratory infections

The absence of vitamin A leads to a lowering of the resistance of the mucous membranes, with the result that infections of the respiratory tract tend to develop. Hence, vitamin A is often called the anti-infective vitamin.

VITAMIN B COMPLEX

ACTION. Vitamin B is not a single vitamin but is made up of several factors, many—though not all—of which are known to have a specific action.

The more important factors in the vitamin B complex are:

1. B_1 FACTOR (also called *thiamine* or *aneurine*). Richest sources are yeast, cereals, peas, beans and eggs.
2. NICOTINIC ACID (*niacin*), mainly found in yeast, meat, liver and fish.
3. RIBOFLAVINE, chiefly found in milk, eggs, liver and kidney.
4. VITAMIN B_{12} (p. 331).
5. FOLIC ACID (p. 331).

DISEASES DUE TO LACK OF THE VITAMIN B COMPLEX

In practice, although diseases may result from a deficiency of any one of the separate vitamins of the vitamin B complex, it is nevertheless more common for diseases to arise when several of the vitamins in this group are lacking at the same time.

1. Beriberi

The disease known as beriberi is supposed to be caused by a deficiency of the B_1 factor (aneurine). It is probable, however, that other factors are involved as well, because pure vitamin B_1 will not always cure the disease whereas an adequate diet, especially in protein, usually does.

Beriberi is very common in such Eastern countries as China, Japan and India where the staple food is polished rice, as the polishing of the rice removes most of the vitamin B and especially the B_1 factor.

The disease is seen in two forms: wet beriberi, which causes a marked oedema with congestive heart failure, and dry beriberi, which causes a peripheral neuritis.

2. Pellagra

Pellagra is common in America and certain parts of Europe, and occasionally occurs in this country. The specific deficiency which causes pellagra is not known, but it is clear that a lack of the nicotinic acid factor plays a large part. Pellagra is often seen in people living on an inadequate diet who have, in addition, a history of chronic alcoholism. Alcoholism increases the metabolism of the body, which in turn increases the body's requirements of food and vitamins. At the same time, however, in chronic alcoholism the amount of food eaten is usually much reduced. This combination of increased need for the decreased intake of the necessary food and vitamins is very prone to cause nutritional and vitamin deficiencies, of which pellagra is one.

The main symptoms of pellagra can be divided into the following groups:

(a) Gastrointestinal. Severe glossitis, stomatitis and diarrhoea.
(b) Skin changes. Symmetrical dermatitis of the face and hands, with characteristic dark pigmentation in the later stages.
(c) Mental. Dementia.

Treatment

Treatment of pellagra mainly consists of the provision of an adequate diet, supplemented by large doses of nicotinic acid and, if necessary, by the other vitamin B factors. Beriberi is treated by giving a properly balanced diet and aneurine.

VITAMIN C (Ascorbic acid)

ACTION. Vitamin C is necessary for the proper growth of the capillary endothelium and for the repair of tissues. The main result of deficiency of this vitamin is haemorrhage from the capillaries.

SOURCES. Oranges, tomatoes, blackcurrant juice, lemons, potatoes and green vegetables.

DISEASES DUE TO LACK OF VITAMIN C

Scurvy is the only disease known to be due to lack of vitamin C, which is often therefore called the antiscorbutic vitamin. Scurvy was at one time a very common disease, especially amongst sailors and infants. Sailors on long voyages used to have to live on a diet lacking in fresh foods, especially fruits and vegetables. Infants fed on the bottle with heated milk also commonly developed scurvy as heating milk destroys all its vitamin C content.

As a result of the recognition of the cause of scurvy the disease is now very rare, especially in the infantile form. Unfortunately, it is still seen in old people living on their own and unable to obtain or afford fresh fruit or vegetables.

There are two main types of scurvy, infantile scurvy and adult scurvy.

1. Infantile scurvy

This, as just mentioned, is now rare owing to the widespread preventive use of orange juice or other source of vitamin C. Breast-fed babies do not develop scurvy because there is sufficient vitamin C present in human milk to prevent the disease. The necessary boiling or pasteurisation of cow's milk, however, destroys practically all the small amount of vitamin C present; as milk is the main if not the sole diet of infants, scurvy will develop in bottle-fed babies unless vitamin C is specially given.

Symptoms and signs

The underlying specific lesion which accounts for most of the symptoms is *haemorrhage*.

(a) Symptoms usually appear about the age of 8 to 10 months and never before 6 months. Scurvy never, as already explained, develops in breast-fed babies.

(b) The commonest complaint is of severe fretfulness in the infant, especially if the limbs, which may be swollen, are touched. The child if old enough to walk is often said to 'go off his feet'. The pain and swelling of the limbs is caused by haemorrhages under the periosteum of the bones.

(c) The gums are swollen, red and spongy. The teeth if present decay and fall out.

(d) Haemorrhages may also occur from the kidneys, bowel or nose. Anaemia is common.

2. Adult scurvy

In adult scurvy the main symptoms are haemorrhages from the nose or into the skin (purpura). Swelling and bleeding of the gums with general debility and anaemia are also commonly present. There is also pronounced delay in the healing of any wound or ulcers that may be present. The bone changes characteristic of the infantile form are not a marked feature of adult scurvy.

Treatment of scurvy

For adults, as for infants, preventive treatment is important in certain conditions. In chronic gastrointestinal diseases necessitating a strict and prolonged dietary regime, care should be taken to ensure that a sufficiency of vitamin C (and, of course, of all other vitamins, too) is given. Extra supplies of the vitamin in the form of ascorbic acid, 100 to 200 mg daily, are often advisable. The treatment of an established case of scurvy is to give large doses of ascorbic acid, 1 to 2 g daily.

VITAMIN D

ACTION. Vitamin D is responsible for the proper absorption of the calcium present in the diet. In its absence calcium is not absorbed from the bowel, and the resultant lack of calcium impedes both the normal growth of bone and the normal activity of nerves and muscles.

SOURCES. The same foods as supply vitamin A, i.e. animal fats, butter, cream, eggs, milk and fish-liver oils. In addition, however, to these food sources of the vitamin, sunlight (or ultraviolet light) has the peculiar property of being able to manufacture vitamin D by its action on the skin.

DISEASES DUE TO LACK OF VITAMIN D

1. Rickets

Before the widespread prophylactic use of cod-liver oil or similar preparations for infants made rickets so much less common in this country, the disease was usually seen in infants brought up in bad hygienic conditions. Here the lack of sunlight combined with a poor diet caused active rickets. It is interesting to note, however, that infants in the tropics, because of the continuous sunlight, even if brought up on a poor diet, rarely develop rickets.

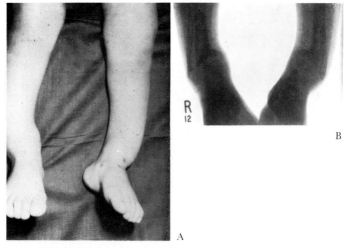

FIG. 12.1 The bowed legs and broad ankles in rickets. X-ray shows the splayed-out lower end of the tibia.

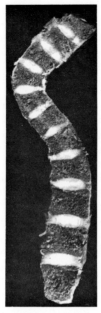

Fig. 12.2   Rickets leading to curvature of the spine.

Rickets is also seen in infants as a complication of chronic gastro-intestinal disease. In this type of disease vitamin D is not properly absorbed from the bowel and this accounts, for example, for the rickets of coeliac disease.

The main changes in rickets are those of disordered bone development caused by the lack of the vitamin, which is essential for normal growth of bone.

Symptoms and signs

(a) These are first noticed, as a rule, at about the age of 6 months; the infant sweats a good deal, especially around the head, whilst respiratory infections are also common.

(b) The wrists and ankles become enlarged at an early stage. The legs become bowed or, alternatively, knock-kneed when the child begins to walk owing to the weight of the body on the softened calcium-deficient bones. The arms, as they are not weight-bearing, are less likely to show such signs.

(c) The skull is softened and enlarged, and the typical appearance is one of a square head with a widely patent fontanelle. The spine may be bowed (kyphosis) or twisted (scoliosis).

(d) The ribs show a characteristic beading ('rickety rosary') owing to the enlarged epiphyseal margins.

(e) All the muscles and ligaments are very flabby and lax.

(f) There may be signs of tetany owing to the low blood calcium. Carpopedal spasms and spasm of the larynx with dyspnoea and cyanosis (laryngismus stridulus) are commonly seen in the tetany of infantile rickets.

Treatment

Vitamin D in the form of cod-liver oil or similar preparations (Adexolin, Radiostoleum) completely restores the bones to normal in early cases. In more advanced cases corrective active exercises may be necessary. If the bony deformities do not disappear under treatment, splints and operations may be employed to try to correct them.

2. Osteomalacia

Osteomalacia means softening of the bones and occurs in adults. Like rickets it may be due to a diet inadequate in vitamin D and calcium, but much more commonly it follows malabsorption of these factors from the small intestine (see p. 234). The long bones and the pelvis become deformed and may fracture.

3. Tetany

Tetany is due to a lowering of the blood calcium. One cause of this is lack of vitamin D, and in these cases tetany accompanies rickets. As, however, other factors—apart from vitamin D—are also involved in the control of the blood calcium (especially the parathyroid glands), tetany has a variety of causes and can therefore occur unassociated with rickets.

Tetany is fully described under Diseases of the Endocrine Glands (p. 453).

VITAMIN K

ACTION. Vitamin K is necessary for the formation of prothrombin, which is normally present in the blood and is one of the essential factors in blood clotting.

SOURCES. Spinach, cabbage, cauliflower and oats. In addition, the bacteria normally present in the bowel can manufacture vitamin K.

CONDITIONS ASSOCIATED WITH A LACK OF VITAMIN K

1. Haemorrhagic disease of the newborn

In the first few days of life, owing to deficient storage of vitamin K in the foetus, there is a low content of prothrombin in the blood. This can lead to haemorrhage if the deficiency is sufficiently severe (p. 353).

2. Obstructive jaundice

Bile salts are essential for the proper absorption of vitamin K, and so in obstructive jaundice there is deficient absorption of this vitamin. In consequence, in prolonged cases of obstructive jaundice a low prothrombin level with resulting haemorrhages may arise.

3. Gastrointestinal and liver diseases

In such chronic diseases of the gastrointestinal tract as sprue and chronic ulcerative colitis, or after extensive removal of the bowel, the resultant deficient absorption of vitamin K from the intestines may lead to prothrombin deficiency and haemorrhages.

Severe liver damage, such as may arise in cirrhosis of the liver or severe cases of hepatitis, can prevent the formation and storage of prothrombin in the liver.

4. Anticoagulant drugs

Certain drugs can destroy the prothrombin in the blood and so lead to a prolonged clotting time. Phenindione and other allied anti-coagulant drugs are very potent in this respect and in medicine are used for the sole purpose of producing a prolonged clotting time in the treatment of venous and coronary thrombosis.

Salicylates have an effect which is similar to but much less powerful than that of the anticoagulant drugs.

HORMONES

Hormones, the secretions of the endocrine glands, are described under diseases of these glands. Many of these hormones have a profound effect on the body metabolism.

1. THYROID HORMONE. Deficiency causes stunted growth and sluggish metabolism (cretinism and myxoedema).

2. PITUITARY HORMONES. Deficiency of the growth hormone causes lack of growth (dwarfism). Excess of the growth hormone causes gigantism and acromegaly.

3. ADRENAL CORTICAL HORMONES. Deficiency causes upset in salt and carbohydrate metabolism (Addison's disease).

4. PARATHORMONE and CALCITONIN. These regulate the flow of calcium to and from the bones.

The remaining hormone which plays a most important part in metabolism is the secretion of the islet cells of the pancreas, known as insulin. As this is so important it is discussed at length under Diabetes Mellitus.

WATER

Water makes up nearly 70 per cent of the total body-weight. It is taken into the body either as fluid or in the solid foods, which themselves contain a considerable amount of water. The amount of water needed in 24 hours is normally about 2500 ml.

Water leaves the body in the following ways:

1. Through the lungs in the expired air.
2. Through the faeces, which contain a small amount of water.
3. Through the skin, in the sweat.
4. Through the kidneys, in the urine.

The amount of water which leaves the body via the skin and kidneys varies; the greater the loss through the skin (as seen in very hot conditions) the smaller the excretion by the kidneys. This is part of the body's mechanism to save water. The excessive loss by the skin in high temperatures is a reaction to cool the body and so prevent a rise in body temperature. In very hot conditions, e.g. stoking in an engine room, as much as 7500 ml of water can be lost in the sweat in a day.

The body also makes use of the above methods of excretion of water (especially by the kidneys) to get rid of waste products. If, therefore, excretion through the kidneys is very severely diminished these waste products can accumulate in the blood stream with serious effects. This is discussed below under Dehydration.

Thirst. This is one of the ways in which the body shows that it requires more fluid. The essential mechanism operates by decreasing the flow of saliva thus causing dryness in the mouth. This sets up the sensation of thirst in the nerves on the back of the tongue. Certain drugs, such as atropine, by producing a diminished flow of saliva, cause thirst. Excess of salt in the food also causes a dryness in the mouth and consequent thirst.

DISTURBANCE OF WATER BALANCE

Deficiency of body fluid gives rise to dehydration while excess fluid causes oedema.

Deficiency in the body—dehydration

Dehydration can be caused by an insufficient intake of water or, more often, by excessive loss of water. Excessive loss of water is seen in the following conditions.

(a) Excessive heat resulting in marked sweating. Dehydration caused through excessive loss of water by sweating is usually seen in stokers or miners, who have to carry out heavy manual work in extremely hot conditions. The loss of water and also of salt (which is present in the sweat) causes stokers' or miners' cramps. Other more serious effects of dehydration are also seen.

(b) In diseases which cause excessive loss of fluid from the body such as:

    (i) Diseases causing severe vomiting and diarrhoea.
    (ii) Very high fevers, especially in hot climates.
    (iii) Diabetes mellitus (owing to the excessive polyuria).
    (iv) Severe haemorrhage and burns.
    (v) In prolonged coma, owing to the lack of fluid intake dehydration may also develop.

Effects of dehydration

In the early stages fluid is withdrawn from the skin and tissues in order to maintain the blood volume, whilst to conserve water the kidneys excrete less urine. If the dehydration is not corrected more serious effects follow. The blood volume is reduced and this leads to deficient circulation, especially through the kidneys, which therefore fail to excrete waste products from the body. Acute renal failure (uraemia) then develops, which if not quickly relieved will prove fatal.

Clinical recognition of dehydration
  (a) The patient is lethargic and dull. Thirst is often, but not always, present.
  (b) The tongue is very dry and leathery in appearance.
  (c) The skin loses its normal elasticity and if pinched remains in a fold.
  (d) The output of urine is markedly decreased and any urine passed is highly concentrated. The specific gravity of a 24 hour specimen is often 1030 or more.
  (e) The blood urea is raised.

The best clinical indications of an *adequate* fluid balance are the 24 hour output of urine, which should never fall below 1000 ml, and the condition of the tongue, which should always be moist.

In most cases of dehydration there is a loss of salt as well as of water, so that often in treating the dehydration salt plus water is given in the form of saline by intravenous infusion. In a case of severe dehydration 3000 to 4000 ml a day are often necessary; in less severe cases approximately 2500 ml.

Excess of water in the body—oedema

Fluid in the body flows from the blood into the tissues or vice versa. There are four main factors which control this flow.

(a) The pressure in the small capillaries and veins tends to force fluid out from the circulation into the tissues. Anything, therefore, that increases the venous pressure tends to force fluid into the tissues. Owing to the force of gravity, increases in the venous pressure are most marked in the lowest parts of the body; as a result the flow of fluid into the tissues is greatest in the most dependent parts. In addition, fluid also quickly collects in the large serous sacs of the body, such as the pleural and peritoneal cavities.

(b) Counteracting this venous pressure, which forces fluid out into the tissues, is the opposite action of the proteins in the blood (albumin and globulin). These proteins have the power, often called the *osmotic power* of proteins, of attracting fluid, with the result that they keep fluid in the blood and out of the tissues.

Normally, these two opposing factors, the venous pressure and the osmotic power of the blood proteins, keep a steady balance of fluid within the body. Any upset in either leads, however, to changes in the water balance.

(c) A third factor which can affect the amount of fluid in the tissues is damage to the walls of the capillaries, in consequence of which fluid may leak through the walls.

(d) Salt is another most important factor in oedema. Retention of salt in the body causes retention of water.

TYPES OF OEDEMA CAUSED BY THE ABOVE FACTORS

Cardiac oedema. In congestive heart failure there are two fundamental causes of oedema. First there is an increase in the venous pressure which tends, when the pressure is great enough to overcome the opposing power of the blood proteins, to force fluid into the tissues. The oedema, as explained above, forms in the most dependent parts of the body, as the venous pressure is greatest in these areas. If there is gross oedema, fluid also collects in the pleural and peritoneal cavities.

Secondly, the kidneys in congestive heart failure fail to excrete salt properly so that salt accumulates in the body. This causes retention of water which in turn causes oedema.

Renal oedema. In chronic nephritis, owing to the continued loss of protein in the urine (albuminuria) and the consequential diminished power of the proteins in the blood to keep fluid out of the tissues, renal oedema develops. In renal oedema the face is characteristically affected, especially around the eyelids. Oedema of the face is hardly ever seen in congestive heart failure, as the increased venous pressure causing the oedema is most marked in the lower parts of the body.

Oedema is also a feature of the acute stage of nephritis. Here, however, the oedema is not caused by the lowered level of blood proteins, but possibly by damage to the lining walls of the capillaries allowing fluid to leak out into the tissues.

Oedema of local venous obstruction. Obstruction to a large vein will cause increased venous pressure behind the vein, resulting in a localised oedema of the area being drained by the affected vein.

Pressure by a tumour in the lungs can cause venous obstruction, resulting particularly in oedema of the face and arms.

A large thrombus in a main vein of a limb commonly causes oedema of the affected limb.

Recognition of oedema

This is usually simple. The affected parts are swollen, and pressure on the swollen area causes 'pitting' of the area owing to the displacement of the fluid. This pitting on pressure distinguishes the solid swelling of a tumour, or just pure fat in the tissues, from the swelling due to fluid.

Difference between oedema fluid and inflammatory fluid

One of the most important changes which occurs in acute inflammation is an increased flow of fluid (exudation) in the inflamed area. When inflammation affects the great lining sacs of the body, such as the pleura and peritoneum, exudation may be very copious, causing a large accumulation of fluid in the chest or peritoneal cavities.

The fluid which collects as a result of inflammation is called an *exudate*, whilst the fluid in oedema is called a *transudate*.

NORMAL GASTROINTESTINAL TRACT

For the proper absorption of food and the correct functioning of the body's metabolism it is essential that the intestinal tract should function normally. In many long-standing and chronic diseases of the gastrointestinal tract there may be deficient absorption of essential foods, vitamins, etc.

1. In *chronic ulcerative colitis* with prolonged diarrhoea severe wasting may occur. Several vitamin deficiencies due to lack of absorption of vitamins and also an anaemia due to lack of iron absorption are often seen too.

2. In *major operations* on the gastrointestinal tract severe anaemia can occur owing to lack of absorption of iron. In addition, in the absence of the intrinsic factor in the stomach which is necessary for proper formation of the red blood cells a pernicious form of anaemia may occasionally arise.

3. In the malabsorption syndrome, which includes *coeliac disease* and *sprue*, there is inadequate absorption of various foods so that there is severe wasting and lack of growth. Calcium and vitamin D are also poorly absorbed in coeliac disease so that bone changes similar to those of rickets may develop. Tetany, as a result of the low blood calcium, may occur too.

NORMAL LIVER FUNCTION AND BILE CIRCULATION

The liver has many important functions in connection with metabolism. Breakdown of proteins, storage of sugar, formation and storage of the essential factor in the development of the red cells and also the formation and storage of prothrombin (necessary for blood clotting) are all functions of the liver.

Liver diseases may thus severely disturb the normal nutrition of the body and lead to wasting, severe anaemias and deficient blood clotting with haemorrhages. It should be noted, however, that the liver has such great reserves that it is only when diseases of the liver are very advanced that any serious interferences with body metabolism are met with.

Bile is essential for the proper absorption of vitamin K, which is required for the formation of prothrombin, which is needed for blood clotting. In obstructive jaundice, where no bile is present in the intestines, a lack of vitamin K develops in the body, which in turn causes a deficiency of prothrombin.

COMPOSITION OF A NORMAL DIET

The essential constituents of a normal diet and the other factors necessary for the utilisation of food and water have been outlined.

It remains to state how much of these different foods, etc. is needed to maintain health. Naturally, the requirements vary with different people according to the amount of energy they expend.

Fundamentally, all food and other essential factors are needed:

1. To repair the normal wear and tear of the tissues and to supply the energy to make the tissues and organs perform their work.
2. To supply sufficient energy to enable the individual to lead a normally active life.

In calculating the food requirements of the body, the amount of energy provided by food can be expressed in terms of *joules*. Weight for weight, fat produces more than twice as many joules as either carbohydrate or protein:

1 gram of fat produces 38 kilojoules (kJ)
1 gram of carbohydrate produces 16 kJ
1 gram of protein produces 16 kJ.

The calorie requirements of an individual will vary according to his age, size and occupation. Thus a sedentary worker may be satisfied with 9000 kJ (9 megajoules) a day while a heavy manual labourer may need over 12,000 kJ (12 MJ).

In converting these calorific requirements into food it is important that certain amounts of each of the individual foods be eaten to secure a balanced diet. A minimum of 70 g of protein foods a day is needed to replace wear and tear in the tissues. During times of stress this may have to be increased.

The amount of fat and carbohydrate in a normal diet varies according to the individual taste for much or little fat and also with the economic status. A high fat diet is more expensive than a high carbohydrate one. In an average diet the fats usually supply from 90 to 150 g and the carbohydrates 300 to 500 g.

A balanced diet must include, however, not only the protein necessary for repairing wear and tear of tissues and enough fats and carbohydrates for energy purposes, but also all the mineral salts mentioned earlier. These will be automatically supplied if all the ordinary foods are eaten, especially milk, eggs, butter, meat, fish cereals, fruit and vegetables. These foods will also supply sufficient vitamins.

At certain periods, especialy in childhood and during pregnancy and lactation, the diet may need supplementing. For children a higher proportion of proteins is needed to allow for growth. For this reason the diet should contain plenty of milk, at least 1½ pints (800 ml) a day being required. Milk also supplies the much needed calcium for growth of bones.

Ample quantities of green vegetables, fruit and cereals are important, both for their vitamin content and for their nutritional value. In infants extra supplies of vitamins A, D and C are essential.

During pregnancy a full diet is essential as the energy requirements increase with the growth of the foetus. Vitamins A, B, C and

D are especially important and should be added to the diet. Iron may also be required.

SOME IMPORTANT FOODS

1. Milk

Milk is of particular value because it contains most of the main items necessary for a normal diet, such as carbohydrates, proteins and fats, minerals and vitamins. The proteins in milk are of high biological value. In addition, milk is extremely easily digested, as is shown by the fact that it forms the staple article of diet for infants.

The vitamins contained in milk are A, B and D. Small amounts of vitamin C are present, but most of this vitamin is destroyed in pasteurisation. This is the only adverse effect of pasteurisation on milk.

The content of minerals in milk is very high, especially of calcium. The iron content is, however, low. The amount of milk recommended for daily consumption is 1 pint (550 ml) for adults and $1\frac{1}{2}$ to 2 pints (800 to 1100 ml) for children.

MILK FOODS

Butter is formed from sour milk in churning, and being almost pure fat has a very high calorific value. Butter contains vitamins A and D. Margarine is a cheaper and artificial substitute for butter, but with added vitamins is of similar value.

Cheese, formed from curded milk, contains a high percentage of protein and fat, and also of vitamins A and B_2. It is a very valuable food in an easily digestible form.

2. Eggs

Eggs have a very high nutritional value, particularly for their proteins and fat. They also contain a high proportion of minerals and vitamins A, B and D.

Eggs are a very valuable food as they are so easily digested, and are particularly useful in illness.

3. Meat

Meat is of especial value because of the important proteins it contains. Properly frozen meat has the same nutritional value as fresh meat. White meat (poultry and game) is more easily digested than red meat, but there is no appreciable difference between the protein content of red and white meats.

Liver, kidney and heart also contain valuable proteins, and, in addition, very high quantities of vitamins B and A.

4. Fish

Fish contains almost as much protein as meat, and also a plentiful supply of vitamins A and D. Herrings particularly supply valuable protein, a large amount of fat, abundant vitamins A and D and also iodine relatively cheaply.

5. Cereals

Mainly because of their cheapness, cereals are the commonest foods eaten throughout the world. They are also very valuable foods, supplying abundant carbohydrate and a fair amount of protein. The drawbacks of a diet consisting mainly of cereals are that the vitamin content is low; minerals, such as calcium, are insufficient, and the quality of the protein supplied is not of very high value, being inferior to that of meat, eggs and fish.

COMMONEST CEREALS CONSUMED

    (a) Wheat. The commonest grain in Great Britain.

    (b) Rice. The staple cereal of eastern countries.

    (c) Barley. Similar to wheat in value; grows in a drier climate.

    (d) Oats. Higher nutritive value than wheat; grows in harder climates.

Modern methods of milling wheat to produce white flour means that valuable fibre is lost with the outer layers of the wheat germ. This fibre is known as bran and should provide important roughage in the diet. Wholemeal bread contains the whole wheat germ and is preferable to white bread in this respect.

Wheat flour contains a particular protein called gluten. In some children gluten prevents proper intestinal absorption of food and leads to coeliac disease (see 'Malabsorption Syndrome'). Wheat flour must be completely excluded from the diet of these children.

6. Vegetables

    (a) *Green vegetables* (spinach, cabbage, brussels sprouts, lettuce, etc.). These are of value in providing roughage in the diet and so preventing constipation. They are also of value in providing bulk in the diet with little calorific value and are therefore used in diets for obesity.

    Green vegetables are, in addition, a useful source of vitamins A and C. However, the practice of cooking vegetables for prolonged periods and then discarding the water results in most of the valuable vitamins present being lost.

    (b) *Root vegetables* (potatoes, carrots, turnips, parsnips). Potatoes provide much energy at low cost and they also contain vitamin C. Carrots contain much less carbohydrate than potatoes, but contain a large amount of vitamin A. Parsnips have a lot of carbohydrate, while turnips and swedes are of little nutritive value except for vitamin C.

    (c) *.Peas, beans and lentils.* These vegetables have a large content of both protein and carbohydrate. They also contain iron and vitamin B complex.

7. Fruits

These supply much-needed roughage and in many cases vitamin C. Oranges and black currants in particular contain a large amount of vitamin C. Fruits are mainly composed of carbohydrates.

Tinned fruits and vegetables. With modern methods of canning, tinned fruits and vegetables retain their natural properties, and especially their content of vitamin C, for many months at least. Tinned fruits are preserved in syrup so that their carbohydrate value is very high. For this reason they must be avoided in cases of obesity and diabetes.

OBESITY

Overeating of food, particularly sugar and other carbohydrate foods, leads to an excessive increase in weight. Obesity is not only disfiguring and disabling; it also offers a hazard to health. It disposes to coronary thrombosis, hypertension, emphysema, gall stones, varicose veins, osteoarthritis, gout and diabetes. Fat people do not live as long as those who are of normal weight. Their activity and enjoyment of life are restricted by their excessive weight.

The cause of obesity is not always apparent. Many people overeat because they are unhappy or bored and they find that eating offers some temporary solace. Sometimes women put on weight excessively during pregnancy, perhaps because they think mistakenly that they must 'eat enough for two' and partly because they tend to stay at home during the last few months with food always available. Obesity tends to run in families. This may be due to a hereditary tendency or it may merely be due to the fact that some families make a habit of overeating.

It is often thought that obesity is 'due to the glands', but this is seldom true. Excessive cortisone, either administered as tablets or occurring naturally in Cushing's disease, leads to obesity of an unusual kind; the face and trunk are obese but the legs and arms are spared. Patients with myxoedema appear plump but this is not real obesity since there is not usually an excess of fat.

Treatment

DIET

The only successful way to reduce weight is to eat less, though patients are usually reluctant to accept this comfortless doctrine, hoping for magic tablets or injections.

In grossly obese patients, complete starvation of solid food will lead to a loss in weight of about a stone (6·5 kg) in 10 days. Fluids are allowed and the patients are best kept under observation in hospital, at least initially. Although hunger may be troublesome at first, strangely the appetite usually subsides after a few days.

A more normal weight-reducing diet is one in which carbohydrates are severely restricted. Sugar, chocolates, biscuits, cakes and jams are forbidden; bread and potato are strictly limited. Protein foods such as fish, meat, chicken, eggs and cheese can be eaten in reasonable amounts, with green vegetables or salads.

Reducing diets appear frequently in magazines and lay journals, varying in calorie content from 800 to 1200 calories a day and all attempting to make attractive the ugly fact that in order to lose weight it is necessary to exert great self discipline.

APPETITE SUPPRESSANTS

Various drugs are available which control hunger at meal time and so help the obese patients to eat less.

Amphetamine (Benzedrine) and dexamphetamine (Dexedrine) are stimulants which help to curb the appetite. Unfortunately, they are habit-forming and must only be prescribed for short periods, if at all. Fenfluramine (Ponderax) 20 mg given two or three times a day for a month will help to reduce weight. Other appetite suppressants include phenmetrazine (Preludin) and diethylpropion (Tenuate). These compounds are effective in reducing hunger in most patients and so make dieting less hard to sustain. But they are also liable to lead to drug-dependence and so are best prescribed for intermittent periods. They are most useful in the first few weeks of a restricted diet. Thyroid increases metabolism and if taken to excess causes tachycardia and loss of weight. It should never be prescribed for purposes of dieting.

EXERCISE

Regular exercise is helpful in preventing obesity but is not success-ful in itself in getting off fat unless carried to extremes unsuitable for patients no longer young.

Success in reducing weight can only be obtained if the patient is aware firstly of the dangers to health in being obese, and secondly that the only way to reduce weight is to eat less.

ANOREXIA NERVOSA

This is a condition in which there is complete aversion to food of any sort. It occurs most often in young women and is a manifestation of a serious psychological disturbance, sometimes of a psychosis.

Although the patient may say benignly that she eats quite a lot, in fact it can be observed that her food is left largely or completely uneaten. If food is eaten, vomiting often follows. The patient becomes more and more emaciated, the periods cease and in severe cases, death from inanition or infection may result.

Hence the situation must be treated seriously and the patient not allowed to starve herself to a dangerous level before medical advice is sought. An assessment of the underlying psychological disorder should be made by a psychiatrist and the patient is best admitted to hospital where encouragement and sympathy at meal times may help to restore the weight to a more normal level. It must be admitted that the ultimate outlook is not good in most cases, since although occasionally the anorexia is brought about by unhappy circumstances which can be rectified, in most cases the personality of the patient herself is unstable or psychopathic.

ACIDOSIS AND ALKALOSIS

The reaction of the blood normally remains constant and is always alkaline. It never becomes acid or death would be the result. Even a slight change in the reaction of the blood leads to profound and serious changes in the body.

Normally there is a complicated mechanism by which the reaction of the blood is kept constant, for although in the process of normal metabolism acids are formed, the body continues to get rid of them in several ways, e.g. carbon dioxide, which is an acid, is washed out in the lungs whilst the kidneys also excrete any excess acid.

Acidosis

Acidosis means the accumulation of excess acids so that the reaction of the blood becomes less alkaline. It rises chiefly in the following conditions.

(a) Diabetes mellitus. In this disease excessive combustion of fats occurs owing to the disturbance of carbohydrate metabolism. As the final result of fat metabolism is the formation of the acid ketone bodies, these may then accumulate in the body (p. 412).

(b) Renal failure. Here the kidneys fail to excrete the acids formed during normal metabolism.

(c) Prolonged diarrhoea, especially the severe acute forms in children. A large quantity of alkali may be lost in the faeces with resultant acidosis.

(d) Severe prolonged illnesses or major operations.

Treatment

It is, of course, essential that the disease causing the acidosis should be treated wherever possible. In addition, however, to any such specific treatment, abundant fluids with salt must be given. This is because in any case of acidosis the body, in an effort to get rid of the excess acids, also depletes itself in various ways of a great deal of fluid and salt.

Excess carbon dioxide causes an increased respiration rate and thus an increased loss of water in the respirations. The kidneys in excreting more acids excrete more urine (fluid) too. Severe illnesses with prolonged pyrexia and the associated sweating also lead to an excessive loss of fluid, whilst the marked dehydration associated with the ketosis of diabetes has already been noted. It is therefore necessary to give abundant fluids, often by the intravenous route. Glucose is also of great value in acidosis.

Alkalosis

The opposite to acidosis, alkalosis, is most usually seen as a result of:

(a) Prolonged vomiting. Here the alkalosis is due to the excessive loss of the hydrochloric acid in the gastric juice. Pyloric stenosis with its persistent vomiting is often accompanied by alkalosis.

(b) Hysterical overbreathing, where the alkalosis is caused by the loss of acid, carbon dioxide.

(c) Ingestion of alkalis, as used in the treatment of peptic ulcer. Nowadays, however, the alkalis in common use (magnesium trisilicate, aluminium hydroxide) are not absorbed into the blood and there is therefore no risk of alkalosis. Sodium bicarbonate in large quantities is the alkali most likely to cause alkalosis.

The main chemical result of alkalosis is tetany, which is discussed elsewhere. The treatment of alkalosis is to remove the cause and to give calcium for the tetany.

13   Diabetes Mellitus

Diabetes mellitus is a disease primarily affecting the metabolism of carbohydrate. It is an extremely common complaint and it can start at any age. The usual age of onset is between 40 and 60, but it has been reported in newborn babies and it can develop in very old people. When it develops in middle age, diabetes may be so mild as to pass unnoticed for many months before it makes it presence felt. In fact, although more than 300,000 people in Great Britain are known to have diabetes, about an equal number have the disease without being in the least aware of it. Many cases are discovered when the urine is tested routinely, for an insurance examination or before an operation, for example. Since undiagnosed diabetes may do harm, every patient admitted to hospital or attending a clinic should have the urine tested to exclude glycosuria.

Diabetes is partly a hereditary ailment so that more than one member of the family may be affected. If either parent has diabetes there is an increased chance that one or other of their offspring will develop diabetes but the risk is not a very great one.

Cause

As has been seen, under normal circumstances carbohydrate foods (such as bread, potato and rice) are broken down in the bowel and absorbed into the blood as glucose. Glucose is then carried to the liver where it is stored as glycogen by the action of insulin. Only enough glucose is left in the blood for the provision of normal metabolism. Hence insulin plays a very important part in regulating how much glucose is available in the blood for energy, and how much is stored away in the liver as glycogen.

Insulin is a hormone produced by special collections of cells in the pancreas known as the islets of Langerhans. The islets of Langerhans pour a lot of insulin into the blood stream after a large carbohydrate meal has been eaten, since large quantities of insulin are necessary to store excessive glucose in the liver.

In diabetes, something goes wrong. Either the pancreas gland does not produce enough insulin, or if insulin is produced, it is rendered ineffective in its action. In either event, there is not enough insulin available, and instead of excess glucose being stored in the liver, it simply accumulates in the blood. When the sugar in the blood rises above a certain level or threshold, the kidneys excrete the excess sugar in the urine. Hence, large quantities of urine are passed to get rid of the excess sugar. This excessive urination soon leads to thirst, while the continuous drain of glucose from the body depletes the tissues of their vital energy supplies. In severe cases, since carbohydrates are no longer available for adequate metabolism, fat is used instead. Improper fat metabolism leads to the formation of toxic ketone bodies and it is the excessive production of these toxic acids (ketosis) which may lead to diabetic coma.

In persons hereditarily disposed to diabetes, persistent overeating and obesity coming on in middle age may lead to the onset of the ailment, perhaps because fat makes the tissues insensitive to the action of insulin. Sometimes the onset of diabetes is precipitated by an infection, by an accident or by pregnancy.

Especially in children, diabetes develops without obvious cause and usually without anybody else in the family with the disorder. More children develop diabetes in the winter months than in the summer and it is thought in these cases that a virus infection might be responsible by damaging the islets of Langerhans. Diabetes sometimes follows mumps, for example. Other viruses, at present unidentified, could have the same effect.

Symptoms and signs

In mild cases coming in middle age (maturity onset diabetes) there may be no obvious symptoms and the ailment is first diagnosed as the result of a routine examination for sugar in the urine.

In more severe diabetes, especially coming on in children or young adults, the symptoms are more pronounced. There are four cardinal symptoms:

1. *Polyuria.* Excessive output of urine occurs during the night as well as in the day. In small children, bed wetting is common.
2. *Thirst.* Consequent on the polyuria and dehydration, there is a constant desire to drink fluid.

TABLE IX

	Young patients	Middle-aged or elderly patients
Onset	Rapid: with loss of weight, drowsiness, polyuria and thirst	Gradual: symptoms slight or absent
Weight	Loss of weight Thin	Usually obese
Urine	Sugar and acetone	Sugar
Coma	Liable to coma if neglected	Coma very unusual
Treatment	Full diet Insulin	Restricted diet. Sometimes tablets

3. There is a *loss of weight*, often despite the fact that the patient is eating well.

4. *Lassitude* and loss of energy occurs; if the diabetes is not diagnosed, this may lead to drowsiness or even coma (see later).

Other lesser symptoms are often present:

(i) Particularly in elderly women who are obese, irritation of the genitalia (*pruritus vulvae*) is caused by local deposition of sugar from the urine. This may be severe and disturbs the sleep.

(ii) Paraesthesia (tingling) may occur in the fingers and feet.

(iii) Aching and cramps are common in the legs.

(iv) Temporary blurring of vision: excess sugar causes changes in refraction in the eyes.

(v) Minor infections such as boils or unhealed cuts are liable to occur.

Diagnosis

The diagnosis is suspected by the clinical picture and confirmed by finding excess sugar (glucose) in the urine and blood.

1. URINE

(a) The output is increased.

(b) The urine is pale in colour but has a high specific gravity (1030 to 1040) due to the glucose contained.

(c) The tests for sugar are positive.

(d) Ketone bodies (acetone) may be present in more severe cases.

2. BLOOD

(a) Normally, the fasting blood sugar is about 4·5 mmol per litre (80 mg/100 ml) and this rises to about 6·5 mmol per litre (120 mg/100 ml) after a meal. In diabetes, the fasting blood sugar may be over 11 mmol per litre (200 mg/100 ml) and even higher after food.

(b) In doubtful cases, a *glucose tolerance test* may be performed. The suspected subject is advised to eat a normal diet on the days preceding the test but must have no food or drink on the morning of the test. He is then given a drink containing 50 g of glucose and blood is taken for the estimation of glucose at intervals of half an hour thereafter. The test takes two and a half hours. Normally the blood sugar does not rise above 10 mmol per litre (180 mg/100 ml) even at the peak level at one and a half hours, and returns to the fasting level of 4·5 mmol (80 mg) at the end of two and a half hours. These levels are exceeded when diabetes is present.

TYPES OF DIABETES

There appears to be two main types of diabetes.

Juvenile onset type

This form of diabetes occurs mainly in children and young adults, though it can come on at any age. The symptoms (thirst, polyuria, loss of weight and lassitude) usually become severe and the patient or his parents are soon obliged to seek medical advice. The urine contains sugar and acetone. Patients of this type need *insulin* and a *full diet*. They do not respond to tablets. They are prone to diabetic coma if they neglect themselves or if they develop an infection such as pyelonephritis or gastroenteritis.

Maturity onset diabetes

These patients are usually middle aged or elderly and symptoms may be absent or mild. In women, pruritus vulvae is common. Thirst and polyuria develop gradually. The urine contains sugar but not acetone. It is very unusual for this sort of patient to go into coma and insulin is not needed. The patient must adhere to a *low carbohydrate diet* in order to lose weight. In most cases, once a normal weight has been achieved, the blood sugar levels return to normal and no sugar can be found in the urine.

In patients of this type who are not overweight and who do not respond to dietary restriction, tablets are available which reduce the blood sugar to a normal range (see later).

TREATMENT OF DIABETES

Treatment will depend on the type of diabetes.

DIABETICS NEEDING INSULIN

In severe diabetes of this type, the initial treatment is best carried out in hospital since patients have to be instructed as to their diet, self-injection of insulin and how to test the urine for sugar. Patients are more likely to co-operate if they understand the nature of their complaint, and although there are many books on diabetes available for the public, nothing can take the place of a friendly and reassuring explanation as soon as possible after diagnosis. This is particularly important in children, when parents must be able to co-operate.

Dietary regime

In normal people the supply of insulin from the pancreas is regulated by the food eaten. If no food is taken, very little insulin is secreted. Following a large carbohydrate meal, the pancreas produces considerable amounts of insulin. In diabetics this mechanism is lost. A fixed amount of insulin is injected each day and hence the diet must not be allowed to vary in quantity. The principles of the diet in patients taking insulin must include:

1. A diet sufficient in quantity to enable the patient to undertake his activities, to satisfy his appetite and to maintain his weight at a proper level. A girl of slight physique leading a sedentary life may require a diet of 2000 calories (8000 kilojoules). A man doing a heavy labouring job may need 2800 calories (11,500 kJ) or more.

TYPE	URINE	TREATMENT
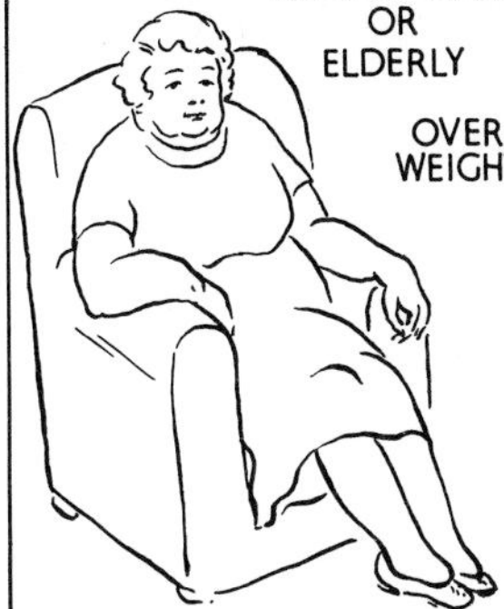 MIDDLE-AGED OR ELDERLY OVER-WEIGHT MILD SYMPTOMS	SUGAR BUT NO ACETONE	MUST LOSE WEIGHT REDUCING DIET 800-1200 calories daily
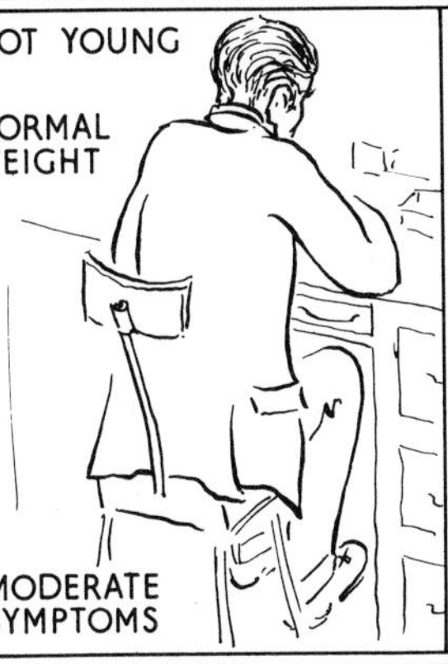 NOT YOUNG NORMAL WEIGHT MODERATE SYMPTOMS	SUGAR BUT NO ACETONE	TABLETS ADEQUATE DIET 1500-1800 calories daily
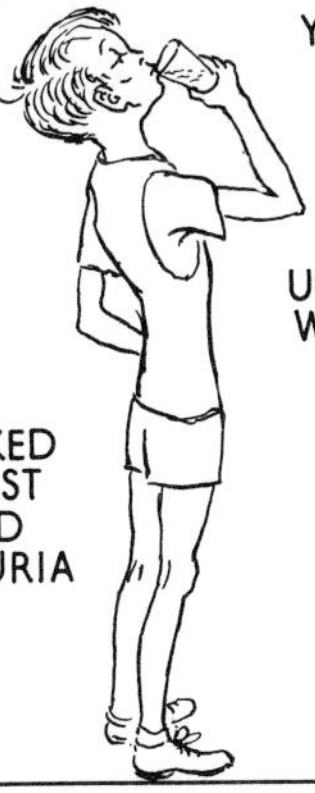 YOUNG UNDER-WEIGHT MARKED THIRST AND POLYURIA	SUGAR AND ACETONE	INSULIN FULL DIET ACCORDING TO SIZE AND ACTIVITY 1800-2800 calories daily

Fig. 13.1   Type of diabetes.

2. The diet must contain an adequate amount of protein (at least 75 g) and carbohydrate (at least 180 g). It must contain fruit and fresh vegetables.
3. Meals must be spaced during the day. Thus, in addition to the three main meals of breakfast, lunch and dinner, there should also be snacks in the middle of the morning, in the early afternoon and at bedtime.
4. Meals must be taken at regular times. Delayed meals may lead to hypoglycaemic attacks (see later).

TABLE X   Specimen outline diet

2200 Calories (8800 kJ)

Breakfast (51 g carb.)
  Egg or alternative
  Bread, 3 oz
  Butter, ½ oz
  Milk for tea or coffee, 2 oz

Midmorning snack (19 g carb.)
  Milk for tea or coffee, 2 oz
  Bread, 1 oz
  Butter, ¼ oz

Dinner (47·5 g carb.)
  Lean meat, 3 oz
  Green vegetables
  Boiled potatoes, 5 oz
  Milk pudding (milk 7 oz, rice ½ oz)

Tea (35 g carb.)
  Bread, 2 oz
  Butter, ½ oz
  Salad, etc.
  Milk for tea, 2 oz

Supper (51 g carb.)
  Cheese, 2 oz or alternative
  Salad or green vegetables
  Bread, 2½ oz
  Butter, ½ oz
  Fruit, one portion
  Milk for tea or coffee, 2 oz

Bedtime snack (20·5 g carb.)
  Milk, 7 oz
  Two cream crackers

A list of alternatives is provided for each item on the diet.

Arranging the diet

A diet is chosen suitable for the patient's size and activities, say about 2200 calories (8800 kJ). This will contain:

230 g carbohydrate	= 920 calories	(3800 kJ)
75 g protein	= 300 calories	(1200 kJ)
110 g fat	= 990 calories	(4100 kJ)

Total   2210 calories (8800 kJ)

Tables and charts are available which set out the composition and calorie values of common articles of food, and so a diet can be composed to suit the tastes of the individual. In practice, many diabetic clinics provide their patients with an outline diet, similar to that shown in Table X, and a list of alternatives. Thus, protein foods are exchangeable. Meat can be exchanged for equivalent amounts of cheese, fish or eggs, for example. Carbohydrate foods are particularly important. Bread can be exchanged for appropriate quantities of

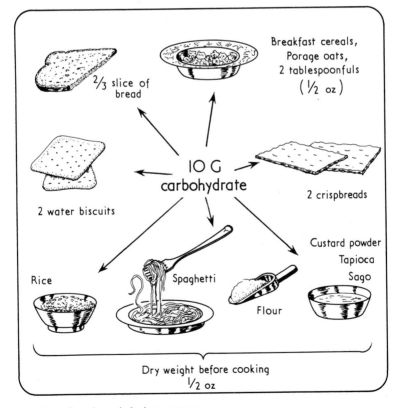

Fig. 13.2   Cereals: carbohydrate content.

potato, water biscuits, fruit or vegetables. Using a portion of 10 g of carbohydrate as a standard, the equivalent values of various common carbohydrate foods are set out in Figs 13.2 to 13.5. Thus it can be seen that once a diabetic patient has grasped the principles of the diet and has learned the food values of the common items of food, the diet can become both interesting and varied. In the early stages, food must be weighed until the patient is confident of his or her ability to

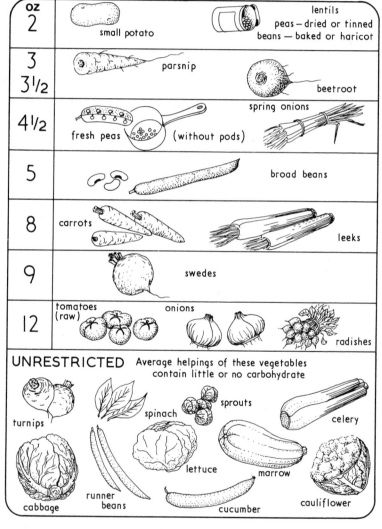

Fig. 13.3   Vegetables, in ounces, containing 10 g carbohydrate and others containing very little carbohydrate.

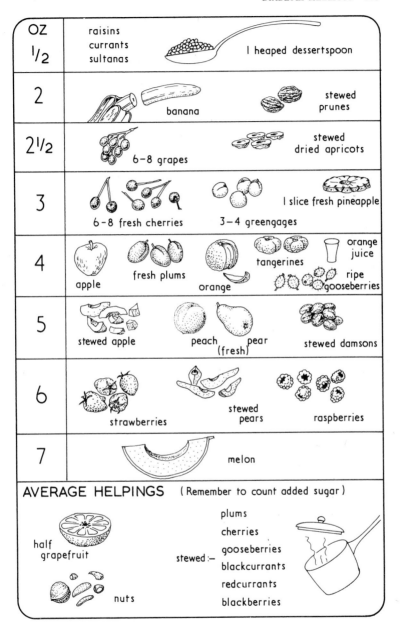

OZ		
½	raisins currants sultanas	1 heaped dessertspoon
2	banana	stewed prunes
2½	6–8 grapes	stewed dried apricots
3	6–8 fresh cherries 3–4 greengages	1 slice fresh pineapple
4	apple fresh plums orange tangerines	orange juice ripe gooseberries
5	stewed apple peach (fresh) pear	stewed damsons
6	strawberries stewed pears	raspberries
7	melon	

AVERAGE HELPINGS   (Remember to count added sugar)

half grapefruit

nuts

stewed:– plums
cherries
gooseberries
blackcurrants
redcurrants
blackberries

Fig. 13.4   Fruit portions containing 10 g carbohydrate.

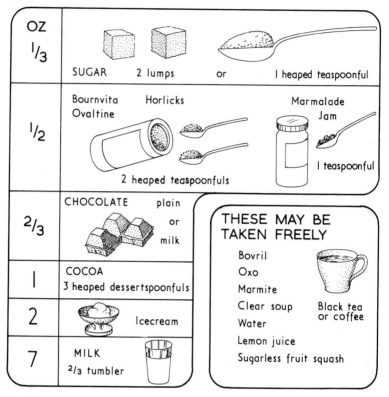

OZ		
1/3	SUGAR 2 lumps or I heaped teaspoonful	
1/2	Bournvita Horlicks Ovaltine 2 heaped teaspoonfuls	Marmalade Jam I teaspoonful
2/3	CHOCOLATE plain or milk	THESE MAY BE TAKEN FREELY Bovril Oxo Marmite Clear soup Black tea or coffee Water Lemon juice Sugarless fruit squash
I	COCOA 3 heaped dessertspoonfuls	
2	Icecream	
7	MILK 2/3 tumbler	

FIG. 13.5   Each item, in ounces, contains 10 g carbohydrate.

recognise the weight of the various food components without need to weigh. Nevertheless, many diabetics prefer to weigh all items of food just to make sure.

Insulin

Insulin is prepared from the pancreas glands removed from cattle and pigs after slaughter. The glands are immediately frozen to prevent the destruction of insulin by the digestive enzymes also present, and insulin is later extracted by special methods.

Insulin is destroyed by the gastric juices with the result that it cannot be given by mouth and has to be administered by subcutaneous injection. Clear insulin, known as soluble insulin, when injected subcutaneously leads to a fall in the blood sugar, but its effect only lasts a few hours. Hence, various forms of insulin have been prepared which prolong its action to last all day. There are now many different types of commercial insulin available, differing from each other in various ways:

SOURCE. Some insulins are obtained from the pig, some from the ox (beef) and some from a mixture of both.

LENGTH OF ACTION. Some insulins act very quickly in lowering the blood sugar but the duration of effect is only a few hours. Other forms of insulin take a longer time to be effective but the length of action is prolonged.

STRENGTHS. Two strengths of insulin are generally available in Europe, 40 units per ml and 80 units per ml. In North America only one strength is used, 100 units per ml.

PURITY. The purest insulins are known as monocomponent because they are freed from every minute impurity (probably harmless) present in previous commercial preparations.

Some commonly used preparations include:

1. Soluble insulin. This is clear insulin and its effects last about 6 hours. In order to control diabetes on its own it must be given at least twice a day. It can be given intravenously in the treatment of diabetic coma. Nuso, actrapid and neutral insulins are less acid than soluble insulin and are alternative preparations. These short acting insulins can be mixed with certain of the longer acting insulins in the same syringe. Thus, soluble insulin can be mixed with isophane insulin: the soluble acts quickly until the isophane begins to exert its effect.

2. The medium insulins, such as isophane or retard, if injected in the morning before breakfast, exert their maximum effect at lunchtime and early afternoon. The effect is less marked overnight and consequently a second injection is often necessary before the evening meal.

TABLE XI   Some insulins available

Preparation	Source	Type of action	Maximum effect	Duration of action
Soluble	Beef			
Nuso	Beef	Short	About 2–4 h	Up to 8 h
Actrapid	Pig			
Neutral	Pig			
Globin	Beef			
Isophane	Beef			
Semilente	Beef	Medium	4–12 h	Up to 24 h
Rapitard	Beef and pork			
Retard	Pork			
Semitard	Pork			
Protomine zinc insulin	Beef			
Ultratard	Beef	Long	6–12 h	30 h or longer
Lentard	Beef and pork			
Monotard	Pork			

3. The long-acting insulins such as lentard or monotard are useful as a single injection in the morning for diabetics easy to control and not needing a large dose.

INJECTING INSULIN

Insulin is prepared in solutions of 40 or 80 units per ml, and the standard insulin syringe (B.S.1619) has 20 marks per ml. Hence, if 40 strength insulin is used, each mark on the syringe is worth 2 units. If 80 strength insulin is used, each mark is worth 4 units. Unfortunately, many syringes with different marking systems are available and can lead to considerable confusion.

New diabetics needing insulin must be fully instructed on the following points:

1. The dose of insulin in terms of units and marks on the syringe.
2. The strength of insulin to be used, 40 or 80 units per ml.
3. The type of insulin or insulins to be used.
4. The technique of giving the subcutaneous injection and the sites suitable for injection. The site of injection should be varied from day to day.
5. The care and sterilisation of needle and syringe.

If through illness the patient is unable to eat his food, he must inject his insulin and take a glucose drink instead of food. He must consult his doctor, but it is dangerous to omit insulin since this will lead to ketosis.

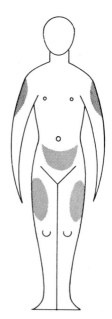

FIG. 13.6   Sites suitable for insulin injections.

Hypoglycaemia

When the blood sugar level falls too low, symptoms of hypoglycaemia occur. Some diabetics, sometimes called 'brittle' or 'unstable', are particularly liable to these attacks despite all precautions. Hypoglycaemia is most likely to occur:

1. When meals are delayed or irregular.
2. When unusual exertion or exercise is undertaken.
3. When the insulin dose is excessive due to unwise attempts to ensure that all specimens of urine are free from sugar.

The earliest symptoms of hypoglycaemia are sweating, mental confusion, a feeling of hunger or weakness, palpitations and trembling. An astute nurse should be on the lookout for these symptoms in a diabetic patient taking insulin, especially before mealtimes. The patient may have a vacant look, he will be pale and sweating, with a rapid pulse. It is most important to institute treatment immediately since otherwise the patient will go into hypoglycaemic or insulin coma. The patient should be persuaded to take a glucose drink without delay, and only if he becomes too stuporous to swallow is it necessary to administer glucose by a stomach tube or by intravenous injection. Every diabetic patient taking insulin should be aware of the early symptoms of hypoglycaemia and must always carry lumps of sugar or glucose sweets to prevent this happening. Diabetics should carry a card or bracelet stating that they are diabetic and if found confused or unconscious must be sent to hospital as an emergency.

When patients are admitted to hospital in hypoglycaemia or 'insulin coma', it is often not known whether the patient is a diabetic. Search should be made for evidence of insulin injections in the thighs or lower abdomen. The patient is usually sweating, with dilated pupils and normal blood pressure. The breathing is quiet and there is no evidence of dehydration or collapse. The urine, if it can be obtained, is free from sugar. This condition should not be confused with diabetic coma (Table XII). Glucose must be injected intravenously and the patient soon comes round. Nevertheless, in some cases who have been allowed to remain in coma for many hours, permanent cerebral damage may result and recovery will not take place despite elevation of the blood sugar level to normal. This danger explains the importance of prompt treatment in the early stages.

Glucagon is a hormone secreted by special cells in the islets of Langerhans and has exactly the opposite effect of insulin. It causes the liver to produce more sugar and so the blood sugar rises. Glucagon is available in a powder form and when dissolved in sterile water, it can be injected subcutaneously. When the blood sugar is low and the patient cannot be given intravenous glucose for any reason, an injection of glucagon (2 mg) subcutaneously will elevate the blood sugar in about 15 minutes. In a comatose patient, there is a return of consciousness and glucose can then be given by mouth.

TESTING THE URINE

Diabetics needing insulin should test the urine three times a day. Unstable diabetics may have to test the urine every day, but mild diabetics may find one or two days a week is adequate. Specimens should be collected before breakfast, before lunch and last thing at night. It is best not to test urine that has been in the bladder for many hours. In the morning, for example, the patient should discard the urine passed immediately on rising and should keep for testing a specimen passed just before breakfast. The urine should be tested with Clinitest or Clinistix and the results recorded on a chart kept for the purpose.

DIABETICS NEEDING TABLETS

Many adult patients who develop diabetes can be controlled without recourse to insulin. These diabetics are not overweight, but they are not thin or wasted. The urine contains sugar but no acetone.

Dietary regime

The diet should just be adequate to maintain weight at the normal standard for the patient's age and height. In practice, most patients in this category require a diet varying from 1500 (6000 kJ) calories to 2000 calories (8000 kJ), which is less than is usual for diabetics taking insulin.

Tablets

Two types of sulphonylurea tablets are in common use to bring down the blood sugar. These compounds stimulate the pancreas to produce more insulin, and this explains why they are ineffective in the more severe type of diabetes where the pancreas is incapable of producing insulin at all.

1. *Tolbutamide* is the weaker tablet, and since it is effective only for a few hours it must be given two or three times a day. The usual dose is 0·5 g (one tablet) three times a day.
2. *Chlorpropamide* is stronger and has a long action, so that it need be administered only once a day. The usual dose is 250 mg (one tablet) each morning.

Both these tablets reduce the blood sugar in mild cases, so that the urine soon becomes free from sugar. They are well tolerated, and only very rarely give rise to toxic effects such as skin rashes, agranulocytosis or jaundice.

Another group of hypoglycaemic agents are the biguanides, of which *phenformin* and *metformin* are available. These often give rise to nausea and vomiting, but they are sometimes used in small doses in combination with the sulphonylureas when these are not quite strong enough on their own.

OVERWEIGHT DIABETICS

These patients usually need neither tablets nor insulin, provided they are willing to reduce their weight by restricting the food intake. Overeating places a strain on the pancreas, and if the supply of insulin is limited diabetes will result. Hence the diet must be so restricted that the patient loses weight. Depending on the degree of obesity, the diet will vary from as little as 800 calories (3500 kJ) a day to 1200 calories (5000 kJ) a day. Once the weight is reduced, the blood sugar falls to normal, the urine becomes free from sugar and the symptoms disappear. The patient must always keep to a diet, though not necessarily as severe as the original one.

Complications of diabetes

The immediate aim of the treatment in diabetes is to keep the diabetic at work, feeling well and free from troublesome symptoms. The ultimate aim is to reduce the risk of various complications which tend to occur after diabetes has been present for many years. It is believed that the incidence of complications can be reduced by keeping the blood sugar level as near normal as possible, and this means careful adherence to the diet and careful adjustment of the dosage of insulin. The diabetic patient should attend his doctor or hospital clinic at regular intervals to ensure that the urine and blood do not contain more sugar than can be avoided. Unhappily, complications, especially in the eyes, kidneys and nerves, can occur even in diabetics who have done their best to keep to their regime. These complications are as follows.

1. *Retinopathy*. Degeneration of the retina at the back of the eye occurs in a high percentage of patients who have had diabetes for 20 years or more. Haemorrhages may occur and may be of sufficient severity to lead to blindness.

2. *Nephropathy (Kimmelstiel-Wilson syndrome)*. The kidneys are damaged by long-standing diabetes and this kidney disease may ultimately lead to albuminuria, oedema of the legs, high blood pressure and uraemia. This is frequently a cause of death in diabetes.

3. *Neuropathy*. Involvement of the peripheral nerves leads to loss of the reflexes, pain in the legs, wasting of the muscles and weakness of gait.

4. *Arteriosclerosis*. Particularly in elderly patients, hardening of the arteries of the legs leads to an impoverishment of the blood supply to the feet. Any minor damage to the toes takes a long time to heal and is prone to infection. This dangerous sequence may lead to gangrene, with consequent amputation of the whole leg. Hence elderly diabetic patients must be urged to look after their feet. They must make sure that there are no holes in their stockings and no nails in their shoes. They must keep the feet warm but avoid roasting them before too hot a fire. They must avoid cutting the toe nails too

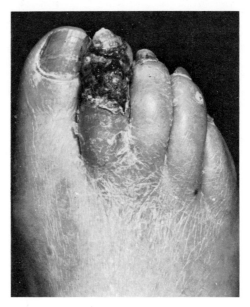

FIG. 13.7 Gangrene of the toe in diabetes.

short or digging into the corner of the toes. It is often best for a regular foot toilet to be undertaken by a trained chiropodist.

5. *Infections.* Diabetic coma is often ushered in by an infection such as tonsillitis, pneumonia, pyelitis, appendicitis or phlebitis. Treatment of the infection must be vigorous and immediate.

6. *Pregnancy.* Diabetic mothers tend to have large babies, often weighing more than 10 lb (4·5 kg) at birth. These babies are sometimes stillborn, and are very oedematous. Since the damage is done in the last month of pregnancy, many obstetricians perform a Caesarian section at the 36th to 38th week to avoid this risk. The diabetes must be carefully controlled throughout the pregnancy, and the mother must take plenty of rest.

Diabetic coma (diabetic-ketoacidosis)

Before the days of insulin, young people who developed diabetes nearly always died in diabetic coma. Nowadays, with earlier diagnosis and effective treatment, diabetic coma is uncommon. Sometimes old people or mentally slow people delay reporting to the doctor when symptoms develop; they become more drowsy and are found in coma. In patients already known to have diabetes, coma is nearly always due to an accompanying infection, such as pneumonia, pyelitis or gastroenteritis. The patient may feel too ill to eat, and may mistakenly omit the usual injection of insulin. The blood sugar rapidly rises, ketosis occurs and coma is often ushered in by vomiting.

TABLE XII

Symptoms and signs	Diabetic coma	Insulin coma (hypoglycaemia)
1. Onset	Gradual. History of severe thirst and polyuria: abdominal pain and vomiting	Sudden. Patient previously well and active, taking insulin
2. Infection	Usually present (e.g. tonsillitis, enteritis, pyelitis)	Not usually present
3. Respirations	Deep, sighing. Breath smells of acetone	Quiet regular breathing
4. Skin	Dry, inelastic. Tongue dry and shrunken	Sweating, moist
5. Blood pressure	Very low; rapid thin pulse	Normal. Full pulse
6. Urine	Sugar and acetone	No sugar or only a trace

Symptoms and signs of diabetic coma

1. At first drowsiness with great thirst and polyuria, followed by unrousable coma.

2. Deep sighing respiration with the breath smelling of acetone.

3. Cold extremities, sunken eyeballs, shrivelled tongue, dry skin and a low blood pressure: these signs are due to dehydration (loss of fluid).

4. Urine contains heavy amounts of sugar and ketones.

Treatment of diabetic coma

The successful treatment of diabetic coma demands constant supervision and close co-operation between nurses, doctors and laboratory staff. The basic requirements are administration of insulin and the adequate replacement of fluid and electrolytes, with frequent monitoring of the clinical state, and the biochemistry of the blood and urine.

A special chart must be kept of the fluid and insulin administered, of the urine passed and the results of the blood tests.

1. These patients are seriously dehydrated, having passed large quantities of urine in the hours or days preceding the onset of coma. Vomiting may have caused further loss of fluid. Fluid must be administered intravenously by drip, and in most cases isotonic saline is given initially. The first litre can be given rapidly, perhaps within half an hour; thereafter, the drip can be run at a slower rate as judged by the patient's progress. When keto-acidosis is very severe, alkaline solutions (sodium bicarbonate) may be administered.

2. The best way to give insulin is by continuous intravenous infusion and insulin can conveniently be added into the saline bottle. Thus 20 to 40 units soluble insulin can be added to each bottle, the amount regulated by the results of repeated blood and urine sugar estimations. A more accurate method of delivering insulin is by means

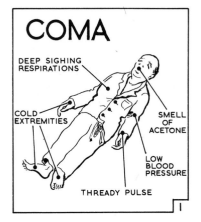

COMA

DEEP SIGHING
RESPIRATIONS

COLD
EXTREMITIES

SMELL
OF
ACETONE

LOW
BLOOD
PRESSURE

THREADY PULSE

1

**URGENCY
ESSENTIAL**

**LABORATORY
ALERTED**

2

**IMMEDIATE
TREATMENT:—**

1 INSULIN

2 INTRAVENOUS
FLUIDS

3 ANTIBIOTICS
FOR INFECTION

3

**AT 2-HOURLY
INTERVALS:—**

TEST URINE FOR
SUGAR AND
KETONES

BLOOD TO LABORATORY

INSULIN AS ORDERED
ACCORDING TO RESULTS OF TESTS

CHECK INTRAVENOUS FLUIDS
AND URINE OUTPUT

4

PATIENT OUT OF COMA

LIGHT DIET
25-30 gm of
carbohydrate
given 4-hourly

INSULIN as ordered

POTASSIUM

LATER
Routine diabetic treatment

5

Fig. 13.8   The treatment of diabetic coma.

of a constant rate infusion pump attached by a fourway tap to the intravenous tube. This can deliver insulin in saline at a steady rate of 6 units every hour and is independent of the rate of the drip.

An alternative method is to give insulin every hour by intramuscular injection, usually 20 units as a start and then 10 units every hour.

3. Whatever the method of administering insulin, regular estimations of the urine tests and blood sugar and electrolytes are essential to guide progress. The aim is to get the blood sugar to a near normal level within 4 to 6 hours.

4. As the blood sugar falls, there is a tendency for the blood potassium to fall too low so that it may be necessary to add potassium (KCl) to the infusion.

5. The onset of coma may have been precipitated by infection. For example, there may be evidence of pneumonia or of a renal tract infection. Appropriate chemotherapy may be necessary, often given intravenously by adding to the drip.

6. Urine should be tested every 2 hours and for the purpose a retention catheter may be needed. The urine is tested for sugar and acetone.

7. Where there has been frequent vomiting, it is best to empty the stomach by using a stomach tube.

PROGRESS

1. As the patient gains consciousness and the blood sugar and electrolytes return to normal, the drip can be maintained at a slow rate. It should not be discontinued until it is clear that the patient is able to take adequate fluids by mouth without nausea.

2. A régime of subcutaneous soluble insulin can be started, usually three times a day for the first few days.

3. A light diet should be given with frequent small feeds. The energy content is not important at this stage.

14 Disorders of the Endocrine System

The endocrine system consists of a series of endocrine glands and special cells which manufacture *hormones* and pass them directly into the blood stream. Hormones are chemical messengers. When released into the blood, hormones are capable of exerting important regulatory effects on the metabolism and function of the cells of the body.

The endocrine system, like the nervous system, helps determine the way in which the body reacts to the environment. The outer world is perceived by our five senses: sight, hearing, taste, smell and touch. These senses relay impulses to the *cerebral neurones*, the cells of the nervous tissue of the brain. The cerebral neurones secrete substances called *neurotransmitters* and these control the hypothalamus.

The **hypothalamus** is composed of groups of special cells lying at the base of the brain. It lies above the pituitary gland and is connected to it by a stalk containing blood vessels and nerve fibres. Under the influence of the neurotransmitters from the cerebral neurones, the cells of the hypothalamus produce a number of hormones which it transmits to the pituitary gland. Some of these hormones stimulate the cells of the pituitary gland (*release hormones*), others prevent them from acting (*inhibitory hormones*). Many of these hormones have been isolated and some are in use. For example, TRH (thyrotrophin release hormone) is used as a test of thyroid function.

The **pituitary gland** produces growth hormone and controls the action of other endocrine glands. The thyroid, adrenal cortex and the gonads are all controlled by the pituitary gland. However, not all endocrine glands are under the influence of the pituitary gland. The parathyroid glands and the adrenal medulla are independent of the action of the pituitary gland. There are many collections of endocrine cells lying in the pancreas (the islets of Langerhans), in the wall of the bowel and in the kidney which produce hormones in response to metabolic changes in the body state, uninfluenced by the pituitary.

Any part of the endocrine system, the hypothalamus, the pituitary

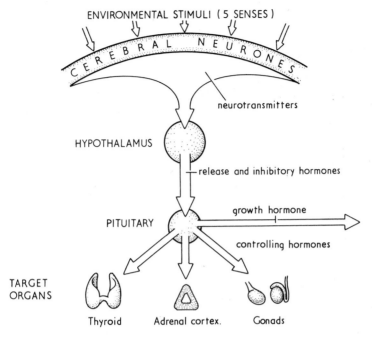

FIG. 14.1 Outside stimuli release neurotransmitters in the brain: these then act on the endocrine system.

or any of the endocrine organs or cells can be affected by a tumour or some other disease. This leads to a change in the hormone pattern of the body, often with profound constitutional disturbances.

PITUITARY GLAND

The pituitary gland lies in a bony cage at the base of the skull (pituitary fossa). It is controlled by the hypothalamus to which it is connected by the pituitary stalk. It is divided into two main divisions, or lobes, the anterior and the posterior.

The hormones of the anterior lobe

1. THE GROWTH HORMONE. An excess of this hormone gives rise to gigantism in young people and acromegaly in older people. Lack of the growth factor causes dwarfism.

2. SEX HORMONE STIMULATORS. These are necessary for the normal functioning of the testicles in the male and the ovaries in the female.

3. ACTH (CORTICOTROPHIN). This stimulates the adrenal cortex to produce cortisone.

4. THYROTROPHIC HORMONE. If this is deficient the thyroid gland lapses into inactivity and fails to produce thyroxine.

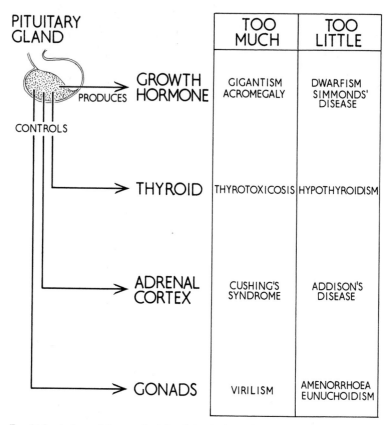

FIG. 14.2 Actions of the anterior lobe of the pituitary gland.

DISEASES OF THE PITUITARY

GIGANTISM

Sometimes in childhood or adolescence, a tumour of the pituitary gland develops with excessive production of growth hormone. Since the epiphyses of the bones have not yet united, tremendous increase in size results with the formation of giants. Several instances of giants reaching 8 or 9 ft are known. In many cases, however, these giants lose their excessive strength and develop signs of increased intracranial pressure (headaches, vomiting, blindness and coma) from growth of the tumour.

ACROMEGALY

Oversecretion of the growth hormone arising after the epiphyses of the bones have united leads to the condition known as acromegaly. There is no increase in height, but nevertheless characteristic changes

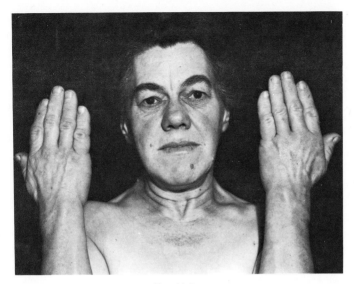

Fig. 14.3.

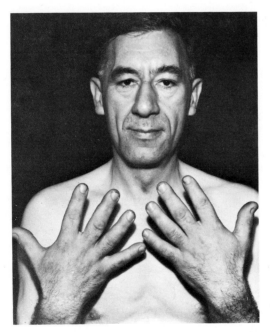

Fig. 14.4.

Figs. 14.3 and 14.4 Two patients with acromegaly. Note the heavy features, the large lower jaw and the broad fingers and hands.

occur in the bones, i.e. the lower jaw becomes massive and the whole contour of the face broadened, whilst the hands and feet become excessively wide, usually being described as spade-like. In addition to the above changes, the skin becomes thick and coarse and the tongue hypertrophied.

If a tumour of the pituitary gland is responsible for the acromegaly, signs of increased intracranial pressure may gradually develop as a result of growth of the tumour. Pressure on the optic tract may lead to restriction of vision.

Diagnosis

X-ray of the skull may show thickening of the bones and enlargement of the pituitary fossa due to a tumour of the pituitary. Growth hormone can be measured in the blood and is found to be higher than normal.

Treatment

Particularly where there is pressure on the optic tract, surgical removal of the pituitary growth should be undertaken. In other cases, radioactive seeds can be implanted into the pituitary fossa through the nose to destroy a pituitary tumour.

Bromocriptine is a drug which acts on the cerebral neurotransmitters and partially suppresses the output of growth hormone by the pituitary. It is sometimes helpful in the treatment of acromegaly.

SIMMONDS' DISEASE (HYPOPITUITARISM)

Simmonds' disease is due to destruction of the pituitary gland, either by a tumour or by necrosis of the gland after a difficult childbirth. As a result the thyroid, the adrenal cortex and the sex glands all fail to function properly. In children absence of the growth hormone results in a failure to grow.

Symptoms and signs

1. Loss of sexual functions with amenorrhoea and atrophy of the genital organs.

2. Marked loss of energy with dull, sluggish mentality. In advanced cases mental changes supervene.

3. Smooth fine skin and loss of axillary and pubic hair. The appearance is one of premature senility, particularly in young people.

4. Very low blood pressure and basal metabolism.

DIAGNOSIS. Where pituitary necrosis has occurred after a difficult childbirth, the diagnosis is suggested by the shrinkage of the breasts and failure to produce milk in the postpartum period. The menses fail to return and the attitude of the mother to her baby shows a lack of interest and initiative. Where the disease is fully developed, the diagnosis is often made from the appearance of the patient. The smooth pale skin and the hairless trunk are very suggestive.

The diagnosis can be confirmed by tests for thyroid and adrenal

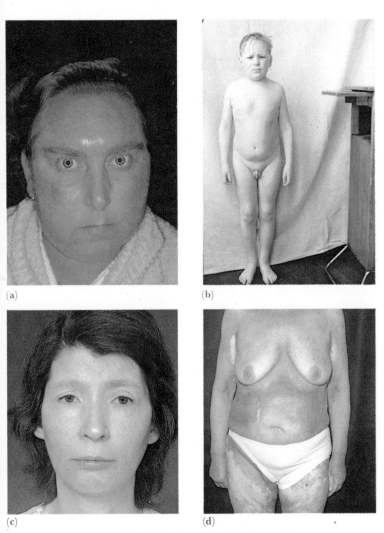

(a)

(b)

(c)

(d)

FIG. 14.5   Some endocrine abnormalities.
(a) Cushing's syndrome (obesity, plethora, hypertension).
(b) Pituitary dwarf. (Age 14½ years, height 50 in., no secondary sex changes.)
(c) Simmonds' disease. (Pale smooth skin, hairless trunk, amenorrhoea.)
(d) Addison's disease. (Brown pigmentation on trunk and limbs.)

function, since both are deficient without pituitary stimulation. There is a poor uptake of iodine by the thyroid gland, and a deficient excretion of cortisone by the adrenal gland (see later).

Treatment

Patients with Simmonds' disease are treated with cortisone tablets (about 37·5 mg daily) which usually leads to marked improvement. In addition to cortisone, other hormone therapy is often needed, such as thyroid, oestrogens and testosterone.

DWARFISM

Destruction of the pituitary gland deprives the growing child of growth hormone and normal sex development. As a result the child never grows up and always retains the hairless body and high-pitched voice of childhood (the 'perpetual Peter Pan').

It should be realised, however, that pituitary diseases account for only a minority of the causes of dwarfism and it is convenient here to classify briefly the main causes of dwarfism.

1. Chronic infection in early childhood
   - (a) Congenital syphilis
   - (b) Chronic nephritis.
2. Metabolic and deficiency diseases
   - (a) Rickets (deficiency of vitamin D)
   - (b) Coeliac disease (malabsorption syndrome).
3. Bone diseases
   - (a) Achondroplasia ('clowning circus dwarf')
   - (b) Fragilitas ossium (p. 477).
4. Endocrine gland diseases
   - (a) Pituitary diseases
   - (b) Cretinism (lack of thyroid hormone in infants).
5. Congenital heart disease.
6. Genetic and familial.
   Stunted stature may be familial or may be transmitted by faulty genes (p. 14).

CUSHING'S SYNDROME

This is due to excessive production of cortisone and is described under the adrenal glands (p. 446). It is sometimes caused by a pituitary tumour. This overstimulates the adrenal cortex by excessive ACTH production.

DIABETES INSIPIDUS

This is the only disease commonly recognised as being due to changes in the posterior lobe of the pituitary. One of the main secretions of the posterior lobe is the antidiuretic hormone which acts on the kidneys and prevents loss of too much fluid. In diabetes insipidus there is a lack of this hormone with the result that these patients pass tremendous quantities of urine which is characteristically very pale and of a low specific gravity. These patients commonly complain of thirst. It should be noted that in diabetes insipidus, as opposed to the other form of diabetes, diabetes mellitus, the urine does not contain any sugar.

Treatment

The deficient hormone is given either by injection (vasopressin) or in the form of a nasal spray.

Two drugs, normally given for other purposes, reduce the output of urine in diabetes insipidus by enhancing the action of the anti-diuretic hormone. These are bendrofluazide and chlorpropamide.

THYROID GLAND

ANATOMY AND PHYSIOLOGY. The thyroid gland is situated in the neck and comprises two lobes, one on each side of the trachea, joined by a middle portion called the isthmus. It is made up of cells which produce one important hormone called thyroxine. The main function of this hormone is to control metabolism in the body. Excess of the hormone leads to a general overactivity of bodily function and produces the condition of thyrotoxicosis (hyperthyroidism).

In most cases of thyrotoxicosis the thyroid gland becomes enlarged, and the term *goitre* is used to describe such enlargement. In addition, however, to toxic goitre, i.e. goitre associated with thyrotoxicosis, enlargement of the thyroid without oversecretion of the thyroid hormone also occurs—non-toxic goitre.

Undersecretion of the thyroid hormone causes a lowering of bodily function, which in adults causes the disease myxoedema and in children cretinism.

One of the main substances required for the manufacture of the thyroid hormone is iodine.

DISEASES OF THE THYROID GLAND

GOITRE

There are various forms of goitre or enlargement of the thyroid:

1. Simple (non-toxic) goitre. This form of goitre is not associated with oversecretion of the thyroid hormone and therefore there are no signs of thyrotoxicosis.
2. Toxic goitre. This type of goitre is accompanied by signs of overactivity of the thyroid hormone. It takes two forms:
   (a) Primary diffuse toxic goitre (exophthalmic goitre or Graves' disease).
   (b) Nodular toxic adenoma.
3. Malignant goitre.

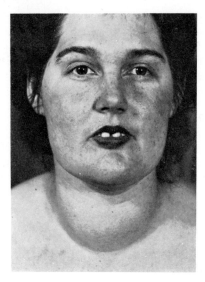

Fig. 14.6   Simple (non-toxic) goitre.

Simple (non-toxic) goitre

This is a common condition, especially in some areas where it is almost endemic. It is believed that in these areas this type of goitre is due to lack of iodine in the water. It is very prevalent in Switzerland, parts of America and in certain regions of England, such as Derbyshire. It is also commonest at certain periods of life, e.g. at puberty and during pregnancy. In most cases little treatment is needed as the goitre usually subsides of its own accord. Preventive treatment has been used in many endemic areas and has definitely succeeded in lowering the incidence of this type of goitre. The treatment consists of adding a small quantity of iodine to ordinary table salt.

In some cases, however, a non-toxic goitre may persist and eventually cause trouble. It may grow so large that it is unsightly: or it may cause pressure symptoms, such as difficulty in breathing and stridor: or it may become toxic in later life and so cause damage, particularly to the heart; whilst finally, there is the possibility of these long-standing non-toxic goitres becoming malignant.

Whenever non-toxic goitre persists into later life the question of its removal by operation must be considered. Any signs of the development of toxic symptoms or, of course, of pressure symptoms will call for operation.

Toxic goitre (thyrotoxicosis)

When swelling of the thyroid gland (goitre) appears in conjunction with oversecretion of the thyroid hormone it is known as

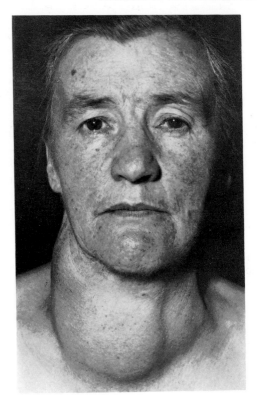

Fig. 14.7   Non-toxic goitre. The goitre was removed because it was causing pressure symptoms.

toxic goitre. There are two main types of toxic goitre, but the symptoms of toxicity are practically the same in both. The diffuse type (which is also known as *Graves' disease*) occurs in younger people and is associated with generalised diffuse enlargement of the gland though sometimes the enlargement is only slight. In the nodular type (which usually occurs in older people) the gland is not diffusely enlarged: instead, one or more adenomata develop causing a nodular goitre. Toxic nodular goitre in particular (probably because it affects older people) is liable to cause atrial fibrillation.

Symptoms and signs of toxic goitre (thyrotoxicosis)
    Thyrotoxicosis is due to oversecretion of the thyroid hormone, the general effect of which is to increase metabolism throughout the body. The symptoms and signs of thyrotoxicosis are as follows.
    (a) Patients usually complain of general nervousness, irritability, being on edge and a feeling of anxiety.
    (b) There is usually continuous loss of weight although the patient

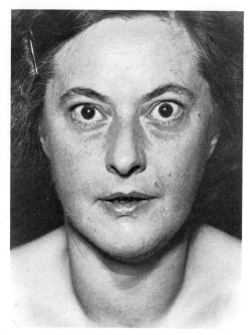

FIG. 14.8   Primary toxic goitre (Graves' disease) showing the characteristic staring, apprehensive expression and the enlarged thyroid.

has a good appetite. This is an important point, as most diseases which cause loss of weight are associated with a poor appetite. (The only other common cause of severe loss of weight with a good appetite is diabetes mellitus.)

(c)   Sweating is usually a marked feature and the patient normally dislikes hot weather.

(d)   There is a fine tremor of the fingers, best seen when the hands are outstretched.

(e)   Exophthalmos. This is a term used for the characteristic protrusion or prominence of the eyes which is most often caused by thyrotoxicosis, and especially by the diffuse type (Graves' disease). A characteristic 'staring' expression is often present. Lagging of the upper eyelid on looking down is also a useful sign.

(f)   Tachycardia. A persistently fast pulse rate is one of the marked features of thyrotoxicosis. In most cases the heart rate is regular, but atrial fibrillation commonly occurs in elderly patients suffering from the toxic nodular form of goitre. In severe cases heart failure may develop, and thyrotoxicosis is in fact one of the known common causes of congestive heart failure.

(g)   Attacks of diarrhoea and vomiting may occur in the more severe cases. The enlarged thyroid gland can usually be seen or felt in the neck.

Diagnosis

In the presence of such typical symptoms as wasting, sweating, tremor, exophthalmos and tachycardia, together with enlargement of the thyroid gland, the diagnosis is easy.

The level of circulating thyroxin can be measured in the blood and is considerably in excess of normal in thyrotoxicosis.

Treatment

Treatment can be divided into two main groups—medical and surgical.

MEDICAL TREATMENT

(a) *Antithyroid drugs.* These drugs reduce the activity of the thyroid gland and are therefore frequently used in the treatment of toxic goitre. The drugs in most frequent use are carbimazole (Neo-Mercazole) and thiouracil. Carbimazole is less toxic than thiouracil and is given in initial doses of 10 mg eight hourly and in maintenance doses of 5 to 15 mg daily. Thiouracil is given in initial doses of 200 to 400 mg and in maintenance doses of 50 to 100 mg daily.

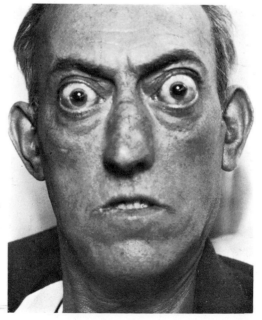

FIG. 14.9   Severe exophthalmos in a case of primary toxic goitre (Graves' disease).

TYPE OF GOITRE	HORMONE SECRETION	SIGNS AND SYMPTOMS	TREATMENT
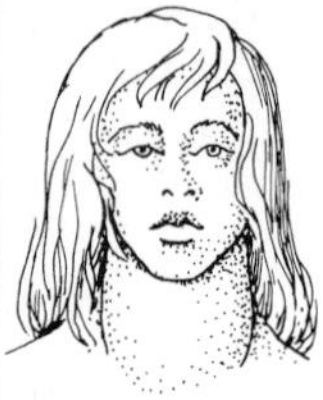 SIMPLE	NORMAL	Sometimes local pressure symptoms	Iodine Thyroxine Removal if persistent

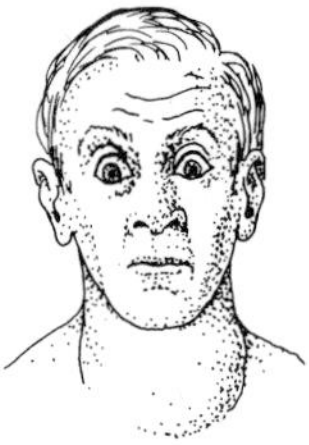
TOXIC
	INCREASED	Irritability
		Loss of weight
		Sweating
		Tremor
		Exophthalmos
		Tachycardia
			MEDICAL
			  Carbinazole
			  Thiouracil
			  Radioactive
			     iodine
			
			SURGICAL
			  Partial
			  thyroidectomy

MALIGNANT	NORMAL	Goitre hard Local pressure symptoms Secondaries	Total thyroidectomy
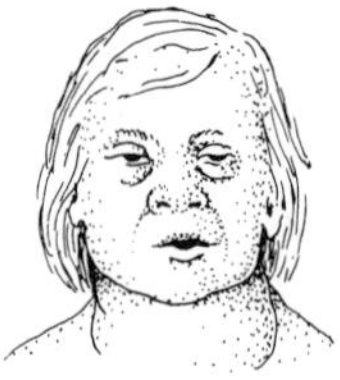 MYXOEDEMA (Hashimoto's disease)	DECREASED	Skin thickening Loss of hair Slow pulse Slow mentality Constipation Fatigue	Thyroxine

Fig. 14.10   Types of goitre.

The main toxic reactions from antithyroid drugs are:

(i) Agranulocytosis, where there is a marked reduction in the number of polymorphonuclear white blood cells. In severe forms this may prove fatal.

(ii) Marked increase in the size of the goitre.

(iii) Drug rashes, often resembling measles.

The main danger is agranulocytosis, and if a patient who is on antithyroid drugs complains of a sore throat the drug must be stopped immediately and a white blood cell count performed to confirm the diagnosis. A sore throat is an early symptom of agranulocytosis (p. 358).

Antithyroid drugs are most useful in patients with thyrotoxicosis where the gland is small and diffuse. As carbimazole (or thiouracil) takes some days to exert its full anti-thyroid effect, it is often combined initially with a beta-blocker such as propranolol which has a more immediate effect in slowing the rapid heart rate.

(b) *Radioactive iodine.* Treatment with radioactive iodine is usually very successful. As, however, it is not certain that after such treatment myxoedema will not develop after a period of 5 to 10 years, radioactive iodine is at present usually given only to older patients with toxic adenoma. Radioactive iodine is also used in the treatment of malignant goitre. Complicated apparatus for adjusting the dose of radioactive iodine is required, so that this treatment is possible only at special hospitals.

SURGICAL TREATMENT

Surgical treatment is probably best in all cases of toxic adenoma (as opposed to Graves' disease). It is also necessary in all cases which have been treated medically and have failed to respond, and in cases where the goitre is causing pressure symptoms.

The aim of surgical treatment is to remove the larger portion of the gland, leaving only enough to prevent the development of myxoedema.

Except for very mild cases, patients with toxic goitre are usually given a preoperative course of carbimazole so as to reduce toxicity and the risk of operation. As carbimazole makes the goitre larger and more vascular, the drug must be discontinued two weeks before the operation and replaced by Lugol's iodine, 5 minims twice a day. If carbimazole is not discontinued before the operation excessive haemorrhage from the gland during the operation is liable to occur.

Malignant goitre

Some cases of toxic goitre, particularly the toxic adenoma, may become malignant. In these cases the goitre is very hard and often painful. Malignant goitre is very likely to cause local pressure symptoms, such as dyspnoea, stridor and dysphagia. Thyroid carcinoma is also liable to spread and so cause secondary growths, which are especially common in the bones.

The treatment is surgical removal of all the thyroid if possible. Treatment by radioactive iodine is sometimes usefully combined with surgical removal of the thyroid gland.

DISEASES DUE TO DEFICIENCY OF THE THYROID HORMONE

It has already been stated that the main function of the thyroid hormone is to control metabolism in the body and that oversecretion of the hormone causes a great increase in metabolism with well-marked physical changes (thyrotoxicosis). Similarly, undersecretion of the thyroid hormone causes a lowering of bodily function which is seen in two diseases, myxoedema in adults and cretinism in infants and young children.

MYXOEDEMA

Causes

1. Removal of the thyroid gland in the treatment of thyrotoxic and malignant goitre. Destruction by radioactive iodine.

2. Primary atrophy of the gland, probably due to destruction of the gland by abnormal antibodies. Sometimes the gland is enlarged (Hashimoto's disease).

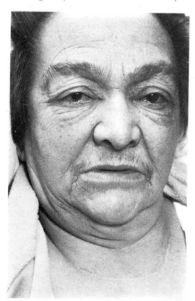 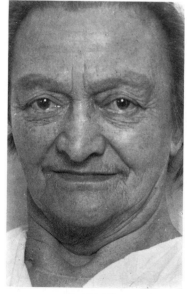

Fig. 14.11.   Fig. 14.12.

Fig. 14.11 Myxoedema showing the characteristic puffy and bloated appearance. The condition developed after thyroidectomy for a toxic goitre. (The scar in the neck is still visible.)

Fig. 14.12 Myxoedema after thyroid therapy showing the marked improvement. (Same patient as Fig. 14.11.)

Symptoms and signs

1. A general increase in weight is an early and fairly constant feature and extreme obesity may eventually develop.

2. Skin changes, with coarse thickening of the skin and a puffiness almost like that due to oedema, are very common. The skin, however, although very puffy does not actually pit on pressure as in true oedema.

3. The hair tends to fall out.

4. The pulse is usually slow.

5. The patients have a very dull and sluggish mentality and often a defective memory. They easily become tired.

6. Constipation is a marked feature.

Diagnosis

The appearance of the patient, the cold extremities, thick voice and slow reactions all suggest the diagnosis. Confirmation can be sought by two blood tests. First, the thyroxin level is below normal: and, second the TSH level is high. TSH is the thyroid stimulating hormone produced by the pituitary gland. In myxoedema an excess is produced by the pituitary in an attempt to stimulate the thyroid gland.

Treatment

Thyroxin or thyroid extract is given orally. The dose of thyroxin is 0·1 mg or less initially, and this is gradually increased as necessary. Signs of overdosage with thyroid extract are excessive loss of weight, tachycardia, sweating and diarrhoea. In elderly patients, the quickened heart action may lead to angina pectoris or even myocardial infarction. Hence the dose of thyroxin must be increased cautiously.

CRETINISM

CAUSES. Cretinism is usually due to an atrophy of the thyroid gland which is itself of unknown cause. It is especially common in districts where goitre is very frequently found, and in many cases the mother has a goitre. Lack of iodine is undoubtedly a factor.

Symptoms and signs

1. The infant is usually normal at birth, but symptoms begin to appear within six months.

2. There is a failure of growth, both physical and mental. If the condition is allowed to continue unrecognised and untreated the child becomes a mentally deficient dwarf.

3. The infant is of very ugly appearance, with a flat depressed nose, dry skin and scanty hair. The hands become thick and spade-

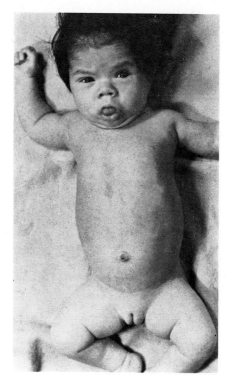

Fig. 14.13   Cretin, aged 8 months. The appearance with the thick protruding tongue is typical, as is also the umbilical hernia.

like. The tongue is very thick, coarse and wide, and is constantly protruded through the open mouth.

4. The abdomen is usually distended (pot belly) and an umbilical hernia is often present.

DIAGNOSIS. Cretinism must be distinguished from the other causes of mental deficiency and stunted growth (see Dwarfism, p. 436).

Treatment

It is most important that cretinism should be recognised as early as possible as early treatment can result in a complete cure. If, however, treatment is delayed too long then some permanent mental deficiency may remain. As in myxoedema, thyroxin is prescribed though naturally in much smaller doses applicable to a child.

ADRENAL GLANDS

ANATOMY AND PHYSIOLOGY. The adrenal or suprarenal glands are divided into two main parts, the cortex and medulla.

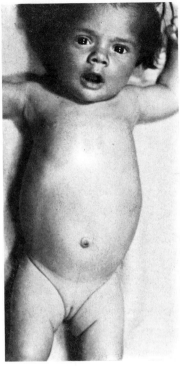 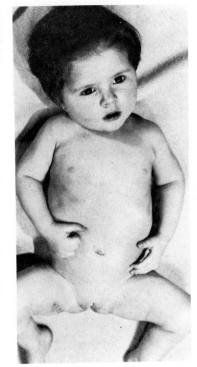

Fig. 14.14.   Fig. 14.15.

Fig. 14.14   Same patient as Fig. 14.13. Three months after starting thyroid therapy.

Fig. 14.15   Same patient as Fig. 14.13. Eleven months after starting treatment; the child's health is now normal.

The cortex

The adrenal cortex secretes many different hormones, which can be classified as follows:

1. CORTISONE. This important hormone has many actions. It plays a part in the control of carbohydrate metabolism and can convert protein into glucose. It affects the output of sodium. It controls the processes of inflammation and allergy, and this property explains its use in the treatment of many diseases.

2. ALDOSTERONE. This hormone regulates mineral metabolism, particularly sodium and potassium. If present in excess the body retains excessive sodium and excretes too much potassium.

3. SEX HORMONES. These include the various androgenic hormones, which have a masculinising effect and also tend to cause bodily growth. The other main sex hormones are the oestrogens.

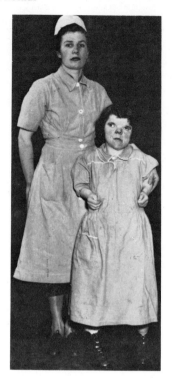

Fig. 14.16   Untreated cretin, aged 36 years.

Corticotrophin (ACTH) is the pituitary adrenocorticotrophic hormone which stimulates the adrenals to produce cortisone and allied hormones.

The medulla

The medulla secretes two hormones, adrenaline and noradrenaline, which have very powerful effects and are used in the treatment of several diseases (p. 458).

DISEASES OF THE ADRENAL CORTEX

1. Addison's disease, which leads to lack of the several hormones which deal especially with the regulation of the various salts in the blood.

2. Hyperplasia or tumours, which lead to overproduction of the hormones.

ADDISON'S DISEASE

Causes
1. Tuberculous disease producing wide destruction of the gland.
2. Atrophy of the gland probably due to destruction by abnormal antibodies.

Symptoms and signs
1. There is profound weakness which, in later stages, may be so severe that the patient is unable to get about. Wasting is also a fairly early feature.
2. There is a characteristic pigmentation of the skin and mucous membranes. Brown patches are often seen on the lips, in the mouth and around the nipples. The pigmentation may also be more generalised and is particularly prominent in areas exposed to sunlight, in areas under pressure from a belt or constricting garment or in scars.
3. Nausea, with attacks of diarrhoea and vomiting, is very frequent.
4. A low blood pressure, often with a systolic blood pressure of less than 100 mmHg.
5. When the blood is examined it will be found that there are many typical changes present. The amount of sodium and chloride is usually diminished and the potassium raised, especially during the acute stages. The fasting blood sugar is often low.
6. The level of cortisol (cortisol is secreted by the adrenal gland) is very low in the blood in Addison's disease and does not rise when ACTH (which normally stimulates the gland to produce cortisol) is injected. This is used as a test in the diagnosis of Addison's disease.

Course
If undiagnosed and untreated, patients with Addison's disease gradually deteriorate and collapse, the so-called acute adrenal crisis. This is often precipitated by vomiting and diarrhoea or a chest infection. The blood pressure falls to dangerous levels, the pulse becomes rapid and thready and the extremities are cold. Death will follow unless treatment is instituted.

Treatment
1. Patients with Addison's disease can be maintained in good health by taking cortisone. The usual dose varies from 25 to 50 mg of cortisone daily. The blood pressure rises to normal, the pigmentation lightens and the patient feels well again.
2. In some patients 0·1 mg of fludrocortisone (Florinef) can be taken daily in addition to cortisone to maintain normal . salt metabolism.
3. TREATMENT OF AN ACUTE ADRENAL CRISIS. The patient's pulse is recorded and charted hourly and frequent blood pressure readings are

taken. The foot of the bed should be raised. Intravenous hydrocortisone is given as soon as possible: 100 mg eight-hourly the first day and 50 mg six-hourly the second day. This dose is gradually reduced. An intravenous saline drip is usually necessary in the initial stages because of the severe vomiting: food by mouth is not usually tolerated, but as soon as the patient can take food a light diet is given.

The prevention of adrenal crisis is most important and the patient should be warned to avoid chills if possible and to obtain prompt treatment for even the mildest infection.

CUSHING'S SYNDROME

This is the clinical picture resulting from excess cortisone. It can be caused in different ways.

1. A tumour of the pituitary gland which produces excess ACTH and so stimulates the adrenal cortex to produce too much cortisone.

2. A tumour (adenoma) of the adrenal cortex which produces excess cortisone.

3. Some forms of lung cancer (bronchial carcinoma) produce excess ACTH.

4. Steroid therapy. Cortisone or prednisone if given in large doses or for over long periods in the treatment of various disorders (p. 456).

Clinical features

1. Obesity affecting particularly the face ('moon face'), the upper back ('buffalo hump') and the trunk, but sparing the limbs.

2. Purple streaks ('striae') can be seen on the lower abdomen and buttocks. Acne on the face and increased hair may occur.

3. The blood pressure is raised.

4. Diabetes may develop with sugar in the urine.

5. Thinning of the bones (osteoporosis) may lead to fractures.

6. Muscular weakness and mental depression occur.

Diagnosis

Normally cortisone is formed and released into the blood overnight, so that the blood levels of cortisone are higher in the morning than in the evening (diurnal variation). In Cushing's syndrome the blood levels of cortisone are very high and are unaltered day or night.

When the diagnosis is confirmed in this way, further investigation is necessary to establish the cause. The level of ACTH in the blood can be measured and will be very high if the cause of the disorder is in the pituitary but will be low if there is an adrenal growth. X-ray of the skull will show if the pituitary fossa is enlarged, which would suggest a pituitary tumour. X-ray of the chest might reveal a bronchial carcinoma. A plain X-ray of the abdomen can be taken to see if there is an adrenal tumour with calcification.

Operation might be indicated either on the skull to remove a pituitary tumour or on the abdomen to remove an adrenal tumour.

Adrenogenital syndrome (virilism)

Here, there is chiefly an excessive secretion of the sex hormones, although the other adrenal cortical hormones may also be affected. For this reason a 'mixed' picture of Cushing's syndrome and the adrenogenital syndrome is often met with.

1. The most prodominant signs are seen in women, who develop masculine characteristics with excessive growth of hair on the face (hirsutism). The voice deepens and muscular development resembles that of a man. The sex organs undergo striking changes, with enlargement of the clitoris. Amenorrhoea is present and acne of the skin is also a feature.

2. In adult males there may be few striking changes, but generally the picture is similar to that described under Cushing's syndrome.

3. In young boys there is very early sex development with growth of hair on the face, enlargement of the penis and pronounced muscular growth—pseudo-sexual precocity.

4. If excessive adrenal activity occurs in intrauterine life it produces in girls the picture of virilism plus pseudohermaphroditism with abnormality of the urogenital organs. The child may be mistaken for a boy. Pre-natal adrenal cortical oversecretion in boys causes marked enlargement of the external genitalia.

Diagnosis

Male hormones (androgens) are excreted in the urine as 17-keto-steroids and these are found in excess.

Treatment

Treatment depends on whether an actual tumour or merely hyperplasia is present. Tumours, which are more likely to be present in adults than in children, are removed. If hyperplasia only is present, as is probable in young children, cortisone is given and this will suppress the activity of the adrenals.

DISEASES OF THE ADRENAL MEDULLA

PHAEOCHROMOCYTOMA

The only disease known to affect the adrenal medulla is a tumour called a phaeochromocytoma. This tumour produces an excess of the normal secretion of the medulla—adrenaline. The main effect of this overproduction of adrenaline is severe hypertension, which characteristically occurs in paroxysmal attacks. During these attacks the patient complains of very severe headaches, sweating and vomiting and the blood pressure is markedly raised.

When the diagnosis is suspected, special chemical tests can be used to detect excessive amounts of derivatives of adrenalin (catecholamines) excreted in the urine. If these are present operation should be undertaken to remove the tumour.

PARATHYROID GLANDS

ANATOMY AND PHYSIOLOGY. The parathyroid glands are four in number and are situated behind the thyroid gland. The main function of the parathyroids is the regulation of the calcium and phosphorus content of the bones and blood. Therefore, to understand the changes that arise as a result of diseases of the parathyroids, it is necessary to appreciate the role that calcium plays in the body in health. The main functions of calcium are:

(a) The formation of bone. (Any disturbance in the level of calcium can lead to improper development of and deformities in the bones.)

(b) The control of the irritability of muscles and nerves.

(c) As a factor in the proper clotting of blood.

The proper absorption and usage of calcium is regulated in three main ways.

1. Vitamin D controls the absorption of calcium from the bowel. Most of the calcium absorbed goes to the bones to help in their proper formation and calcification. Lack of vitamin D, as one would expect, leads to marked changes in the bones (rickets in children and osteomalacia in adults).

2. The parathyroid hormone (parathormone) regulates the flow of calcium between the bones and the blood. Excessive secretion of the hormone causes a withdrawal of calcium from the bones into the blood with the result that the bones become soft, spongy, deformed and liable to fracture. On the other hand, deficiency of parathormone leads to a low level of calcium in the blood, which causes one form of the clinical syndrome known as *tetany*. (As there are many different factors which cause tetany this disease will be described later.)

3. Calcitonin is secreted by the parafollicular cells of the thyroid gland. It opposes the effect of parathormone and increases deposition of calcium into the bones from the blood.

DISEASES OF THE PARATHYROID GLANDS

Tumours of the parathyroid glands may lead to overproduction of parathormone (parathyroid hormone). Underproduction is usually due to damage of the glands (which lie behind the thyroid gland) during operation on the thyroid.

TUMOURS

Tumours of the parathyroid gland are rare. They lead to oversecretion of the parathyroid hormone which produces a very characteristic clinical picture known as *osteitis fibrosa cystica* or *hyperparathyroidism*.

Systems and signs

These may be divided into three main groups due to:
1. Excessive calcium in the blood.
2. Changes in the bones.
3. Increased excretion of calcium by the kidneys into the urine.

Excessive calcium in the blood. This usually causes weakness and loss of appetite and weight. Generalised muscle and joint pains are common. In severe cases there may be nausea and vomiting.

Changes in the bones. Owing to the excessive removal of calcium from the bones as a result of the overactivity of the parathyroid hormone the bones become soft, deformed and liable to fracture. Large cysts may occur in the bones.

Excretion of calcium into the urine. Because of the presence of excessive calcium in the urine renal calculi develop, and in severe cases blockage of the kidneys may occur with signs of renal damage and uraemia.

DIAGNOSIS. The diagnosis is usually made on the above symptoms and signs and by estimating the amount of calcium in the blood, which is markedly raised above normal.

Course and treatment

Unless the condition is treated the patients usually become bed-ridden owing to the bony deformities, and they usually die from renal failure. The treatment is to explore the parathyroid glands and remove the tumour. If this is done early a complete cure can be effected.

INJURIES DURING OPERATION ON THE THYROID GLAND

The condition which most commonly affects the parathyroid glands is accidental injury or removal of the parathyroids during operations on the thyroid gland. The main effect is to produce a deficiency of parathyroid hormone which results in tetany. In most cases, however, the tetany is transient and responds to large doses of calciferol which raise the blood calcium level.

TETANY

In the discussion on the action of the parathyroid hormone we saw that undersecretion of this hormone can lead to a low blood calcium level and so to the condition of tetany. Tetany presents a clinical picture with characteristic symptoms and signs that develop owing to lowering of the blood calcium; it can be caused in several different ways.

1. *Undersecretion of parathyroid hormone.* This cause is rare and is usually the result of injury to or accidental removal of the para-thyroids during operations on the thyroid gland.

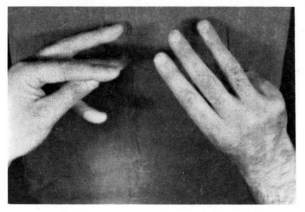

FIG. 14.17 Tetany showing the characteristic position of the hands in carpopedal spasm.

2. *Lack of vitamin D*. It was mentioned previously that vitamin D is necessary for the control of absorption of calcium from the bowel. If vitamin D is lacking, various diseases result, especially the condition known as rickets, which may also be associated with tetany.

3. *Alkalosis*. Normally, the reaction of the blood is kept at a constant level. If the blood should become too alkaline the calcium becomes altered and is not available to the body, i.e. a deficiency of calcium results with consequential development of tetany. Alkalosis can arise in several ways, e.g.

    (a) From loss of acid owing to persistent vomiting in cases of pyloric stenosis. The gastric secretion contains hydrochloric acid and if this is continuously depleted by persistent vomiting alkalosis can result.

    (b) Excessive overbreathing leads to loss of the acid, carbon dioxide, and a resulting alkalosis with tetany. This type of tetany is commonest in hysteria.

    (c) Excessive administration of large doses of alkalis (especially sodium bicarbonate) as self medication for 'indigestion'.

Symptoms and signs

1. Painful cramps occur in the hands and feet. The hands take up a characteristic attitude with the thumbs pressed into the palms and the fingers hyperextended. This attitude is known as *carpopedal spasm*. Pressure on the arms will bring on the carpopedal spasms and this reaction is referred to as Trousseau's sign.

2. Convulsions, which are particularly common in children.

3. Laryngeal spasm. Sudden spasm of the larynx occurs causing cyanosis and stridor. This laryngeal spasm is called *laryngismus stridulus* and is particularly seen in the tetany of rickets.

4. Chvostek's sign. Tapping on the branches of the facial nerve in the face produces twitching of the muscles of the face. This is due to the irritability of the nerves which is present in tetany.

5. There are the signs of the disease, e.g. rickets in children, pyloric stenosis and hysteria, which is associated with the tetany.

Treatment

This will depend on the cause, but relief of spasm can be obtained by slow intravenous injection of calcium gluconate. When the parathyroid glands are not functioning prolonged treatment with vitamin D (calciferol) will be necessary. The normal dose varies from 1 to 5 mg daily and regular estimations of blood calcium levels are necessary to regulate the amount.

THYMUS GLAND

The thymus gland plays an important role in the foetus and in infancy since it is a factory for lymphocytes. In the adult these are produced in the lymph glands and the spleen. The thymus secretes a hormone which prepares the lymphocytes for the production of all the various antibodies necessary to combat infections later in life. The gland gradually atrophies in childhood and seems to play no part in adult life.

The rare disease, myasthenia gravis, is sometimes associated with an enlarged thymus or a thymic tumour, but the association is not understood. Removal of the thymus is often successful in relieving the symptoms of this disease.

THE USE OF HORMONES IN CLINICAL MEDICINE

Hormones are used not only to replace the natural hormones where these are deficient, but also in the treatment of other disorders.

CORTISONE AND ALLIED STEROIDS

Cortisone is one of the most important steroid hormones produced by the adrenal cortex. These steroids control the processes of inflammation and allergy, and so cortisone is often prescribed to suppress excessive inflammatory or allergic reactions. Unfortunately, in most diseases in which cortisone is beneficial, relapse occurs when the drug is discontinued. Furthermore, if these steroids are given in too large a dose or for too long a time, serious side effects may be noted. In particular, retention of salt occurs with subsequent oedema and hypertension. Since the isolation of cortisone, many similar compounds have been synthesised which have less tendency to lead to salt retention.

1. Cortisone

This is effective when given by mouth or by intramuscular injection. Its main use is to replace the natural hormone in conditions where the adrenal cortex is not functioning.

(a) *Addison's disease.* Cortisone is life-saving in this condition. The usual dose is one and a half tablets (37·5 mg) daily, and this is sometimes supplemented by fluorohydrocortisone (Florinef), a powerful salt-retaining steroid.

(b) *Simmonds' disease.* Lack of stimulation from the pituitary gland leads to atrophy of the adrenal cortex. Cortisone must be taken daily.

(c) *Total adrenalectomy.* This operation of removing both adrenal glands is performed in certain cases of breast cancer and Cushing's disease. Large doses of cortisone must be given during the pre-operative and postoperative stages, and maintenance doses of cortisone must be continued for life.

2. Prednisolone

This is a synthetic compound with properties similar to those of cortisone but less likely to lead to salt retention. Many such steroids are now available (e.g. prednisone, triamcinolone, dexamethasone), and their main use is to suppress excessive inflammatory or allergic reactions. They do not remove the cause of these reactions, though they relieve the effects, much as an umbrella keeps one dry but does not stop the rain.

(a) *Rheumatoid arthritis.* Where the condition is active and has failed to respond to safer remedies, prednisolone (or similar compound) may prove helpful in relieving the pain and swelling in the joints and in permitting more mobility. The dose should be as low as possible to avoid unwanted effects.

(b) *Rheumatic fever.* In severe cases which have responded poorly to salicylates, steroids should be employed. Often large doses are needed in the initial stages to bring down the temperature and relieve joint swelling.

(c) *Asthma.* Prednisolone can be used in resistant cases and is strikingly successful in relieving respiratory wheezing and dyspnoea.

(d) *Ulcerative colitis.* Prednisolone is sometimes helpful in suppressing the inflammation and ulceration of the colon in this condition, though often the improvement is not maintained despite continuation of therapy.

(e) *The nephrotic syndrome.* Especially in children, steroid therapy can be successful in reducing the oedema and albuminuria. High dosage of prednisolone is necessary.

(f) *Blood diseases.* Steroids can lead to a remission in haemolytic anaemia and in purpura.

(g) *Allergic states,* such as drug allergy, hay fever, dermatitis, or angioneurotic oedema. Prednisolone should only be used in very severe conditions that have failed to respond to antihistamines.

(h) *Collagen diseases.* Steroids must be employed in large doses and may be life-saving in these diseases.

3. Hydrocortisone

This is also a natural hormone like cortisone. It is available for intravenous injection and is usually given in a dose of 100 mg in an intravenous drip for emergency treatment in cases of collapse due to acute adrenal insufficiency, as sometimes occurs in Addison's disease, or in adrenalectomised patients who omit to take their routine cortisone tablets.

4. Corticotrophin (ACTH)

ACTH is the pituitary adrenocorticotrophic hormone which stimulates the adrenals to produce cortisone. Hence, unless the adrenals are damaged, the effect of ACTH is similar to that of cortisone. It has to be administered by intramuscular injection, and is sometimes used where oral steroid therapy has given rise to gastric symptoms. The daily maintenance dose is from 20 to 40 units.

Hydrocortisone, prednisolone, and other steroids are also available for *local treatment* to relieve inflammation in specific areas:

(a) Eye drops, for acute inflammatory eye conditions.

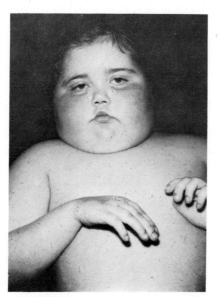

FIG. 14.18   Nephrotic syndrome treated with large doses of prednisolone to protect the kidneys. The bloated moon face is due to prolonged steroid treatment.

(b) Ointments or sprays, for local application in skin conditions such as eczema or pruritus ani.

(c) Intra-articular injections, especially of the knees in rheumatoid arthritis or osteoarthritis.

(d) Retention enemas for ulcerative colitis.

Toxic effects of steroids

1. Retention of salt, leading to oedema and high blood pressure. Patients taking prolonged courses of steroids should avoid salt in the diet.

2. Conversion of protein to carbohydrate, leading to increased blood sugar. This may precipitate diabetes. Diabetic patients taking cortisone may need more insulin.

3. Reduced resistance to infection, due to suppression of inflammatory reactions which normally offer protection. Tuberculosis, if present, can spread very rapidly in patients on steroid therapy. A chest X-ray should be taken to make sure there is no evidence of pulmonary tuberculosis. Similarly, patients with a peptic ulcer should be given cortisone with caution as healing of the ulcer may be delayed and perforation has been known to occur.

4. Acne, obesity, and thinning of the bones (osteoporosis) occur with excessive dosage. In fact, Cushing's syndrome is due to excessive cortisone and can be caused by injudicious therapy.

5. Adrenal collapse. When cortisone is given, the natural secretion of the gland is suppressed and the gland becomes inactive. Hence, if cortisone treatment is stopped suddenly, collapse due to adrenal insufficiency is likely to occur. This could lead to a fatal outcome, particularly if any operation is undergone. Therefore steroid therapy must always be discontinued gradually.

Patients taking steroids are given a blue card warning them that it is dangerous to stop their tablets without medical advice, and urging them to report to the doctor if they get abdominal pain, since this might be due to peptic ulceration.

ADRENALINE (Epinephrine) AND NORADRENALINE

Adrenaline and noradrenaline are the two secretions of the medulla of the adrenal gland.

Actions of adrenaline

1. Constricts the arterioles of the skin and mucous membranes.

2. Relaxes the smooth muscle of the bronchioles of the lungs.

3. Raises the blood sugar by releasing glucose from the liver into the blood stream.

4. Increases the rate and force of the heart.

Uses of adrenaline

1. To stop bleeding from mucous membranes, as in epistaxis; gauze plugs soaked in adrenaline are used. Adrenaline is also used

in local anaesthetic solutions to constrict the vessels and so reduce the amount of bleeding.

2. Because of its action in relaxing spasm of the bronchioles, adrenalin or its derivatives have been used in various inhalers in the treatment of asthma. Unfortunately, its action on the heart can be dangerous and its overuse has led to many deaths. It has been replaced by salbutamol which is much safer in this respect.

3. In anaphylaxis and other severe hypersensitivity reactions, subcutaneous injections of 0·5 mg adrenalin may offer immediate relief.

4. In cases of cardiac arrest due to asystole, adrenalin injected directly into the heart may start the heart beating again.

OESTROGENS

Oestrogens are the hormones secreted by the ovary and are responsible for the normal female development. Many synthetic and natural preparations are available for clinical use, including stilboestrol and oestrone (premarin).

1. **Menopause.** In the majority of women, ovulation ceases around the age of 50. The periods become less frequent and finally cease. The menopause is often associated with constitutional symptoms due to a falling off of oestrogens from the ovaries. Hot flushes are a sudden suffusion of the face and body, often associated with free sweating. Emotional instability, irritability of mood and depression may occur. When hot flushes, sweats and mood disturbance are severe, courses of oestrogen, such as oestrone, may be prescribed, usually for a month at a time and offering great relief of these troublesome symptoms.

2. **Contraceptive pill.** The use of oral contraceptives has steadily increased since their introduction in the early 1960s and nearly 15 per cent of married women use this form of birth control. The pill contains synthetic oestrogens and progesterones which in combination prevent ovulation without leading to break-through bleeding between cycles. Some preparations contain both compounds together, to be taken for cycles of 20 to 22 days. Others contain the oestrogen alone for the first 15 or 16 days after cessation of menstruation, followed by the combination for a week to complete the course. The oestrogen used is usually either mestranol or ethinyloestradiol, but there are a number of different progesterones.

If taken regularly and according to instruction, oral contraceptives are a completely effective form of birth control, but they have disadvantages:

   (a) Nausea, headaches and breast discomfort may occur especially during the first few cycles.
   (b) There is an impairment of glucose metabolism with a tendency to diabetes. Diabetic patients may find their insulin requirements need increasing when they start the pill, while actual

diabetes may develop in those hereditarily disposed to the ailment.

(c) Oestrogens disturb the blood-clotting mechanism and so the pill disposes to venous thrombosis and pulmonary embolism, as indeed does pregnancy.

(d) Amenorrhoea may follow discontinuation of the pill, and may persist for many months.

3. **Suppression of lactation.** If a mother has to give up breast feeding her baby for any reason, stilboestrol can be given. It suppresses the formation of milk and relieves the breast engorgement.

4. Stilboestrol is given for the maintenance treatment of **carcinoma of the prostate.** It inhibits the growth and spread of the cancer and relieves the symptoms.

ANDROGENS

Androgens are male hormones secreted mainly by the testicles but also by the adrenal cortex. They are responsible for the maturation of the male secondary characteristics after puberty, and are effective in building up protein. They are sometimes used:

1. In the treatment of osteoporosis to strengthen the protein structure of the bones.

2. In certain forms of jaundice when skin irritation is troublesome. It has been found that androgens relieve the itching.

OTHER HORMONES

Other hormones have been described in the appropriate sections.

1. Antidiuretic hormone (vasopressin) in the treatment of diabetes insipidus.

2. Thyroxine in the treatment of myxoedema and cretinism.

3. Insulin for the treatment of diabetes mellitus.

4. Glucagon for the treatment of hypoglycaemia.

15 Diseases of Joints, Bones and Connective Tissue

JOINTS

Disease of the joints can be due to a number of causes. *Rheumatoid arthritis* is a constitutional ailment of unknown origin, primarily affecting the joints but also other systems of the body as well. *Osteoarthritis* is a degenerative condition of individual joints. *Gout* is a metabolic disorder leading to severe joint damage. All these complaints are loosely referred to as forms of 'arthritis'; they are very common and a source of a great deal of disability.

RHEUMATOID ARTHRITIS

Rheumatoid arthritis is a widespread and chronic condition which ultimately can be so severe as to render patients disabled or even bedridden though most cases run a milder course.

The parts of the bones which form a joint are covered by smooth firm cartilage, lubricated by a thick viscid fluid. This fluid is secreted by the synovial membrane. The synovial membrane encloses the joint space and is formed of epithelial cells. It is these cells which secrete the synovial fluid into the joint.

In rheumatoid arthritis, the synovial membrane becomes thickened and inflamed and the cartilages are eroded. The synovial membrane may invade the joint space and the whole joint becomes swollen and painful on movement.

It seems likely that rheumatoid arthritis is due to a disorder of the immunity system, perhaps started by a virus infection. Abnormal antibodies (the *rheumatoid factor*) are found in the blood of most patients with rheumatoid arthritis and it may be that these abnormal antibodies are responsible for the inflammatory changes in the synovial membrane and the cartilage.

Symptoms and signs
1. The disease is two or three times as common in women as in men, the average age of onset being about 40; but it can occur in children (Still's disease) or in the very elderly (senile rheumatoid).

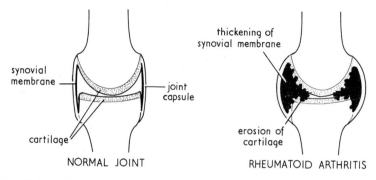

Fig. 15.1   A joint affected by rheumatoid arthritis.

2. It tends to run a chronic progressive course, despite remissions when the symptoms subside. Some cases are very severe and lead to crippling within a few years. Others run a mild course and only cause slight disability.

3. The main effect is on the joints. The fingers are often the earliest affected, giving rise to pain and stiffness especially on first getting up in the morning. The feet, ankles, knees, wrists, elbows and shoulders also become involved, and later the spine. The affected joints become swollen and tender with thickening of the surrounding tissues and restriction of mobility. Pain may disturb sleep, and getting about becomes an effort. In severe cases, the joints may become fixed and deformed so that the patient is unable to look after herself and may become bedridden. Fortunately, only a small proportion of cases progress in this relentless fashion.

4. Even in the early stages there are signs of general constitutional symptoms. There is a feeling of exhaustion and a loss of weight. The temperature may be raised. There is nearly always some anaemia and the sedimentation rate is raised.

DIAGNOSIS. Diagnosis is usually easy; characteristic features are swelling and pain affecting several joints (particularly the hands and feet), general ill-health and a chronic course with remissions. Osteoarthritis, the other common form of arthritis, tends to affect only single joints and the general health is not seriously disturbed.

The blood can be tested for the rheumatoid factor which is positive in the majority of cases. A strongly positive RA (rheumatoid arthritis) test means that the ailment is very active.

Treatment of rheumatoid arthritis

There is no specific cure for rheumatoid arthritis and so medical supervision has to be regular and prolonged.

GENERAL MEASURES

In the acute phase, when the joints are swollen and painful and the temperature raised, bed rest is essential. A firm back support should be used during the day and a cradle should take the weight of the bed clothes off the affected limbs. The legs must be kept straight and a pillow behind the knees must be forbidden if flexion deformities are to be avoided. When the acute pain and swelling have subsided, active exercises should be undertaken, usually under the guidance of a physiotherapist, and the patient is allowed up for increasing periods.

The diet should have a high protein content with plenty of milk and eggs. Anaemia is difficult to correct and iron may have to be given.

LOCAL MEASURES

Acutely painful joints should be immobilised in light plastic splints or even plaster of Paris. In more chronic cases, injection of prednisolone into the joint leads to relief of pain and subsidence of swelling. Particular involvement of an individual joint may require the advice of an orthopaedic surgeon. Wax baths may be beneficial in reducing stiffness in the hands and feet and as movements are easier to perform under water, special warm baths may be helpful. Remedial exercises should be maintained when the patient has left hospital.

DRUGS

Calcium aspirin is probably the best available drug for most patients with rheumatoid arthritis. Usually 600 mg three times a day

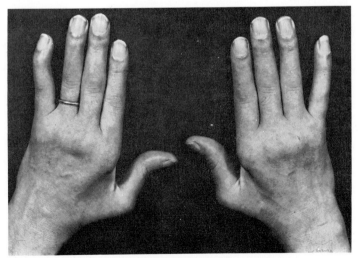

FIG. 15.2   Early rheumatoid arthritis of the hands, showing the characteristic swelling and deformity of the joints.

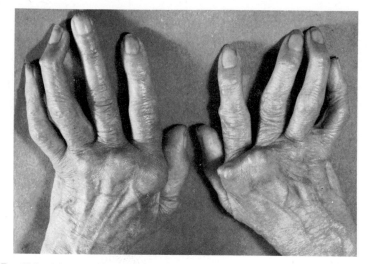

FIG. 15.3   Advanced rheumatoid arthritis of the hands, showing the gross deformity and the typical position of the hands.

is sufficient to relieve the nagging joint pains and the stiffness, but prolonged usage can lead to gastric pain and even haematemesis.

2. Phenylbutazone (Butazolidin) is effective in relieving the joint pain in rheumatoid arthritis, especially in old people. When given at a dose of 100 mg three times a day, toxic effects are rare but when this dose is exceeded, blood disorders (such as agranulocytosis), skin rashes and haematemesis can occur.

3. Indomethacin (Indocid) has an effect similar to phenylbutazone but is more likely to give rise to gastric irritation.

4. Steroids. Prednisolone (p. 456) soon relieves the pain and stiffness in the joints but the disadvantages of prolonged usage in the end outweigh the benefits. For this reason steroids are now seldom used in rheumatoid arthritis, except in the form of a local injection into a swollen joint.

5. Gold salts (Myocrisin). After initial small doses of 10 mg to make sure there is no reaction, gold injections of 50 mg can be given weekly to a total of 1 g. This course of injections usually leads to a gradual amelioration of symptoms, and can be repeated after an interval of a few months. Gold may cause toxic reactions leading to severe dermatitis, agranulocytosis or nephritis. The urine should be tested for albumin before each injection and frequent blood counts taken.

6. Chloroquine and hydroxychloroquine (Plaquenil) may be useful in the long term treatment of rheumatoid arthritis but have to be given for several months to achieve improvement. Unfortunately, toxic effects on the eyes may occur unless there is careful supervision.

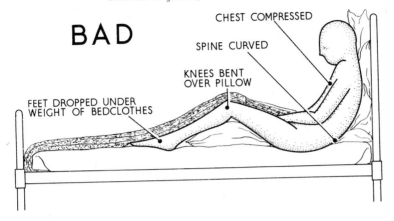

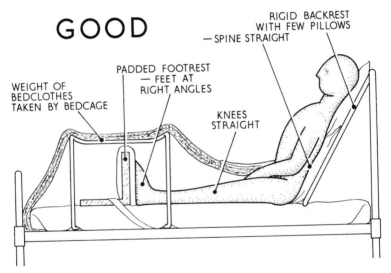

Fig. 15.4   Bed posture in rheumatoid arthritis.

CHRONIC CASES

Surgical intervention may be necessary on individual joints. The joint can be opened in the theatre and the thickened synovial membrane removed (*synovectomy*). This is successful in relieving pain and restoring some mobility to the joint.

When the patient is unable to undertake his usual occupation, he may be eligible for various training schemes and rehabilitation courses. Every effort should be made to enable patients to maintain their independence and if possible to sustain some wage earning capacity, and not to feel abandoned.

Ankylosing spondylitis

This condition appears to be similar in many respects to rheumatoid arthritis but it affects the spinal column and is much commoner in men than in women.

Signs and symptoms

1. It begins with constitutional symptoms of loss of weight and general malaise.

2. There is usually low back pain, associated with restriction of mobility of the spinal column and diminished chest expansion.

3. As the disease progresses, the spine becomes more fixed and rigid ('poker' back). The head is held in a fixed position and chest expansion is so restricted that breathlessness may result on exertion. The patient complains of persistent back pain and severe limitation of movement.

4. X-ray of the spine shows that the vertebrae have fused into one rigid bony column ('bamboo' spine).

Treatment

Treatment is symptomatic. As with rheumatoid arthritis, phenyl-butazone or prednisolone may help to reduce the discomfort. Deep X-ray therapy often relieves pain and increases mobility, but unhappily this treatment has been shown to lead to leukaemia in some cases.

GOUT

Gout, like diabetes, is a disorder of metabolism. It is an upset of the metabolism of certain types of protein called purines, which are present in the tissue cells. These purines break down to uric acid and in gout such excessive amounts are produced that deposits of uric acid and urates settle in the joints and cartilages.

Symptoms and signs

1. Gout often occurs in people who have taken alcohol in excess and have lived on rich foods.

2. Acute attacks of severe pain in the joints occur. The big toe joint is characteristically affected, becoming swollen, red and extremely tender.

3. The patient is very irritable and restless from the severe pain.

4. In between the acute attacks lesser degrees of pain and discomfort in the joints occur, and a chronic arthritis of the affected joints develops.

5. Characteristic tophi occur in the lobes of the ears and around the finger joints. These are nodules of soft cheesy urates which often ulcerate.

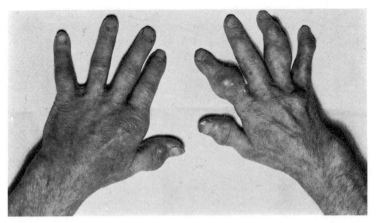

FIG. 15.5   Chronic gout showing the appearance of the hands with swelling and deformity of the joints.

Treatment

1. IN THE ACUTE STAGE. Colchicum is the best drug for relieving the pain of acute gout. It can be given either as a tincture in 15 minim doses or in tablet form (0·5 mg) every four hours. It can also be combined with salicylates to advantage. Phenylbutazone (Butazolidin) has also proved effective in the treatment of acute gout in 400 to 600 mg doses daily. The danger with phenyl-butazone is its toxic effects, particularly agranulocytosis (p. 358). In very severe attacks of gout, cortisone and allied drugs have proved very effective.

The affected joint should be protected from injury by a bed cradle and by wrapping in warm wool.

2. IN THE CHRONIC STAGE. Allopurinol (Zyloric) is a drug which prevents excessive breakdown of purines to uric acid. If taken regularly, it prevents attacks of gout by keeping uric acid levels in the blood normal.

It is important for gouty patients not to be overweight and a reducing diet should be planned accordingly. Alcohol should be taken only in moderation.

OSTEOARTHRITIS

This is an extremely common form of arthritis mainly seen in people over 40 years of age. It is often called a degenerative, as opposed to an infectious, joint disease. The exact cause is unknown, but there are several factors which may play a part in producing the disease. Trauma, often only trivial, may initiate the arthritis, and strain from obesity, which is commonly present with this disease, is also important. The weight-bearing joints of the lower limbs are most frequently affected, especially the knees and hips. In these patients degenerative changes in the terminal finger joints may also cause the nodular swellings (*Herberden's nodes*) which are so often seen.

This form of arthritis differs from the other type common in adults (rheumatoid arthritis), in that the disease remains a local affection of the joint and causes little general constitutional disturbance. The patients complain of pain and swelling of the joint with limitation of movement, so that getting about may be difficult.

The best treatment is rest, with calcium aspirin to relieve pain. Reduction of weight is very important when the patient is obese. Heat applied to the joint is sometimes helpful and when the pain is not relieved by these measures, intra-articular injections of hydrocortisone or prednisolone are particularly effective, especially for the knee. Physiotherapy may be helpful in strengthening muscle movement and in regaining movement when the joint pain has subsided.

Particularly with the hip joint in older patients, surgical replacement of the joint by an artificial joint restores mobility and relieves pain when the arthritis was previously incapacitating.

OTHER TYPES OF ARTHRITIS

1. Traumatic arthritis

Injury to a joint is one of the commonest causes of arthritis, and this form is fully described in surgical textbooks. Trauma, even of a trivial nature, may also cause a predisposition to other forms of arthritis as will be seen when osteoarthritis is discussed.

2. Specific infective arthritis

Arthritis caused by known specific organisms is usually classed as infective arthritis. There are many different forms of this type of arthritis, and as some of them are rare only the more common forms will be mentioned.

(*a*) *Acute septic arthritis.* Pyogenic organisms such as streptococci, staphylococci and pneumococci may gain entrance to a joint either by direct invasion or by blood stream infection. Usually one joint only is affected; the result is acute severe inflammation with swelling, tenderness and pain in the joint. Pus may be present.

The general condition is, in most cases, that of a severely ill toxic person with high fever and often with rigors. The treatment is an intensive course of one of the antibiotic drugs such as penicillin, tetracycline or chloromycetin. If the condition does not rapidly improve surgical drainage by aspiration or incision into the joint is necessary.

(*b*) *Tuberculous arthritis.* This form of arthritis is usually seen in young adults and tends to affect one joint only, such as the hip or elbow joint. The tuberculous infection may spread into the surrounding muscles and tissues to form an abscess. This abscess has several special features in that it travels to the surface to break down and form a chronic sinus. Because it is unlike the abscess due to a pyogenic infection, of which increased local heat is always a feature, a tuberculous abscess is often called a '*cold abscess*'.

The diagnosis of tuberculosis as the infective agent is most important as for this form prolonged rest with streptomycin is necessary. X-ray examination of the joint is very valuable in determining the diagnosis.

(*c*) *Gonococcal arthritis.* The gonococcus often causes a generalised arthritis affecting several joints, including the knee, elbow and temporo-mandibular. Generally there is a history of a recent attack of gonorrhoea, and blood tests may be positive for the gonococcal infection. General constitutional symptoms, including fever, are present. Penicillin is given, which has a very good effect. Later, active massage and heat treatment are given.

(*d*) *Syphilitic arthritis.* Syphilis does not often cause a direct infection of the joints, any involvement of the latter usually being due to spread from syphilitic disease of bones or a result of syphilitic neurological diseases (see Charcot's joints).

Congenital syphilis, however, often causes a chronic swelling in both knee-joints (Clutton's joints).

3. Joint neuropathies

In some diseases of the central nervous system the sensory nerves from the joints and muscles are affected, leading to loss of the sensation of pain. Because they cause no pain, repeated trivial injuries or strain may then be incurred without being noticed, with consequent extensive damage to the joints. The arthritis produced is a form of osteoarthritis, except that it is much more severe, resulting in almost complete destruction of the joint. This is grossly swollen and can be moved into many abnormal positions without any pain.

Charcot, the great French neurologist, was the first to describe this form of arthritis in neurological disease and so it is usually called 'Charcot's joint'. Generally Charcot's joints occur in tabes dorsalis, due to syphilis. They sometimes occur in diabetes and in the less common disease, syringomyelia.

4. Deficiency diseases and arthritis

In scurvy haemorrhages occur around the joints, causing swelling and pain. In rickets arthritis is not common, the ligaments and bones being primarily affected.

INTERVERTEBRAL DISCS

The intervertebral discs lie between the bodies of the vertebrae to permit mobility of the spinal column. The discs act as cushions and they are composed of a tough outer rim of cartilage and fibres enclosing a soft compressible pulpy centre. Under conditions of considerable strain, the outer rim is weakened and the centre prolapses out to form a bulge. This is known as a prolapsed disc. The prolapsed disc may bulge into the vertebral canal and so compress the spinal canal and the nerve roots lying in it. Thus a prolapsed cervical disc may press on the nerves to the arms while a prolapsed lumbar disc may affect the sciatic nerves to the legs.

Prolapsed lumbar disc

This very common disorder is often the result of heavy lifting or unwonted exercise such as digging the garden. The patient may be seized with sudden severe pain across the lower back ('lumbago' as it used to be called). He can walk only with extreme discomfort and may have difficulty in straightening himself. The pain may pass into the buttock, down the back of the thigh and into the leg due to pressure on the sciatic nerve ('sciatica'). In other cases, the patient may suffer a series of milder attacks of back pain, until the back becomes continually stiff and painful. X-ray of the spine shows narrowing of the space occupied by the disc between the vertebral bodies.

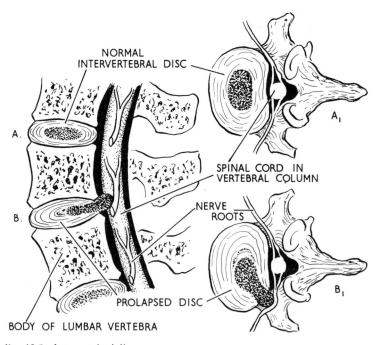

Fig. 15.6 Intervertebral discs.

Treatment

The best treatment in the acute case is rest in bed on a firm mattress supported by boards. Soluble aspirin can be given to relieve pain, and sometimes traction is applied to the legs by means of weights hung over the end of the bed. Most patients respond to simple rest and analgesics, and can gradually be restored to activity by slow stages. In the more chronic cases a spinal support or surgical corset can be worn; this offers support to the back and prevents the patient from making movements which might exacerbate the discomfort. In rare cases pressure on the spinal cord may require surgical intervention; the prolapsed part of the disc is then removed.

Prolapsed cervical disc

The onset may be sudden with severe pain in the neck passing down into the arms. The patient usually holds the head to one side and is afraid to make a movement which might bring on the pain. In elderly patients the condition may develop more gradually, with symptoms of pain, tingling and numbness in the arms and fingers.

Treatment

In the acute phase rest in bed is essential, with the head and neck placed in a comfortable position by the use of several firm pillows. Later, the neck can be immobilised by a plastic or rubber collar which can be worn when the patient is up and about. Analgesics such as aspirin may be needed in the acute phase, and neck traction is some-times helpful.

CONNECTIVE TISSUE

Collagen disease

Collagen is protein material and is the most important component of connective tissue. In a group of rare diseases, known as collagen diseases, disintegration of collagen fibres occurs. Since collagen fibres are widespread throughout the body, particularly in the skin and blood vessels, these diseases give rise to many varied manifestations. The presence of antibodies in the blood suggests that these ailments are due to a disorder of the immunity system. The body forms antibodies against its own collagen tissues which are thereby destroyed.

Disseminated lupus erythematosis

This disease occurs mainly in young women and is characterised by severe constitutional changes.

1. There is often a raised temperature and a high sedimentation rate.
2. A red skin rash appears on the cheeks and the trunk.
3. There may be pleurisy or pericarditis.

4. The kidneys may be involved with protein and red cells in the urine, suggesting nephritis.

The diagnosis is suspected by the clinical features and confirmed by finding an antinuclear factor (ANF) in the blood.

Treatment

Steroids in large doses such as prednisone 60 mg daily, suppress the symptoms but do not necessarily prolong life if the kidneys are seriously affected.

Polyarteritis nodosa

This ailment is commoner in men than women and usually comes on later in life. Widespread inflammation of small arteries give rise to constitutional features of sweating, malaise and tachycardia. Thrombosis of these small arteries can damage any organ in the body and can lead to complications such as coronary thrombosis, nephritis or neuritis.

The lungs are commonly affected, giving rise to recurrent attacks of breathlessness and patchy pneumonia.

The disease may run a protracted course and particularly when the kidneys are involved, may end fatally.

The diagnosis is made by the clinical features and a high sedimentation rate. A biopsy can be taken from a muscle in the thigh and examination under the microscope may show typical changes in the small arteries in the muscle.

Treatment

Steroids will suppress the symptoms and prevent further thromboses.

Temporal arteritis

This ailment is commonest in elderly women and is due to inflammation of the arteries, particularly of the temporal and ophthalmic arteries.

The illness starts with malaise, temperature and head pains over the scalp and the temples. There is often mental confusion. Most importantly involvement of the ophthalmic arteries may lead to loss of vision.

The diagnosis is usually obvious on clinical grounds but can be confirmed by performing a biopsy of the temporal artery. The surgeon ties the artery and removes a small segment for examination under the microscope. Typical changes of inflammation in the artery are found.

Treatment

Steroids must be given immediately since this not only relieves the symptoms but also protects the eyes.

Polymyalgia rheumatica

This is a disease of the elderly characterised by malaise, fever and tenderness and stiffness in the muscles. The sedimentation rate is very high. The condition responds to steroids.

Systemic sclerosis (scleroderma)

This is a chronic ailment in which there is a gradual hardening and tightening of the skin, ultimately leading to disabling contractures of the limbs. Treatment is of no avail.

FIBROSITIS—RHEUMATISM

Fibrositis and muscular rheumatism are terms used to describe recurring pains and stiffness in the muscles or in the back, various parts of the body being involved from time to time. The disease does not progress and often such vague symptoms are attributable to emotional upsets. In the absence of any precise cause for the discomfort, treatment is symptomatic. Heat and massage may be helpful, and aspirin can be prescribed.

DISEASES OF THE BONES

Diseases of the bones are of much greater importance in surgery than in medicine. This is because the most common bone lesions are injuries, tumours and infections, all of which come under the scope of surgical diseases. Many of the diseases of the bones which are seen in medicine are rare and only a brief mention of the more important and interesting of these diseases will be made.

1. The changes in the bones in acromegaly, gigantism, rickets osteomalacia and in the rare but interesting disease of the parathyroid glands known as osteitis fibrosa cystica have all already been described.

2. *Osteoporosis* means thinning of the bones and is due not only to lack of calcium but also to a deficient protein structure on which the calcium is laid down. It is very common in old age and in bed-ridden patients, and can be caused by excessive cortisone. It gives rise to pain in the back and down the legs, and X-ray may reveal actual collapse of the thinned vertebral bodies.

Since exercise strengthens the bones, it is important not to allow these patients to stay in bed too long. Extra milk and cheese should be given in the diet, and calcium lactate may be taken as well. Oestrogen hormones may also be prescribed.

3. *Osteomalacia* means softening of the bones due to lack of calcium in the bones. It is due to (a) lack of vitamin D in the diet (p. 396), (b) malabsorption of food and vitamins due to disorders of the bowel (p. 234). The bones are liable to fracture, particularly in the pelvis. Early symptoms are those of pain and muscle weakness. The gait is waddling. The condition usually responds to high doses of vitamin

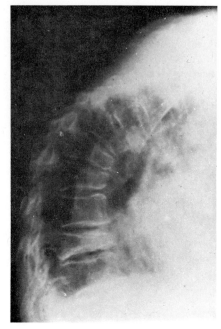

FIG. 15.7   Osteoporosis of the spine, showing compression and collapse of several vertebrae.

D or calciferol. The fractures heal and there is a marked improvement in muscle strength.

4. Fracture of a bone resulting not from any injury but from disease in the bone is known as a *pathological* fracture. The commonest cause of pathological fractures is malignant secondary deposits (*metastases*) which have spread from a primary malignant growth in some organ or tissue to the bones by way of the blood stream. Carcinomas of the prostate, breast and thyroid gland are particularly liable to give rise to secondary deposits in the bones with consequential necrosis (destruction) of the bone.

5. In *multiple myelomatosis* there is widespread invasion of the bones by deposits of myeloma cells. The condition is progressive and fatal. The patient usually complains of severe pains in the bones and a profound degree of anaemia is often present. Spontaneous fractures are common.

6. *Osteitis deformans*, otherwise known as *Paget's disease* of the bones, is perhaps one of the most common bone diseases. The cause is unknown, but it leads to progressive thickening and deformities of the bones, especially the skull, tibia, femur, spine and pelvis. The disease occurs after the age of 40, and men are more frequently

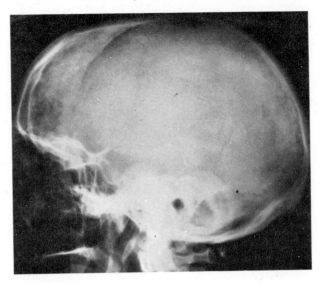

Fig. 15.8   X-ray of a normal skull.

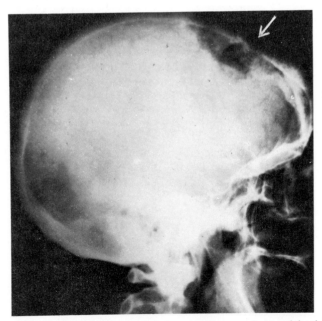

Fig. 15.9   Secondary deposits in the skull from a primary carcinoma of the thyroid. The bone is being eaten away by the malignant tissue.

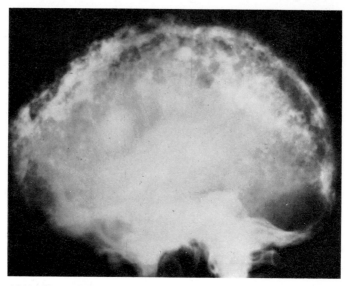

FIG. 15.10   X-ray of the skull in Paget's disease, showing the marked thickening and sclerosis of the bone.

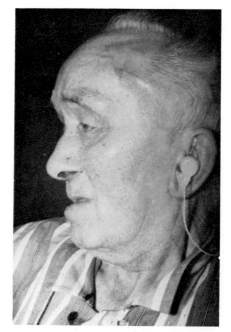

FIG. 15.11   Paget's disease showing large skull. This often leads to deafness.

affected than women. The head becomes enlarged so that an increasing size in hats is needed. The legs become bowed and thickened and the spine curved so that the height is reduced. X-ray examination reveals the typical thickening of the bones. In severe cases, injections of calcitonin usually relieves symptoms of pain.

7. In *achondroplasia* abnormality of the bones in fetal life leads to short limbs, normal trunk and large head. These people are usually dwarfs and are characteristically very good humoured. Most of the dwarf clowns seen in a circus are examples of achondroplasia.

8. In the rare bone disease known as *fragilitas ossium (osteogenesis imperfecta)* the extraordinary fragility of the bones results in recurrent fractures, leading to gross deformities. This disease occurs in infancy and is due to a hereditary defect in bone development. Many of these patients have characteristic blue sclerotics of the eyes.

16 Diseases of the Skin

In a general textbook of medicine it is impossible to give a comprehensive account of all skin diseases. It is therefore intended to mention here only the commoner of the diseases of the skin that the nurse is likely to meet with in a general hospital.

Before dealing with the individual skin disease a brief word on the general terms used in describing different types of skin lesion is perhaps useful:

1. *Macules* are flat spots which are not raised above the skin and are usually red or brown in colour.
2. *Papules* are small raised skin lesions.
3. *Vesicles* are very small blisters filled with clear serous fluid.
4. *Bullae* are large vesicles.
5. *Pustules* are vesicles filled with pus instead of serous fluid.
6. *Wheals* are areas of skin swollen by oedema so that they are a white colour with a red margin.
7. *Scaling* is caused by dead epithelium of the skin flaking off, usually as a result of inflammation of the skin.
8. *Weeping* in skin lesions arises when there is marked exudation of serum or lymph from the skin. It is usually the result of acute or subacute inflammatory lesions.
9. *Crusts* or *scabs* usually result from the drying up of the serum in weeping lesions.

Many other terms are also used in skin diseases, but these are generally self-explanatory.

GENERAL PRINCIPLES OF TREATMENT

In addition to the various specific treatments used in diseases of the skin there are certain general principles applicable to most skin lesions.

1. Remove the cause

It is essential to remove the cause of the skin disease if possible, e.g. stop any drug which may be causing the skin eruption, remove any offending articles either in the diet or coming in contact with the skin, or kill any parasite.

2. External applications

External applications play a large part in the treatment of skin diseases. The following are the applications most commonly used.

(a) POWDERS. These are used on slightly moist areas to dry the skin. They are also useful in preventing friction on the skin. Talc and zinc oxide are powders in frequent use.

(b) LOTIONS. Lotions are widely used, particularly for weeping lesions. Calamine lotion is a very commonly used preparation. Lotions are best applied by dabbing them on with lint. Sedatives, e.g. phenol, to allay itching may be combined with the lotion, as also may antiseptic preparations, e.g. ichthyol.

(c) CREAMS AND LINIMENTS. These are mainly used in weeping and inflamed areas of skin. They should be smeared on or applied on gauze.

(d) OINTMENTS AND PASTES. These preparations are applied when there is no excessive weeping. Pastes are most useful for subacute slightly moist lesions, while ointments are preferred for the more chronic scaling lesions. When ointments or pastes are applied, the removal of the old application should be effected by swabbing with cotton-wool soaked in oil in order to prevent damage to the under-lying skin. Ointments and pastes should be thickly applied and as little covering as possible used. Lassar's paste is a most effective and frequently used paste.

(e) POULTICES. Boric and starch poultices are mostly used in skin diseases for removing thick crusts. Fomentations are used for septic skin lesions.

3. Cold, heat and radiation

These are all frequently used in the treatment of diseases of the skin. Cold, usually in the form of carbon dioxide snow, is used in the removal of warts and naevi; heat, often in the form of a cautery, is also used to remove warts and naevi, whilst radiation in various forms, such as ultraviolet light, thorium X, superficial X-rays and radium, is used in a wide variety of skin diseases.

4. Antibiotics

Antibiotics, e.g. the tetracyclines and neomycin are used in the treatment of skin diseases due to infection. Streptomycin is given for tuberculosis of the skin. Because sensitisation is very likely to develop, penicillin and chloramphenicol are not used for local application.

5. Steroids

Cortisone and allied steroids are given with good effect in several severe skin diseases such as exfoliative dermatitis, dermatomyositis and disseminated lupus erythematosis. Steroids are also used in the form of sprays, creams and ointments for the treatment of local areas of eczema, sensitivity dermatitis and pruritus.

SKIN DISEASES DUE TO STREPTOCOCCAL AND STAPHYLOCOCCAL INFECTION

IMPETIGO

Impetigo is a very common skin disease, which is most frequently met with in infants and young children. It is caused by infection of the skin by staphylococci or streptococci.

Features of the eruption

1. The eruption usually starts on the face, especially around the mouth and behind the ears, and may spread to the scalp.

2. Vesicles form in the first stage, which later develop into crusts of a yellowish colour. These crusts are typically described as having a 'stuck-on' appearance.

Treatment

Impetigo is very contagious and can spread rapidly in a nursery or ward. Children affected must be isolated until cured, and a careful watch kept for new cases.

Loose crusts can be removed by simple bathing, but starch poultices may need to be applied where the crusting is very thick. An antibiotic cream such as neomycin or tetracycline should then be applied to the decrusted areas and this usually leads to healing in a few days. In extensive cases a swab should be taken to establish the organism responsible and the appropriate antibiotic given by mouth.

SYCOSIS

Sycosis is an infection of the hair follicles of the beard region by the staphylococcus. Sycosis is, with impetigo, often included in the term *barber's rash* because infection is often acquired at the barber's.

Features of the eruption

1. The common sites are the upper lip and chin, but in severe cases the lesions rapidly spread all over the beard region.

2. There is generalised redness of the area with small pustules surrounding each hair follicle. A weeping pustular rash soon develops.

3. The condition is very liable to become chronic and resistant to treament.

Treatment

Sycosis is very resistant to treatment and relapses are very prone to occur necessitating prolonged therapy. During the active stage shaving is stopped, the hair being kept short by clipping. As many as possible of the pustular hair follicles are removed.

An antibiotic ointment such as neomycin is applied to the affected areas and also to the nose as this is often the source of the infection.

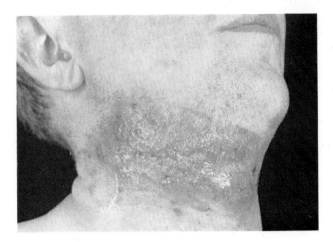

Fig. 16.1   Sycosis.

Since the organisms tend to become resistant, the ointment should be changed at intervals.

Furunculosis (boils)

Furunculosis, caused by infection of the hair follicles with staphylococci, is usually seen in debilitated people. Furunculosis is particularly prone to be found together with diabetes. Areas subject to irritation such as the back of the neck are frequent sites. The typical lesion is the presence of multiple boils. In severe cases the boils may become carbuncles.

Penicillin usually clears up the condition. The general health of the patient must be attended to, and the urine should always be examined for the presence of sugar.

SKIN DISEASES DUE TO ANIMAL PARASITES

SCABIES

Scabies is a very common contagious skin disease caused by the female parasite the *Acarus scabiei* (itch mite). This parasite burrows into the skin where it lays its eggs. The eggs hatch out, and then the small mites in their turn burrow through the skin, causing the typical eruption.

Close contact with an infected person is necessary to spread infection. Furthermore, the acarus usually burrows at night. Infection is therefore usually contracted by sleeping with an infected person.

Features of the eruption

1. The typical eruption is the burrow which is commonest in the

webs of the fingers, and on the wrists, axillae and buttocks. The acarus may often be seen, with the aid of a hand lens, as a tiny white speck at the end of the burrow. In some cases, if the point of a needle is inserted into the burrow, the acarus will adhere to the needle and the mite can then be identified under the microscope.

2. Owing to the severe itching, at night especially, a red papular eruption with scratch marks is always present. Secondary infection is also very liable to occur, with the result that impetigo is often present too.

3. Scabies is very liable to affect several people in the same household as it is a contagious disease.

Treatment

The usual treatment is with benzyl benzoate emulsion, which is applied all over the body from the neck downwards, the patient having first had a hot bath and thoroughly scrubbed all the lesions to lay open the burrows. The benzyl benzoate emulsion dries in about ten minutes. A second application is often applied on the next day.

PEDICULOSIS

Three kinds of lice infect man—the head, the body and the crab lice. Infestation with lice occurs through lack of cleanliness.

1. *Pediculus capitis* (head louse). Infestation with head lice is particularly common in children, especially girls. The eggs of the louse, the nits, become firmly attached to the hairs. The lice feed on blood, and the bites of the lice cause severe persistent itching; the consequent scratching generally results in infected lesions, such as impetigo. The cervical glands of the neck are usually enlarged.

There are many successful forms of treatment for head lice. Gamma benzene hexachloride (lorexane) is effective when massaged into the scalp. The hair should be combed after 24 hours. A week later, the hair should be washed and the treatment repeated.

2. *Pediculus corporis* (body louse). Infection with body lice is usually confined to people who neglect proper cleanliness, and is particularly common in tramps or in overcrowded conditions with a lack of proper hygiene, e.g. in camps in time of war. The body louse lives in the seams of the underclothes and feeds by biting the person. The itching leads to severe scratch marks, particularly on the shoulders. The bites of the lice are seen as small red macules.

Apart from the severe irritation and secondary skin infections caused by body lice, these parasites transmit such important diseases as typhus and relapsing fever.

The treatment consists of the application of 10 per cent DDT powder to the underclothes. Hot ironing of the seams of the clothes will kill off all the lice. The provision of adequate water supplies for washing and laundering in all camps is an essential preventive measure.

3. *Pediculus pubis* (crab louse). *Pediculus pubis* generally affects the pubic region and anus, but also affects the axillae. Infestation is most frequently acquired during sexual intercourse. Severe irritation, with scratch marks, occurs as a result of the bites of the lice.

DDT powder or emulsion thoroughly applied to the affected parts is usually very efficacious; so also is benzyl benzoate, applied as in scabies.

DISEASES DUE TO FUNGI

Fungus infections of the skin are very common. The stomatitis seen in infants and known as *thrush* is due to a fungus infection.

INTERTRIGO

A fungus (monilia) is often responsible for the condition known as intertrigo. This is a moist papular red eruption commonly seen in areas of friction, e.g. under the breasts in women, and in the groins, axillae and natal cleft.

Nystatin ointment or cream is effective in clearing up the infection. In prevention, frequent bathing and keeping the areas as dry as possible by the use of powder are important.

RINGWORM

Ringworm or tinea is due to various fungi, which may affect the skin, hair or nails.

1. Ringworm of the skin

Ringworm usually affects such sites as the feet, groins, beard region and hands.

(a) *Ringworm of the feet* is extremely common and causes a sodden white maceration of the skin between the toes. Infection is probably spread through bath mats or wet floors in bathrooms. The commonly seen thickened skin (hyperkeratosis) of the heel is also due to ringworm infection.

(b) *Ringworm of the groins* (*Tinea cruris*) is usually referred to as 'dhobie itch'. It causes a red inflamed irritating eruption in the groins, which often spreads to the natal cleft. Like all ringworm infections it usually flares up in hot weather owing to the increased sweating.

(c) *Ringworm of the beard* (*Tinea barbae*) is usually contracted at the barber's and is the third type of 'barber's rash' (the other two being impetigo and sycosis). The lesions may be dry, red, scaly and ringed in appearance, or suppurative, with purplish nodules. In both types the hairs break off, leaving stumps.

(d) *Ringworm of the hands and the body* is usually in the form of red scaling lesions which heal in the centre, thus giving the characteristic ringed or circular outline from which the disease gets its name.

Ringworm of the feet and groins is treated by the application of salicylic and benzoic acid ointment (Whitfield's) or any of the many preparations available for the purpose (Mersagel, Mycozol, Tineafax). Every care must be taken to keep the parts as dry as possible. Underclothes and socks must be thoroughly boiled, and care should be taken to prevent reinfection in swimming baths and from wet floors.

Ringworm of the body and hands is similarly treated with Whitfield's ointment or such preparations as Mersagel or Tineafax. In resistant cases dithranol (Cignolin) ointment is used, but this preparation is irritating and also stains the clothes.

Ringworm of the beard may be treated by X-rays, which remove all the affected hairs, and by the use of salicylic and benzoic acid ointment.

2. Ringworm of the scalp

Ringworm of the scalp is usually seen in children. It causes a scaling bald patch on the scalp, the hairs in the affected patch breaking off just above the level of the scalp and leaving well-marked stumps. The affected hairs when examined in a dark room with Wood's light show a characteristic green fluorescence.

There is also another variety of ringworm infection of the hair which does not cause the scaling bald patches just described, namely 'black-dot' ringworm. Here a circular bald patch is seen in which the hairs are broken off close to the scalp, giving rise to the 'black-dot' appearance. In some cases of ringworm, suppuration may occur, resulting in swollen inflamed areas in which pus is present.

Ringworm of the scalp is treated by X-rays or by the antibiotic griseofulvin.

3. Ringworm of the nails

Ringworm of the nails is a very resistant infection causing rough cracked nails and scaling. There is also another type of fungus infection which causes chronic paronychia of the nails in women who constantly have their hands in water. In this form of fungus infection the nail folds become red, swollen and septic.

More recently ringworm can be successfully treated by giving the antibiotic griseofulvin (Grisovin, Fulcin) in daily doses of 1 to 2 g. Treatment may have to be continued for months till all the infected hairs or nails have been shed.

OTHER COMMON SKIN DISEASES

ACNE VULGARIS

Acne vulgaris is a skin disease which is extremely common about the age of puberty, but rarely arises after the age of 30.

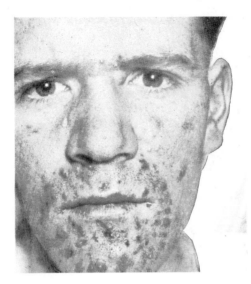

Fig. 16.2   Acne vulgaris.

Features of the eruption

The face, chest and back are the sites usually affected. The typical lesions are *blackheads* (comedones), red papules and pustules. In severe cases with much postule formation scars may develop with consequential permanent damage.

Acne occurs most frequently in people with greasy skins (seborrhoea), and dandruff (scurf, seborrhoea sicca) of the scalp is also usually present. In some cases diet may aggravate the condition, especially overindulgence in carbohydrates.

Treatment

Patients with a tendency to acne suffer from greasy skin and must therefore be discouraged from using greasy preparations on the skin. In the treatment frequent washing of the affected parts to remove the excessive grease is necessary. The application most commonly used is a sulphur lotion (often combined with calamine lotion), which must be applied for a long period. It is also essential to express as many blackheads as possible, either by hand or by the use of a special comedo extractor.

The diet should be regulated where necessary and any dandruff present must also be treated.

In resistant cases a course of chemotherapy such as tetracycline or co-trimoxazole can be given by mouth.

ACNE ROSACEA

Acne rosacea is another very common form of acne, but here the condition usually occurs after the age of 30 and is particularly common in women or in people continually exposed to the weather.

Features of the eruption

1. In acne rosacea, in contrast to acne vulgaris, there are no blackheads. The eruption characteristically starts as a redness and flushing of the nose and cheeks, which occurs particularly after hot meals or drinks. A history of dyspepsia is very common in acne rosacea, and strong tea and alcohol are predominant factors.

2. The redness and flushing of the face become permanent and dilated vessels can clearly be seen. Red papules are also frequently present, and secondary infection may lead to pustular formation.

3. In very chronic cases in men, marked enlargement and hypertrophy of the nose (*rhinophyma*) result.

Treatment

The dyspepsia must be treated and the diet adjusted. Strong tea and alcohol especially must be avoided. In some cases the dyspepsia is associated with a lack of hydrochloric acid in the gastric juice (achlorhydria), and here dilute hydrochloric acid (2 ml before meals) is useful.

Calamine lotion with the addition of 2 per cent sulphur is a very effective local application. Other useful applications include lead or ichthyol combined with calamine lotion.

PSORIASIS

The very common skin disease known as psoriasis usually starts in adult life and is very chronic, recurring over a period of many years at irregular intervals. The cause of the condition is unknown, but in many cases there is a strong familial factor. Especially where it occurs on exposed areas of the skin, psoriasis can be a source of great unhappiness.

Features of the eruption

1. The sites characteristically affected are the extensor aspects of the elbows and knees, the scalp and the trunk. The hands, particularly the nails, may also be affected, but rarely the face.

2. The typical lesion is a red papular eruption surrounded by scales which when scraped off have a silvery colour. The lesions are dry and infection rarely develops. Itching is not a feature.

3. The extent of the lesions varies considerably, from a small patch on a knee or elbow to large confluent patches covering large areas. The patches often have a circular ringed outline.

4. Psoriasis of the nails causes deep pitting in some cases, whilst in others it causes separation of the nails from the nail beds, the nail ultimately breaking off.

Chronic psoriasis is sometimes associated with arthritis involving the distal inter-phalangeal joints of the fingers and the sacro-iliac joints.

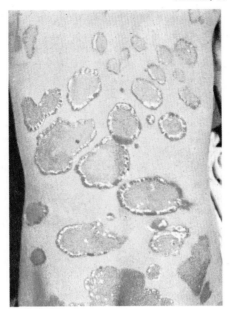

FIG. 16.3   Psoriasis.

Treatment

The presence of psoriasis on exposed areas of the skin is a source of social embarrassment, especially when shedding of scales occurs. It should be emphasised to the patient and relatives that psoriasis is not contagious and that the lesions can disappear. An active life is to be encouraged, though during an acute phase with extensive lesions, a period of bed rest may be beneficial.

Various applications may be used on the skin and most patients have favourite preparations that suit them. Calamine cream is a bland and soothing preparation for mild cases and various cortisone preparations, such as betamethasone (Betnovate) are helpful, though these must be used sparingly because of the danger of causing secondary skin infection (pustular psoriasis).

In more chronic cases, crude coal tar preparations are effective in suppressing active areas of psoriasis but they have a pervasive smell. Dithranol paste is another effective agent but is messy and time consuming to apply.

Methotrexate is an imminosuppressive drug which can inhibit the formation of psoriasis and can be administered orally or by intravenous or intramuscular injection. Although it can be very effective in severe cases, it can lead to toxic effects on the liver.

Impressive improvements in widespread psoriasis have been reported with PUVA (blacklight) treatment. The patient takes tablets of tripsoralen which sensitises the skin and two hours later is exposed to intensive longwave ultraviolet rays. The treatment is only available in special centres, it is expensive and there may be long-term dangers of inducing skin cancer.

ECZEMA

The term *eczema*, or *eczematous dermatitis*, is used to describe several varieties of skin condition which have, however, a number of common features. The exact cause or causes of eczema are imperfectly understood. In many cases eczema can be attributed to external irritants, e.g. soaps, dyes, polishes, chemicals, plants, foodstuffs, etc. Why eczema should develop in some people from contact with such substances is unknown, and it appears that there must be some other internal factor present which renders eczematous patients very sensitive to mild irritants. In support of this theory is the fact that various forms of eczema are associated with the allergic diseases like asthma and hay fever.

Features of the eruption

The many and various types of eczema have different individual features, but in most cases the skin lesions have the following general characteristics:

1. The lesion usually starts as a diffuse reddening or erythema of the skin.

2. Vesicles form on this erythema.

3. Weeping usually occurs owing to serum exuding from the vesicles, and crusts may form.

4. The condition usually becomes chronic, and in this stage dry scaling lesions with thickening and pigmentation of the skin lichenification) develop.

5. Eczematous lesions usually itch.

TYPES OF ECZEMA

It is impossible in the space available to give more than a few of the commoner types of eczema.

1. *Infantile eczema.* This form is very common in infants, particularly males under the age of 2. The face is especially affected, the eczema being weeping and crusted. Itching is usually severe.

2. *Flexural eczema* (Besnier's prurigo). Besnier's prurigo usually follows infantile eczema and is associated with asthma. The flexures of the elbows and knees are particularly prone to be affected, hence the term *flexural eczema*. The face and neck may also be affected. The lesions are usually of the chronic, thickened, lichenified type. Most but by no means all cases tend to improve after puberty.

3. *Varicose eczema.* This form is extremely common, occurring in elderly people with varicose veins and ulcers.

4. *Eczema of the hands and feet.* Eczema of the hands and feet produces a vesicular eruption which is commonly likened to sago grains in the skin. Chronic forms are very frequent in which the skin, owing to its inelasticity, becomes cracked and deep fissures

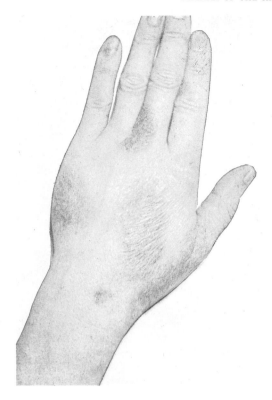

Fig. 16.4   Eczema.

form. Eczema is one cause of a vesicular dermatitis of the hands which often goes under the name of *cheiropompholyx*. Cheiropompholyx may also be caused by external irritants (soap detergents used in cleaning, polishes, dyes, chemicals, etc.) and by fungus infections (ringworm).

Treatment of eczema

The first essential is to remove any irritant which may possibly be causing the eczema. In prevention the use of barrier creams or glycerin preparations by people who continually use strong soaps or cleansing powders is very valuable. The patient's resistance must be built up and any septic focus or disease must be treated.

Local treatment is most important and the particular application depends on the stage of the eczema. In the acute weeping stage a lotion is used such as calamine or lead lotion. These should be applied on gauze or lint and as little covering as possible used. Sedatives, e.g. 1 per cent phenol or 2 per cent tar, may be added to the lotion to allay the itching. In the less acute stage an oily liniment is preferred, e.g. calamine liniment, to which 2 per cent ichthyol may be added. In the chronic stages pastes are the most useful applications, and zinc paste with the addition of tar as a stimulant, or crude coal tar itself, is commonly used.

In infantile eczema it may be necessary to prevent the child scratching the lesions by means of cardboard splints. White's tar paste is a useful application for infantile eczema and is best applied on a mask of butter muslin.

In all cases of eczema soap and water usually aggravate the skin so that their use must be forbidden as far as possible.

In severe cases of eczema which do not respond to the above measures hydrocortisone by local application in a 1 per cent ointment is often given with dramatic effects. Local application of hydrocortisone has the great advantage that it does not cause any of the side effects seen when hydrocortisone and allied drugs are given systemically. Unfortunately, in some cases after cessation of treatment, the condition may relapse.

SEBORRHOEIC DERMATITIS

Seborrhoeic dermatitis is a very common inflammation of the skin which particularly affects the scalp, backs of the ears and flexures.

Features of the eruption

1. Seborrhoeic dermatitis of the scalp in the mildest form causes the well-known condition of a scurfy head (*dandruff*). In more acute cases red weeping crusted lesions develop. The scales and crusts in seborrhoeic lesions have a typical greasy appearance.

2. Seborrhoeic dermatitis of the face produces red or yellow greasy scaling patches; it particularly affects the eyebrows, sides of the nose and ears.

3. Seborrhoeic dermatitis of the flexures mainly arises in the axillae, groins and front of the chest under the breasts. Red follicular papules are usually seen at the edge of the weeping erythematous dermatitis.

Treatment

Frequent shampooing of the scalp to remove all the scales is necessary, and a lotion containing salicylic acid is applied. In acute cases with much crusting starch and boric poultices are first used to remove the crusts.

The preparation selenium sulphide (Selsun) has also proved very effective in the treatment of seborrhoeic dermatitis of the scalp. One or two teaspoonfuls are applied to the scalp and warm water added to make a lather. The lotion is allowed to remain in contact with the scalp for five minutes, after which the hair is thoroughly rinsed. Selsun is applied twice weekly for two weeks.

For seborrhoeic dermatitis of the face and body, crusts are first removed and a soothing calamine lotion applied. In the subacute and chronic stages when the lesions are comparatively dry a sulphur and salicylic ointment is used.

URTICARIA (Nettle-rash)

The characteristic lesion in urticaria is the wheal, with pale oedematous centre and red margin similar to that caused by the sting of a nettle, hence the name 'nettle-rash' (Fig. 16.5).

Causes

Urticaria can be caused by a wide variety of different agents:
1. Following injection of serum.
2. By food, particularly shell fish, strawberries, eggs, etc.
3. By drugs, e.g. phenobarbitone, quinine, penicillin, etc.
4. By bites of insects.

In some cases the direct cause of the urticaria is unknown, and in many of these cases the urticaria is an allergic manifestation in a sensitised person. In the chronic recurring attacks of urticaria it is particularly difficult to ascertain the exciting cause.

In addition to the ordinary form of urticaria known as simple urticaria, another type called angioneurotic oedema or giant urticaria is not uncommonly seen. Here there is gross swelling of the mucous membranes, especially those of the eyes, lips and mouth, in addition to the ordinary skin lesions.

Treatment

A careful search must be made for any exciting factors. In the recurring cases which have no obvious cause a prolonged investigation may be required; nevertheless, even then in many cases, despite

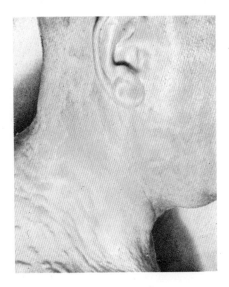

Fig. 16.5   Urticaria.

a diligent search, it may not be possible to find the exciting factor. Antihistamine drugs are very useful in relieving individual attacks. In angioneurotic oedema, adrenaline injections have a dramatic effect in relieving the gross swellings. In very severe attacks (particularly in angioneurotic oedema) which have not responded to the above treatment, cortisone and allied steroids (e.g. prednisolone) are usually given with a very beneficial effect in most cases.

ERYTHEMA NODOSUM

Erythema nodosum consists of a localised eruption with general constitutional symptoms.

CAUSE. The exact cause of erythema nodosum is still in doubt, and it is probable that the disease is either a specific fever or a manifestation of sensitisation to various organisms, particularly streptococci and tubercle bacilli. In some cases active tuberculosis or rheumatic fever have followed attacks of erythema nodosum, while in others there is associated sarcoidosis (p. 184).

Symptoms and signs

1. The onset is acute with the general constitutional symptoms of fever, including headaches, malaise and, particularly, joint pains.

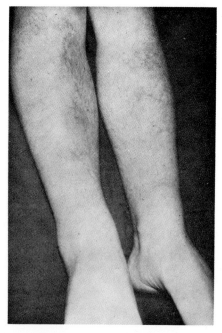

FIG. 16.6   Erythema nodosum. The raised red areas are hot and painful.

2. The localised eruption is usually on the front of the legs and consists of raised, indurated, red, tender nodes.

3. The red swellings gradually change colour like a bruise, becoming purple and yellow.

Treatment

The patient should be nursed in bed till all symptoms and signs have disappeared. This usually takes about fourteen days. No specific treatment is required as the condition subsides of its own accord. Signs of streptococcal infection, sarcoidosis or tuberculosis are carefully looked for and an X-ray of the chest is usually taken.

ERYTHEMA MULTIFORME

CAUSE

Unknown. The disease affects males much more often than females.

Symptoms and signs

1. The onset is often sudden with general constitutional upset including fever, headache, malaise and sore throat.

2. Skin rash. This often resembles measles, but usually appears on the face and the extremities. Sometimes blistering occurs.

3. Eye and mouth lesions occur, particularly conjunctivitis and stomatitis.

4. Inflammation of the genital area with ulceration is usually present.

Course and treatment

The disease has a tendency to recur from time to time. It is believed that erythema multiforme may sometimes occur as a toxic reaction to certain drugs or as an allergic condition. Severe forms of erythema multiforme with blistering and ulceration are often known as Steven-Johnson's syndrome. Cortisone or its allies are given with good effect.

TUBERCULOSIS OF THE SKIN

There are very many different types of tuberculous skin lesion, and it is possible here to mention only the more important forms.

Lupus vulgaris

Lupus vulgaris is the main type of skin tuberculosis. It is a chronic and slowly progressive lesion which usually starts on the face and neck. The characteristic lesion is the 'apple-jelly' nodule, which is composed of miliary tubercles. As the skin lesion spreads it causes severe ulceration of the skin. The mucous membranes of the nose and mouth are frequently affected, and in these cases the ultimate effect of severe lupus is serious deformity of the nose and mouth with ulceration and scarring.

Syphilis in the tertiary stage may cause severe deformity of the face with ulceration similar to that caused by lupus vulgaris. In syphilitic cases, however, the common deformity is destruction of the bridge of the nose, producing the well-described 'saddle-nose,' whereas in tuberculous lesions the tip of the nose is mainly affected.

Another type of skin disease which has to be distinguished from lupus vulgaris is *discoid lupus erythematosus*. Discoid lupus erythematosus is also a chronic and progressive disease, commonest on the face and causing fine scarring. In these cases, however, no deep ulceration is present, and the characteristic lesion is a red scaling patch which leaves a fine scar in the centre when the lesion heals. Sometimes the local condition spreads to the whole system, when it is known as disseminated lupus erythematosus.

Lupus vulgaris is treated by a prolonged course of chemotherapy as for all forms of active tuberculosis (p. 182), and in some cases also by calciferol.

Bazin's disease (erythema induratum)

Bazin's disease is another form, most frequently seen in young women, of tuberculosis of the skin. Hard subcutaneous nodules develop on the back of the lower half of the legs. The nodules, which are purple in colour, may break down, forming ulcers which leave deep scars when they heal. In many of these cases there are signs of tuberculosis elsewhere, particularly tuberculous glands.

ALOPECIA AREATA

Alopecia means loss of hair, and may be caused by a variety of conditions. The common form of senile baldness, which affects men particularly, is well known. Loss of hair may also occur in young men where there is a strong hereditary factor. Seborrhoea capitis (dandruff) too is an important factor in causing early loss of hair. Ringworm of the scalp causes bald scaly patches, but this variety is usually met with in children.

Alopecia areata is a common form of baldness which occurs in young people and is rare after the age of 40. The cause is unknown, although endocrine disturbances or anxiety states are supposed to play a part. In many cases the onset is abrupt, with a bald patch developing overnight. The skin in these patches is completely smooth, with no scaling or inflammation. In some cases complete loss of hair may result, affecting all parts of the body.

Most cases of alopecia areata recover completely after varying lengths of time. Any possible causative factor must be investigated and the general health built up. Regrowth of the hair may be hastened in many cases by the use of ultraviolet light.

Appendix

POISONS AND CONTROLLED DRUGS

The increasing use of powerful, addictive and potentially dangerous drugs has made it important for every nurse to understand the legal restrictions on the supply, storage and use of such drugs. The Poisons Act requires strict control of certain specified poisons and describes the records to be kept, the type of container to be used and the information that must appear on the label.

The Poisons List has two main schedules, one referring to common poisons such as household disinfectants, and the other to poisons and drugs which can be supplied to the public only by qualified pharmacists. In hospitals these drugs are supplied from the pharmacy for individual patients on medical prescription and can only be provided from ward stocks on a signed order from Sister or nurse-in-charge. Drugs specified in these schedules must be stored in the ward in a locked poison cupboard apart from other drugs and the key must be kept on the person of the Ward Sister or deputy. Poison cupboards are inspected at intervals by the hospital pharmacist. Examples of drugs in these schedules are:

1. Certain preparations of atropine and belladonna
2. Barbiturates
3. Codeine
4. Colchicum
5. Digitalis and digoxin
6. Mersalyl
7. Antihistamine drugs
8. Sulphonamides
9. Phenylbutazone (Butazolidin)
10. Anti-depressants such as amitriptyline
11. Chlorpromazine (Largactil)
12. Meprobamate (Equinal)
13. Hypoglycaemic tablets such as tolbutamide, chlorpropamide and phenformin
14. Oestrogens and androgens.

CONTROLLED DRUGS

Controlled drugs are those liable to misuse and addiction and their use is regulated by the Misuse of Drugs Act.

Some common medicines, such as cough linctuses, contain only small and harmless amounts of controlled drugs and may be obtained without prescription (Schedule 1). Schedule 2 enumerates important drugs which can be dangerous or addictive if misused and includes such drugs as:—

Morphine	Pethidine
Omnopon	Cocaine
Nepenthe	Methadone (Physeptone)
Heroin	Amphetamines (Benzidrine and Dexidrine)

Prescriptions relating to these drugs must be signed by the doctor with his full signature, the date and the number of doses to be given. One of the persons concerned in the administration of these drugs must be a State Registered nurse and each dose must be checked before administration by a second nurse. A record of each dose given is made in a special register. The entry must state the name of the patient, the date on which the drug was given, the name of the drug, the dose and the time at which it was administered. Both the person giving the drug and the witness must sign the register, which must be kept for two years after the date of the last entry.

Controlled drugs must be stored in a special cupboard which must be kept locked and the key kept by a State registered nurse. The drugs must be checked at frequent intervals. Fresh supplies can be obtained only on a signed medical order, and the pharmacist supplying the drugs is given a receipt after checking the drugs with the nurse.

THE METRIC SYSTEM AND THE IMPERIAL SYSTEM

The old Imperial system of measures has been replaced by the Metric system. However, since the Imperial system is still occasionally used, equivalents are included for guidance.

WEIGHTS

Metric system	Imperial system
1 mg = 0·001 g	60 grains (gr.) = 1 drachm (ʒ i)
50 mg = 0·05 g	8 drachms = 1 ounce (℥ i)
100 mg = 0·1 g	16 ounces = 1 pound (lb)
500 mg = 0·5 g	14 pounds = 1 stone (st.)
1000 mg = 1 g	
1000 g = 1 kg	

The abbreviation for milligrams is mg; for grams, g; and for kilograms, kg.

VOLUME

1000 ml = 1 litre	60 minims (min.) = 1 fluid drachm (fl. dr.)
A millilitre (ml) is the same as a	8 fluid drachms = 1 fluid ounce (fl. oz)
cubic centimetre (cm³)	20 fluid ounces = 1 pint

METRIC DOSES WITH APPROXIMATE IMPERIAL EQUIVALENTS WEIGHTS

1 mg = $\frac{1}{60}$ gr. (grain)	250 mg = 4 gr.
10 mg = $\frac{1}{6}$ gr.	1 g = 15 gr.
15 mg = $\frac{1}{4}$ gr.	4 g = 60 gr. (1 drachm)
30 mg = $\frac{1}{2}$ gr.	30 g = 1 oz
60 mg = 1 gr.	1 kg = 2·2 lb
100 mg = $1\frac{1}{2}$ gr.	

VOLUME

1 ml or 1 cm³ = 15 minims	550 ml = 1 pint
4 ml = 1 drachm	1 litre = 35 fl. oz
30 ml = 1 fl. oz	

APPROXIMATE VALUE OF DOMESTIC MEASURES

1 teaspoon = 4 ml = 1 dr.	1 eggcup = 30 ml = 1 oz
1 dessertspoon = 8 ml = $\frac{1}{4}$ oz	1 teacup = 150 ml = 5 oz
1 tablespoon = 16 ml = $\frac{1}{2}$ oz	1 tumbler = 300 ml = $\frac{1}{2}$ pint

Domestic measures vary widely and are too inexact for measuring medicines unless so stated.

CONVERSION FAHRENHEIT TO CENTIGRADE TABLES (APPROXIMATE)

Fahrenheit	Centigrade	Fahrenheit	Centigrade
86	30	99	37·2
87	30·5	99·2	37·3
88	31·1	99·4	37·4
89	31·7	99·6	37·5
90	32·2	99·8	37·7
91	32·8	100	37·8
92	33·3	100·2	37·9
93	33·9	100·4	38
94	34·4	100·6	38·1
95	35	100·8	38·2
96	35·5	101	38·3
96·2	35·7	101·2	38·4
96·4	35·8	101·4	38·5
96·6	35·9	101·6	38·7
96·8	36	101·8	38·8
97	36·1	102	38·9
97·2	36·2	102·2	39
97·4	36·3	102·6	39·2
97·6	36·5	103	39·4
97·8	36·6	104	40
98	36·7	105	40·6
98·2	36·8	106	41·1
98·4	36·9	107	41·7
98·6	37	108	42·2
98·8	37·1		

SI UNITS (Système International d'Unités)

The internationally agreed version of the metric system is known as the Système International. Its use will ensure that quantities expressed in metric units will be stated in the same manner in different disciplines. Metric units are already used for drug dosages and this principle has been extended to expressing the results of laboratory tests.

There is an additional SI unit called the mole, which is the measure of the amount of substances present in solution. It can be estimated by dividing the number of grams present per litre by the molecular weight of the substance. Thus the molecular weight of glucose is 180 so that a blood glucose of 180 mg per 100 ml is expressed as 10 mmol/l (10 millimoles per litre).

SI units in nutrition

The energy value of food is expressed in joules instead of calories:

$$1 \text{ calorie} = 4 \cdot 2 \text{ kilojoules (kJ)}$$

APPROXIMATE VALUES

$$800 \text{ calories} = 3500 \text{ kJ } (3 \cdot 5 \text{ megajoules, MJ})$$
$$1000 \text{ calories} = 4000 \text{ kJ } (4 \text{ MJ})$$
$$1500 \text{ calories} = 6000 \text{ kJ } (6 \text{ MJ})$$
$$2500 \text{ calories} = 10,000 \text{ kJ } (10 \text{ MJ})$$

Calorie intake is referred to as energy intake. A low calorie diet is referred to as a controlled energy diet.

Index